METABOLIC MAN

TEN THOUSAND YEARS
FROM EDEN

METABOLIC MAN

TEN THOUSAND YEARS FROM EDEN

by

CHARLES HEIZER WHARTON, Ph.D.[1]

WinMarkPublishing[2]
5575 South Semoran Blvd.
Suite 120
Orlando, FL 32822

[1]Affiliate Faculty, Institute of Ecology,
The University of Georgia, Athens, GA 30602

[2]Ed Maull, Publisher—ed@metabolicman.com
Fax 407/281-9727

Library of Congress Cataloging-in-Publication Data

Wharton, Charles Heizer
 Ten thousand years from Eden : metabolic man / by Charles Heizer Wharton.
  p. cm.
 ISBN 0-9706560-0-9
  1. Nutrition. 2. Food habits. 3. Human evolution. 4. Human ecology. I. Title.

QP141 .W445 2001
612.3'9--dc21   2001035353

1st Edition 2001

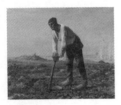

Cover painting is "Man with a Hoe"
by Jean-Francois Millet. The painting was done
between 1860 and 1862 as an oil on canvas.
The original hangs in the
J. Paul Getty Museum in Los Angeles, CA.

Edwin Markham was so impressed
by this world famous painting of a brutalized
toiler that he wrote an epic poem titled
"The Man with the Hoe".

The first four lines which follow are courtesy
of Doubleday Page and Company, who published
Markham's work in 1899.

"Bowed by the weight of centuries he leans
Upon his hoe and gazes on the ground.
The emptiness of ages in his face.
And on his back the burden of the world."

WinMarkPublishing
5575 South Semoran Blvd.
Suite 20
Orlando, FL 32822

Table of Contents

Acknowledgments

I owe a debt of gratitude to many individuals and organizations that have enabled me to observe animals and humans in a variety of natural and artificial environments, especially Harold J. Coolidge, Executive Director of the Pacific Science Board of the National Academy of Sciences, William and Lucy Mann and Ernest Walker of the National Zoological Park, Fairfield Osborne of the New York Zoological Society, William Hamilton Jr. of Cornell University, Louis and Mary Leakey, Marshall Hertig, the Coolidge Foundation, the Caesar Kleburg Foundation, the U.S. Army's Medical Team from Walter Reed Hospital and the International Health Division of the U.S. Public Health Service.

Others have given valuable comments and assistance on the manuscript, especially Sherry Rogers, M.D., Pat Connolly of the Price-Pottenger Nutritional Foundation, Joseph Heckman (ATTRA), Rudolf Wiley, John Lawder, David Watts, Richard B. Allcy, Katherine Milton, Boyd Eaton, William Wolcott, Frank Golley, Jim Fowler, Thomas Murray, Ann Louise Gittleman, Richard Lord, Neal Spruce and Edward Goldsmith.

Finally, my heartfelt thanks goes to Ed Maull of the Center for Aging Control for his unflinching support and insistence that I write this book. For the tedious job of getting the manuscript into presentable form, I must acknowledge the work of Vera Sawyer, Gina Hunkins and Walita Olson.

Forenotes

Thank you for the wonderful experience of reviewing *Ten Thousand Years From Eden*. Reading this book was as experiential as educational for me. I felt as though I was transported through the eons of time to various campfires entranced by the tribal historian storyteller telling me all that had been before my time. The story of humanity was my story, and yours! I rushed home from work each day to get back to the next chapter of this chronicle. We must try to reclaim the Eden we have disassembled through the last 10,000 years and this book is the inspiration to start making a difference right now by our daily choices and activities.

The encyclopedic second half of the book is overwhelming, but what a gift to have so many of the great researchers analyzed and served up to us to help us choose the appropriate servings of REAL FOODS to put on our plates. You so graphically illustrate Dr. Price's message, the best diet for each of us is the diet of our ancestors, and here in the melting pot America, for each of us this is biochemically, metabolically individualized and you supply the information to help us sort this out, having extracted all that you have gleaned from the various researchers. Thank you!

Marion Patricia Connolly
Curator, Price-Pottenger Nutrition Foundation

Ten Thousand Years From Eden is a fascinating, easy-to-read, yet highly-documented book whose theme could not have been more heretical.

The author shows that in the ten thousand years since we gave up being hunter-gatherers, our health, in spite of the incredible achievement of modern science and technology-based medicine, has seriously deteriorated. The main reason, and there are many others, is that our modern diet is so atrocious.

The author goes on to document the work of no less than five physicians and eleven other researchers which has made a real contribution to human health in particular by explaining why and how we should change our diet. In this way, this book provides a most valuable guide for those who realize that modern medicine alone is not sufficient for keeping us in good health.

Edward Goldsmith
Founder of the internationally-respected journal, *The Ecologist,* and editor of its Special Issues. World-renowned environmentalist and author or co-author of thirteen books on global ecology. Awarded Honorary Right Livelihood Award (known as the Alternative Nobel Prize, 1991, Stockholm); Chevalier de la Legion d'Honneur, 1991.

If you've been fortunate enough to join Dr. Charles Wharton in the field, you realize that he is a scientist who possesses a rare insight into the workings of nature. This, coupled with his keen ability to observe, his academic excellence and, above all, his obvious love of life on earth, it's no wonder that his interest in human nutrition has emerged.

Dr. Wharton has lived a life in the wild for many years, from the equatorial forests of Southeast Asia to the mountains of North Georgia. He speaks from experience, not theory. Having personally known "Chuck" for over forty years, I am constantly impressed with the enthusiasm he continues to exhibit when pursuing new areas of knowledge.

When I seek guidance while planning an educational program for one of my ecological parks or want to define new educational messages for the next century, I turn to Chuck. Now, his insight into the natural history of human nutrition will definitely influence my food intake. After all, Dr. Marlin Perkins of Wild Kingdom also stated on many occasions, "You are what you eat."!

I have traveled to many parts of the world, before and after co-hosting "Wild Kingdom," to places that are essentially unchanged. Here, where a few groups of aboriginal humans who are ecologically attuned to nature still live, Dr. Wharton's insights are especially relevant to my experience. If is difficult to observe undisturbed nature without realizing that there are certain undeniable laws that govern its domain.

Proper nutrition is one of those. Our fuel comes from the sun and the soil and always has. As we overcrowd and begin to think that we can control natural systems, it is even more important for us to realize that we are part of nature and, just as every other life form, are the result of millions of years of successful adaptation that has undeniably perfected our physical, chemical and biological selves.

If we are an intelligent species, we will honor our past while we plan for the future. There is probably nothing more important for us today than to learn to respect nature's laws and abide by them. Many civilizations have disappeared when these laws have been unknown or ignored and they have exceeded the capacity of the land to support the nutritional needs of their people. Who is to say that the situation facing our civilization today is an exception!

Jim Fowler
Co-host, Host, "Mutual of Omaha's Wild Kingdom."
Wildlife correspondent, NBC "Today Show."
Host, "Jim Fowler's Life in the Wild" TV series.
Board Member, The Explorer's Club.
Host, Animal Planet's, "Animal Encounters" TV series.
Author, "Jim Fowler's Wildest Places on Earth."

Foreword

Dr. Wharton brings a long-awaited gift to us by putting in historical perspective the evolution of man's dietary habits and then continuing into present time with a synopsis of the individual interpretations of how man should choose his food. I first became aware of the power of food when I met people and reviewed their medical records who had reversed cancers with mere diet after everything that high-tech medicine had to offer had failed. Naively excited that this was the answer for everyone, I detailed the plans in several books so that anyone could follow them. And epidemiologists at Tulane Medical School published (Carter, J., *et al., Journal of the American College of Nutrition,* 1993) the results of people who had followed the macrobiotic diet, showing they had more than tripled their survival from cancer.

As fate would have it, a charming attorney was dropped in my lap with leukemia, whose journey was to teach me that there is no monopoly on ways to control cancer. This diet plan, although diametrically opposed to the former diet, was likewise the subject of research (Gonzalos, N., *Nutrition and Cancer,* 1999), showing it more than quadrupled survival from cancer. And another book was born. Luckily, current sophisticated blood tests, like lipid peroxides, glutathione, natural killer cells, 8-OH,dG, and others negate the need to guess and play the waiting game, for they indicate if one is on the right diet plan for him.

Meanwhile, after 30 years in medical practice, I have had the privilege of watching thousands of people discover the power of the plate. There is no question we are all biochemically unique and to complicate that, our needs change as we adapt to the environment. Dr. Wharton's *Ten Thousand Years From Eden* gifts us with the much needed perspective of a biologist/ecologist/nutritionist. We need to know how it all began, what our journey has been, and what the current hypotheses are in order to make our best plans for the future. I commend him in succeeding with that task.

Since medicine is just beginning to appreciate the power of whole foods, it will be a long time before metabolic typing becomes practiced. But for those who are already ahead of the pack, this book opens the gates for a new journey.

Sherry A. Rogers, M.D.
Diplomat of the American Board of Family Practice
Diplomat of the American Board of Environment Medicine
Fellow of the American College of Allergy, Asthma, and Immunology
Fellow of the American College of Nutrition
Sarasota, FL
2001

Preface

The "Garden" of Eden can be thought of as representing the natural world where man was born and nurtured as just another participant, along with all the other plants and animals interacting together in ecologically sound ways. Our exodus from Eden began a long pilgrimage, largely away from the balanced natural ecosystems of the past. In searching for our own individual sources of health and energy, we can draw on the lessons of this prehistoric and historic journey and bring to bear, finally, our intellectual prowess as large brained primates, to see how each of us fits into the environments of today. For our European ancestors at least, the epitaph of Eden began 10,000 years ago with the inception of sedentary agriculture. The slaying of Abel, a pastoral herder, by Cain, a soil-tiller, symbolizes a giant step away from our past. The herbivorous mammals, herded by pastoral peoples like Abel, enabled humans to derive nutrients from otherwise inedible herbs. This way of life was closer to the concept of living with nature, a legacy of our years in Eden. To the many sick and hungry throughout the world it must seem that those peoples still working happily and traditionally with nature are blessed beyond measure.

In Yeat's beautiful poem, The Song of the Wandering Aengus, his subject catches, at dawn, a little silver trout. When he lays it on the floor and goes to blow his fire aflame, it becomes a glimmering girl who calls him by his name and then runs away, into the glowing brightness of the day. Aengus becomes old with wandering the earth in search of this lost love. I often wonder if this is not a metaphor for the things in nature that we deem most precious and often elusive, our lives becoming an endless quest for the wonders of the natural world that we encounter and cannot always understand.

To understand nature and our own place within it, even how we eat to live, requires that we follow rules laid down through the ages, rules to be followed whether by chemical elements, grains of sand or living organisms. All must participate and, whether we are aware of it or not, nature is in control. Long before us, native Americans embraced the concept of the material and spiritual unity of all things, living or not, honoring and revering all components of their environment, even rocks. This acknowledgement and respect for a universal guiding power has been the basis for the successful survival of many ancient human cultures, relicts of whom still live in remote regions of the earth.

It is fundamental that man is not exempt from a controlling force in nature, the edicts of which we call "natural laws." He once lived in Eden's worldwide. But then, in certain special environments, he encountered tiny, storable packets of nutrition—the seeds of certain grasses—and agriculture was born. Creating his own personal ecosystem almost at will began to erode a relationship that had nurtured him for millions of years, for now he could break the ecological bonds that balance the abundance of animals, to overwhelm the earth with both his numbers and his technology.

From the catastrophic events, wars and pestilence that followed, some have wondered at the silence of God. But maybe God is not silent. Maybe these disasters that befall mankind are messages that we've been too preoccupied to hear, that we've ignorantly violated rules of nature laid down through millions of years of evolution. God has spoken through the all-powerful language of creation. Our disobedience has not gone unnoticed. Perhaps our most grievous error was to sever our umbilical from the local community of soil, plants and animals that had nurtured us for millennia. Of the several penalties issued for this transgression of natural law, the most insidious is degenerative disease.

But there is hope. If we can recognize our own personal and humbling relationship with nature through reconsidering our lifestyle, in particular, our individual metabolic response to the food we eat, we have one last chance to balance the scales that weigh life and death in this modern age. Deep down, we may all have a feeling that something fundamental has gone wrong. Edna St. Vincent Millay may have been trying to express our deep need for our original environment in her poem:

> *Earth does not understand her child,*
> *Who from the loud gregarious town,*
> *Returns, depleted and defiled,*
> *To the still woods, to fling him down.*

Earth cannot count the sons she bore:
  The wounded lynx, the wounded man
Come trailing blood unto her door;
  She shelters both as best she can.

Introduction

"Eden . . . was just a place where human beings lived the way all humans lived before the rise of civilization. . . . We are all exiles from Eden. We have been exiled to civilization."

—Kalman Glantz and John Pearce

The roots of our health go as far back as the primates in tropical forests. We are both nature's child and civilization's victim. When we view the crags and ice fields of the mountains, stand among towering trees, gaze across a vast desert, hear the roar of crashing water or even catch a little silver trout, we may be subconsciously seeking to recapture the essence of the Eden in which we once lived with all the other life forms spawned by the thin and fertile crust of our planet.

As a child of nature, we were punished if we disobeyed nature's rules. As exiles from the wild, we not only idolize material icons but we have forgotten, or never learned, the inexorable laws of the natural world in which we evolved. As victims of the overwhelming speed of our civilization, we have not taken enough time to understand the brain and body with which we are endowed. We are so preoccupied with our maladies and medicares that we miss the basic perspective of how it all came to be. There is a collective wisdom in society, but it is not focused on us as individuals.

Longer ago than I like to think, before I was formally dedicated to the field of vertebrate ecology, I was obsessed with a curiosity about wild environments and the living things that called them home. Forced to feed and care for strange mammals, birds and reptiles in captivity brought me face to face with the fact that the foods eaten by individual species had everything to do with whether they lived or died. Kept under appalling conditions for wild creatures, subject to loud artificial noises and tiny, restrictive cages, they would generally survive if properly fed: it was their food that made the difference.

I was also impressed with the fact that, with most wild creatures, the individuals of each species resembled each other so closely that, to my eyes at least, they looked alike, especially if those of a given age were compared. Furthermore, their dietary preferences seemed to vary even less than their appearance. The tiny primate, the tarsier, would *always* eat small lizards and insects.

I also noted that in remote areas most humans tended to look alike. The color of hair, eye and skin, stature and bodily proportions were remarkably similar. When I returned to the United States, the change was startling, for here was every conceivable color, bone structure, size and proportion. Although I knew that this variation was due to a mix of genetic types the dietary significance of this did not immediately sink in.

Years later, I began to see evidence that not only do we not look alike, but also some of us are each apparently different in our food requirements. This was not evident in "primitive" cultures, which not only resembled each other physically, but also ate the same foods. In fact, their foods seemed downright monotonous. In spite of my experience with feeding captive wild creatures, it wasn't obvious to me at that time that this "monotonous" diet was actually exactly what people *should* be eating in order to stay healthy and be able to propagate their culture. I failed to realize that, through a close partnership with nature, they had developed a way of life that not only enabled them to survive and reproduce, but made no permanent change in the soils, plants or animals with which they lived on the most intimate terms.

I originally thought that this book would deal only with means of determining our highly individualized body chemistries or "metabolic types." I soon realized that this might be putting the cart before the horse. How we eat as individuals might be better accepted if we could see the human in perspective with the earth's environments in which we lived for literally millions of years and with the less-than-natural environments in which we later found ourselves.

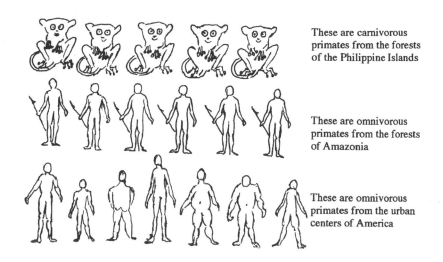

These are carnivorous
primates from the forests
of the Philippine Islands

These are omnivorous
primates from the forests
of Amazonia

These are omnivorous
primates from the urban
centers of America

Figure 0.

Lessons From The Wild

Wild animals engage in a lifestyle that includes eating what is available in the natural environment in which they live. Generally, they eat the same things day after day and year after year. Since they have evolved hand-in-glove with nature, so to speak, they are healthy and seldom if ever overweight. Because of their diet and infrequent gene exchange with distant populations, they reproduce what appear to be carbon-copies of their well-adapted selves. Their physical evolution is dictated primarily by changes in their natural environment.

In contrast, human lifestyles in wealthy and technological nations may include eating anything dictated by taste, custom, transport or advertising. Some humans do not eat the same things, even one day to the next. Since they no longer live in the same environment where they evolved, they are likely to be unhealthy and overweight. Because of their diet and frequent gene exchange with distant populations, they often reproduce widely different copies of not-very-well-adapted offspring. Their physical evolution is dominated primarily by changes in their cultural environment.

As most of us know, small groups of indigenous peoples live today in total dependence on the natural world around them, as in the Kalahari Desert, the Amazon basin and around the Bering Sea. The story of the change that began ten thousand years ago applies principally, in this book, to our European ancestors. The man with a hoe depicts the plight of those whose fate was to wrest their daily bread from the soil—all they had left of a once-diverse and verdant natural system.

Many of the world's other peoples either attempted to remain in their Edens or discovered clever ways to adapt to a diversity of environments where they happened to live: wet marshes, mountain slopes and arid grasslands.

Actually, up until comparatively recent times, from 5,000 to as late as 500 years ago, most of the world was still hunting and gathering their foods. North and South America, most of Africa and much of Asia and Australia were characterized by hunter-gatherer cultures. Other larger populations have lived for millennia among the terraces and ricefields of the world where, by imitating nature's own cycling of organic matter, they could live sustainably and in harmony with their local supply of soil, water and life forms. There's no telling how long the New Guineans have worked their mountain slopes, the Amazonian Indians their garden plots in forest openings or the tribes of Borneo have practiced shifting cultivation. And, from about 8,000 years ago the domestication of horses, cattle, camels and reindeer have made it possible for humans to thinly populate vast areas of steppes, prairie, desert and tundra in Asia, and savannas, and even desert in Africa. In these environments nomadic groups adapted to the carnivore niche, living principally on meat, milk products and blood from their tended herds. As we will see in Chapter 8, Weston Price found, as late as the 1930s, that quite a few human cultures still maintained a sustainable way of life in a variety of coastal, mountain and tropical habitats, fortunately out of reach of commercialized foods.

Now, mostly in cities, affluent or not, the past century has seen a rapid deterioration of health and, probably, much of the joy of living. In search of causes, we may need to reassess the impact of industry and technology on modern life, especially the easy availability of foods grown elsewhere, the use of chemicals, the processing and refining of our foods and their advertisement through profit-motivated media. This implies that cultural change now dictates physical change. The most viable solution would seem to be to find our own rewarding personal lifestyle and, for eating at least, our own personal nutrition. Here is where Part II can assist.

Part I

The book is in two parts. Part I is designed to give a perspective of how humans must eat and live, beginning with our fundamental quest for energy through our foods and following our prehistoric genesis from jungle-dwelling primates to our rapid expansion into most of the earth's ecosystems.

After having stumbled onto agriculture, we developed traditional ways of eating which eventually culminated (for advantaged nations, at least) in a complete loss of our earliest relationships with land and sea. We end up with both successful and failed genetic attempts to adapt to locally available foodstuffs and life styles. For many of us, our major communication with nature is a trip to the local supermarket, mowing the grass or maybe a fall drive to look at the leaves. Our enormous medical expenses attest that we have lost our once healthy relationship with life-giving soils and traditional ways. A new paradigm is necessary and one has appeared: a search for an individual or personal style of eating and perhaps a lifestyle based upon your heredity and your nutritional or biochemical needs.

Some interesting facts and theories regarding your background in time should emerge from reading Part I. *The Fire of Life* looks at the birth of the elements in the fiery cauldrons of space to yield the rocks, water and atmosphere from which such diverse organisms as giant sequoias, dinosaurs, whales and people derive what can be regarded as a sacramental energy exchange, all recycling the same elements in accordance with natural laws. In *Our Primate Heritage* we examine the theory that food choices may have played an important role in the evolution of the human brain and that human gut proportions are adapted to unusually rich wild foods, absorbed primarily in the small intestine. Individuals (and perhaps regional groups) have gut lengths twice that of others, suggesting adaptation to either plant or animal based diets. *Early Man* tells us that humans have spent 99 percent of their time on earth hunting and gathering food, and that the physiology of most Europeans dates back, at least from 11,000 to 19,000 years ago, to pre-agricultural Paleolithic hunter-gatherers. Hence the Paleolithic diet described by Boyd Eaton and associates is applicable to modern man. We are startled to learn the high value that primitive societies placed on fat and how meat hungry Australian aborigines will abandon the carcass of a kangaroo that is too lean: humans can become ill by denying themselves fatty foods. In this section, Greenland Ice Cores tell us that 11,000 years ago there was a sudden and seemingly permanent rise in world temperatures which coincided with the rapid spread of man, the advent of agriculture in the northern hemisphere and the demise of the great Ice Age mammals such as mammoths and ground sloths.

It is startling to consider that agriculture may have been the greatest tragedy to befall the human race, and, in the *Agriculture* chapter, we see new significance in the story that Cain, a tiller of the soil, slew Abel, a pastoral representative of the more ancient hunter-gatherers, who became followers, then herders of hoofed mammals. We find that the domestication of plants sets the stage for the haves and have-nots of the world, and that the discovery of the giant seeds of certain grasses in the Middle East began the slow deterioration of man's original relationship with the natural world where he had evolved for millions of years. We see that the fate of the former Fertile Crescent where European agriculture was born, is now an ecologically destitute object lesson for mankind. We realize that, in spite of technology, most of the world cannot survive out of context with the relationships imposed by the local ecosystems where they live. By this same token, we ourselves need a strong sense of bioregional awareness.

The *Staff of Life* chapter zeroes in on what we ate for hundreds of years prior to emigration to the New World, introducing the healthful values of the age old processes of fermentation and stewpots on the hearth. The fact that 41 percent of 2.5 million Englishmen were rejected as unfit for service as early as World War I, tells us that something went terribly wrong with our nutrition early in the twentieth century. Now that many of us in affluent nations can buy anything we want to eat from a worldwide smorgasbord of foods, we come to realize that to survive, if not to age more slowly, we need some way to identify just who we are as metabolic individuals.

In *Sustainable Agriculture* we find that cash crops are destroying the relationship of man to his local soils, suited only to a subsistence mode of cultivation. We review the many ingenious methods by which man has developed a sustainable agriculture such as by clever irrigation or fantastic efforts at terracing steep mountains. Other societies emulate the structure and function of natural ecosystems with wetland rice paddies, the most exciting of which is the Japanese "Aigamo method" using ducks, rice and fish, a system which is spreading like wildfire in the Orient. Our own organic farming is a growing effort towards sustainability, with widespread benefits.

Our look at *Gardens* examines those horticultural efforts epitomized by the Javanese and Mayan gardens that simulate nature's own organization. Importantly, we observe that in our own local history, our break with the soil began with the exodus of many Americans to towns, away from the intimate relationship they once had with their gardens and general environment. Their subsequent dependence on the local supermarket has led us to a national "non-diet," supplanting the traditional diets that had sustained us through our early, more rural years.

This theme is expanded in *Traditional Eating* when we look at the worldwide research of men like the famed dental authority Weston Price, who, found crooked teeth and facial deformities uniformly in the second generation of people who had abandoned their traditional foods for the refined starches and sugars of "civilization." There was the physician Sir Robert McCarrison who compared the unhealthy English diet with both the best and poorest of Indian subcontinent diets. Then Pottenger came along, working with his famous 900 cats to discover that, in carnivores at least, eating cooked meat or drinking pasteurized milk (versus raw meat and milk) utterly destroyed his animals over time. We also learn why we must soak or ferment grains and soak beans overnight (and throw out the water); that many vegetables contain substances (phytates, protein enzyme inhibitors and lectins) which are designed by plants to inhibit inopportune sprouting and possibly to discourage potential seed eaters. Since only fermentation will reduce these substances in soybeans, mothers may be concerned, since soy protein isolates are primary ingredients in many infant formulas. Also, improperly cooked kidney beans can suppress a child's growth (as few as 5 raw kidney beans can make you ill). This chapter reviews the phenomenon of vegetarianism, and concludes that vegans (no animal protein) may be playing God with their nutrition. However, it is not well known that protein rich legumes, nuts and seeds are prominent dietary components in food pyramids for much of the world, for vegetarians, Asians and Mediterraneans in particular.

The *Tomato* chapter deals with the fact that humans cannot detect the nutrition of a food by sight, smell or taste, but many "dumb" animals can. A tomato may look like a tomato, but its nutrient content is unknown to you or to the store manager. Florida tomatoes have eighteen times more calcium than those from Massachusetts and some tomatoes have fifty-three times more copper than others do. Some spinach is quite low in iron while that grown on other soils has eighty-three times as much of this metal.

In the *Genetics* section, we confront the fact that iron appears to stimulate bacterial and viral growth and thus may harm patients with infections. Here also, is the realization that modern high calorie foods have pushed the menarche of our young girls closer to twelve than the fifteen it once was: (it was reached at seventeen by European girls in the eighteenth and nineteenth centuries). We look at evidence that protection against malaria has been a trade-off with such afflictions as cystic fibrosis and violent reactions from eating fava beans. While we have adapted somewhat in 8,000 years to the protein gluten of grains, in some parts of the world celiac disease is still a downside effect of agriculture. Celiac disease and food allergies in general may damage the intestinal wall, preventing the absorption of vital minerals and vitamins, thus weakening the immune system. The chapter also takes a look at how the brain's primary pleasure centers may have arisen to influence food choices and our lifestyle in general. Thus, we may use the sensory input of TV to activate ancient limbic centers that we share with most other vertebrates. Here we also examine the theory that the complexity of food gathering and an intensely cooperative social life may have led to the larger brains of early savanna-dwelling humans. And we see that this brain may be as much a pharmacy as a computer. The section closes with the idea that what an individual eats, drinks and breathes may be the only sensible way to win the gene wars against aggressive new microorganisms, especially since our minds and bodies were designed for a different and more stable world.

The concluding section of Part I, the *Supermarket* deals with our everyday visits to the grocery store. It leaves us with the disturbing thought that foods on most of the shelves contain substances deleterious to our health. Evidence is cited that, if regularly ingested, additives such as MSG and Aspartame may eventually destroy enough brain cells to materially affect our lives, and that "hydrolyzed vegetable protein" contains three of these dangerous toxins that interfere with calcium channel physiology. The effect on the eyes and hypothalamus of young animals is particularly threatening, although these additives have been eliminated from most baby foods.

Part II

Part II seeks to outline the "new" and perhaps ultimate paradigm in human care: considering each of us as an individual in sickness or in health. The expression "One man's meat is another man's poison" goes back to Roman times. There is a factual basis for this assumption, although most of the data are empirical observations or anecdotal. From this was born the phrase "treat the patient who has the disease not the disease who has the patient." Even some mainline medical specialists are endorsing such a principle. The cancer specialist Robert Nagourney is credited with saying "We've come to realize that response of cancer patients to chemotherapy is not the function of drugs used, but a function of the patient." There is no "average patient"—the drug must be matched to the patient and his tumor as you would fit shoes or eyeglasses. (Life Extension, 2000.)

In "the old days" the family doctor knew much about each individual family member, including their genetic background. Today, it is largely the practitioner of "alternative," "complementary," or "integrative" medicine that assumes this role. Evaluating the individual with his distinctive metabolic and hormonal quirks is a vital part of alternative medicine.

Recognition of individualized health care through diet, vitamin-mineral supplements and herbs may be central to the forthcoming "major ideologic struggle between mainstream and complementary medicine" as Robert Atkins (1999) puts it. Even that bastion of mainstream medicine, the AMA, has devoted an issue of its publication to alternative medicine. (Whittaker, 1999.)

It seems that the public now recognizes that there are alternatives to traditional surgery and prescription drugs for many maladies. In 1997 46.3 percent of Americans visited alternative practitioners, spending $27 billion, much of which was not covered by insurance.

Spokesmen for alternative or integrative medicine are numerous. Physicians like Jonathan Wright, Andrew Weil, Robert Atkins, Julian Whittaker, and Sherry Rogers are to be commended for their leadership in focussing our attention on wellness instead of sickness.

Part II seeks to guide our search for a nutritional regimen that will support a healthy, happy lifestyle, and slow the aging process at the same time. It asks you to consider your genetic background, since even powerful vitamin-mineral supplements have little effect, if you have inherited defects in utilization and absorption of food. From this information and from laboratory tests, you can determine if you have any severe food allergies that may be overloading your immune system and even producing autoimmune disease.

You may need to test yourself for toxic substances such as heavy metals and hormone disrupting chemicals in the environment, particularly those that disrupt the levels of sex hormones such as estrogen. Some foods may contain seventeen times more synthetic estrogen that needed to stimulate breast cancer cells.

In defining your own personal nutrition and lifestyle, you certainly should try to determine what many of the authors in Part II call your "metabolic type." This will tell you what foods and supplements to ingest for optimum health. Several simple do-it-yourself tests using coffee or niacin are explained. "Ideal" ratios of carbohydrate, protein and fat are listed and you can compare these with the food pyramids from Part I (Asian, Mediterranean, vegetarian) in *Traditional Diets* and with the USDA food pyramid in the final chapter.

If you don't wish to drastically change your diet or experiment on yourself, several organizations are discussed who will, on the basis of a questionnaire and simple lab tests, provide you with your nutritional or metabolic type, recommended diets and even exercise programs.

You will read that many common diet plans by physicians and scientists may or may not suit your metabolism.

Part II, following an introduction to metabolic typing, begins with a brief look at the biochemical basis for your individual nutrition and explains why and where certain vitamins and minerals "plug in" to the energy-yielding "machinery" of the cell. This chapter sheds light on why everyone can't take the same vitamins and minerals, just as the ratio of carbohydrate, proteins and fats will be different whether you are a "fast" or "slow" oxidizer. Watt's advice underscores the dangers of self-dosing and megadosing, especially with minerals such as calcium.

Hopefully you will be intrigued to read the summaries of the research and writings of at least 16 different authors who have contributed to the concept of individualized nutrition. Here are some highlights from these contributors:

> Your genetic heritage can be as destructive to your health as poorly chosen foods. Some males have small intestines twice as long (herbivores?) as others (carnivores?) and some individuals may have twelve times more insulin-secreting cells in their pancreas than others (Roger Williams).
>
> The vegetarian diets of East Indian gurus may be right for Asians but wrong for many Caucasians. Simple tests with niacin will give a pretty good idea of your metabolic type. A high meat/fat diet will cure some cancers while juice and raw vegetable therapy will heal others (William Kelley).
>
> Sniffing a certain vitamin can give some people a good clue as to their metabolism. Eighty percent of neuroses, including schizophrenia, can be cured by diet and supplements (George Watson).
>
> Foods with the highest content of the anti-aging nucleic acids (from RNA) are canned sardines, pinto beans and lentils (Benjamin Frank).
>
> Are you a blue-eyed coastal dwelling Nordic, a short-gutted meat and fish eater? Did you know that a quarter pound of chocolate can throw your calcium-phosphorous ratio below the level of immunity to dental decay for 32 hours? (Melvin Page).
>
> If you're heavy-set with a potbelly, the adrenal is probably your dominant gland. If you are a thyroid gland dominant, you crave sweets and caffeine but you should eat an egg sandwich to stimulate the weaker adrenals and balance your system (Elliot Abravanel).
>
> If you're a fast oxidizer, you need a protein-rich breakfast avoiding large doses of vitamins C and B; if a slow oxidizer, you can forego breakfast but need high levels of these vitamins. Only 2 percent of people have perfectly balanced metabolisms and can more or less

eat in accordance with their whims (John Lawder). All stocky, weight lifting mesomorphs are not fast oxidizers and do not need high protein diets (Neal Spruce).

The highest and lowest deviations from a blood plasma pH of 7.46 are inmates at mental institutions. Most (75 percent) men and all diabetics are alkaline. Steak and potatoes are not for them (Rudolf Wiley).

The "jolly fat man" is an overly possessive pitta type (Deepak Chopra).

If you are a slow oxidizer, to rush out and buy calcium supplements is the worst thing that you could do. Fast oxidizers are more suited to cold climates and hence thrive on high protein diets (W. L. Wolcott).

Symptoms are to be treasured as nature's messages. Macrobiotic diets are good for cancer patients during the first few months, then diets should be shifted towards more balance (more meat and fat). Terminal cancer patients may need their vegetables twice cooked to pablum consistency (Sherry Rogers).

Too much calcium or excess vitamin A might cause osteoporosis, especially if certain other minerals such as copper are lacking. The overactive adrenals of the fast oxidizer decrease the stimulating minerals (sodium, potassium) (David Watts).

Skin, eye and hair color and even personality may indicate internal dietary needs. Three meals a day burn up 10 percent more calories than two. Cutting calories too low lowers the metabolic rate to starvation mode, increasing fat storage enzymes up to fifteen times (Ann Louise Gittleman).

Raw, cold vegetable foods may hinder metabolic function of the sleek thyroid or pituitary dominant types. The athletic adrenal types need aerobics, not weight training, while sleek fast oxidizers need weight training (Jay Cooper).

Many of the authors in Part II offer evidence to support the premise that each of us, with our distinctive individual blend of nervous, hormonal and metabolic systems, are entitled to individualized health care. At the very least, Part II should provide evidence that the structure and function of each physiology should be given equal consideration with their diagnosed disease.

Eating right, for you as an individual, could be a major step in helping you achieve the maximum longevity allowed by your genetic blueprint. First, by preventing premature senility and death from unnecessary deterioration and disease and secondly, by slowing the aging process. Almost everyone would concede that normalizing body chemistry through diet removes or alters factors that stress the body's glands, tissues and cells and interfere with their repair.

Another current health concern is weight control. This book is not intended to be critical of any of the many current diets in vogue. However, a certain percentage of people on any one of them will achieve better health and weight loss either because the diet in question is suitable for their own biochemistry, or because most of them offer common sense rules that we all need to follow. A correct metabolic diet is no "fad"—it is a long-lasting, pill-free, weight-normalizing approach to human health.

It is best done with the cooperation of your physician, especially those who are into alternative or integrative medicine. Barring that, consult the best other health practitioner that you can find.

At the same time, bear in mind that there is no substitute for exercise, adequate pure water intake, pure air and minimal environmental toxins and stresses. And then, maybe the search for health will not be the fastest-growing, failing business in America as Emanuel Cheraskin was fond of saying.

PART 1

AN ECOLOGIST LOOKS AT HUMAN NUTRITION

CHAPTER ONE

The Fire of Life

"Perhaps the concept most central to all of science is energy. The combination of energy and matter makes up the universe: matter is substance and energy is the mover of substance. . . . It comes to us in the form of electromagnetic waves from the sun and we feel it as heat; it is captured by plants and binds molecules of matter together; it is the food we eat and we receive it by digestion."

—Paul G. Hewitt

Why do we fear lions, cobras and great white sharks? Because they kill to obtain energy in concentrated packets—the bodies of other animals. Water and air are cheap; food is not. While the energy of green plants comes from limitless solar radiation, the animal world owes its enormous diversity to the fact that it exploits not only the energy from the entire plant world, but also the energy from every conceivable type of animal life. There are specialists, such as sharks and tigers and rabbits, but bears, raccoons and humans are generalists.

Until agriculture came along, our search for energy dominated and defined our lives and, to procure it, we had to adapt to the world's environments. Now, 10,000 years later, our energy sources have been augmented to the point where we have the power to try to fit the world's environments to us. Our quest for energy could still be our Armageddon, either in a planetary sense, from hydrogen bombs, or as omnivorous humans trying to eat in an increasingly complex, technological society.

1

Energy must surely be the most astounding fact of the universe. It is apparently interchangeable with mass at subatomic levels. The energy holding the protons of an atom's nucleus together is beyond belief, the magnitude revealed by a quick look at the physics behind the fission and fusion of our atomic and thermonuclear bombs. Here, a reduction of a tiny (less than 0.1 percent) bit of mass by either splitting or fusing the nuclei of atoms yields an incredible amount of explosive power with much heat and light, whether from nuclear bombs or the internal furnaces of the stars. Conversely, enormous energy, such as generated in an exploding supernova, will take the lightest element, hydrogen, and begin fusing nuclei together until each of the successively higher elements is formed. These will eventually solidify and become rocks. Of the heavier elements, iron is remarkable.

Iron has the most stable and strongest nucleus of all the elements and is least reactive in planetary furnaces. Its atoms tend to accumulate at gravitational centers and, being abundant, form metallic masses such as occupies the center of the earth. Iron, however, reacts so well with oxygen, that life has incorporated it in red blood cells, as the major carrier of oxygen to all parts of the bodies of vertebrate animals.

The purpose of delving into all this is to help us understand that we evolved using the elements generated in the fiery furnaces of space, where matter and energy have interacted throughout the known universe. An ulterior motive is to introduce the tenets of deep ecology, which holds that, along with religions in both the Old and New Worlds, we are indeed one with the universe. We were formed from matter and energy within it, and we must abide by the eternal laws of nature. If you wish to say that these are also God's laws, many will certainly concur. As Fritjof Capra says, "Human beings can choose whether and how to obey a social rule; molecules cannot choose whether or not they should interact." In the developed countries of the world we can choose how to eat and live, but we cannot choose to ignore the molecular interactions within our cells. To do so is to violate nature's rules, and if we choose to ignore those rules, disease and a short life will be the result. Physically, we can be nothing more than what we eat, drink and breathe. And we have found out that even our mental health depends on the molecular interaction from our choices of proteins, fats and carbohydrates. And this choice must be guided by all the knowledge we can muster of our own biochemical individuality.

Let's take a brief excursion into how it all came to be. While we talk glibly about foods and minerals, it needs to be put in perspective how we and the other fellow energy seekers came to be the favored children of the earth. It is really the story of energy, since it is energy that enables the cells of our bodies to perform their function. If the brain cells cannot perform their function, you feel lousy, you attack your mother-in-law, or you simply won't enjoy this glorious world. If liver cells cannot do their job of detoxifying the formaldehyde from your rugs or do not supply sufficient antioxidants so your cells' P53 gene can suppress tumors, you might have cancer.

Genesis 1:3 says: "And God said, let there be light; and there was light." And indeed there was. Science confirms that, whether it was the Big Bang itself or an exploding supernova, there was an incomprehensible brilliance in the heavens. Light is visible energy, and from the energy of its source the universe was born, first gases, then solid things.

From some initial source of energy, life as we know it emerged and eventually gained knowledge of itself and the universe that bore it, ultimately seeking a spiritual awareness and identity with the unity of the cosmos. This surely must be the grandest story ever told. It is the new creation story proposed by the eco-theologian Thomas Berry and, in its acceptance, the story so simply told in Genesis is expanded and glorified beyond measure.

Since energy so involves hydrogen, we can begin the story here. Hydrogen is the lightest element with a single proton in the nucleus encircled by a single, lonely electron. I find it barely comprehensible that everything we are and see originated with hydrogen. I find it equally incredible that over 10 billion years later, the reactions in our own bodies that give us the bulk of our energy to move and live again involve the almost nothing atom of hydrogen. This is done by separating hydrogen into its component parts: the nucleus and the electron. This "electron transport system" as it is now called, is vividly pictured in modern prep-school texts. (BSCS, 1998.)

The hydrogen atom is the simplest and lightest of the ninety odd elements created with the enormous heat generated in the explosion of giant stars, such as supernovas. Eventually, the far-flung matter aggregated into other stars, sometimes with companion planets. Space is still filled, even billions of light years away, with the energy radiated from hydrogen, oxygen and other elements from such explosions out there, elements so vital to life on earth.

The vertebrate body is made from ten of these major elements, and eight or so trace elements. Because of the unique configuration of its outer electrons, the element carbon is the building block of life, as we know it. It and two other common, light nonmetallic elements (hydrogen and oxygen) compose the basic energy molecule (glucose) and, along with nitrogen, provide most of the bulk of all living things. Carbon is at the root of cell energy, just as surely as it is when a log burns in your fireplace. Since carbon atoms attract oxygen atoms much more than oxygen attracts oxygen or carbon attracts carbon, this affinity (oxidation) yields energy and, in the case of wood, coal or oil, the oxygen "burns" the carbon. (Ideally, the end results are carbon dioxide and water given off into the air).

Most of the other elements in our cells are metals, oddly enough. Some of these, such as calcium, lend strength to bones and teeth, while others are vital components of enzymes, which cause all sorts of thing to happen throughout the body. But how did all these elements become us?

Most of the elements heavier than hydrogen wound up in the rocks of planet Earth which, on weathering, became soil. Extracted from the soil by plants, these elements, now called "minerals," are passed along the food chain from plant-eater (herbivore) to meat-eater (carnivore). Some of us, including bears and raccoons are able to eat both kinds of foods (omnivores). Man, as we shall see, is an omnivore, with some of us leaning toward herbivore and others of us leaning toward carnivore. Our theme is to find out where each of us stands in available food chains.

Originally, the elements that eventually became us came from the rocks of the primordial earth. Now, however, due to weathering, volcanism and life itself, three vital elements are conveniently available to us from the air (atmosphere) rather than from soil.

In fact, there could be no plants growing on land or animals crawling about among them, until an envelope containing these elements in gaseous form was evolved. And this in itself is an amazing story. While most of our sister planets have envelopes of gas surrounding them, earth is unique in the elements making up its gas layer. Our atmosphere contains a balance of gases, characterized by much oxygen, lots of methane (source of nitrogen) and almost no carbon dioxide. This makeup, according to James Lovelock and Lynn Margulis is apparently the signature of life. According to Lovelock's Gaia theory, life forms on land and in the oceans have devoted 3.5 billion years to creating and maintaining this balance of gases that we breathe.

Again, it comes back to hydrogen. In those seas billions of years ago, primitive bacteria sought to build the same energy-rich compounds and carbohydrates that we use today. But to do so they needed free hydrogen. They could not break water down to release it until the ancestors of the blue-green algae invented a new process, photosynthesis, which used the energy of visible light to split water molecules into oxygen and hydrogen. This was a milestone event in the history of life. The problem was that free oxygen was toxic to early life. It remained for certain blue-green bacteria to evolve the second great invention: the use of this oxygen (as an electron receiver) to break down organic molecules such as sugar in a type of controlled combustion yielding carbon dioxide, water and a great deal of energy (that formerly held the sugar molecule together).

Keeping in mind that oxygen wants to grab electrons (oxidize) from anything it can—from iron (causing it to rust) or wood (causing it to burn)—it was necessary for life to stabilize the amount of oxygen in our atmosphere. Which it did at roughly 21 percent. If it dropped below 15 percent, nothing would burn, while above 25 percent everything would burn. (Capra, 1996.) Incidentally, I have read that oxygen in cities can drop to as low as 18 percent.

This delicate balance of atmospheric gases is essential for terrestrial life as we know it (and much aquatic life as well). It took from 1.5 to 3.5 billion years to accomplish, until land life emerged, 400 to 450 million years ago. Now we can understand why Lovelock and Margulis postulated that no surface life could possibly exist on the planet Mars, since its atmosphere has little oxygen, much carbon dioxide and no methane and thus cannot sustain life.

To sum it up, "air" provides us with major elements (oxygen, carbon and nitrogen). Add some from atmospheric fallout (sulfur, iodine) and others, principally metals (calcium, magnesium, sodium) from rocks and waters of the earth, and you have the ingredients to construct all living things.

It is humbling and awesome to realize that the largest organisms that ever lived, the giant sequoia trees, the great whales of the sea and the dinosaurs, all derived from elements found in the air, water and rock that originated in fiery cauldrons of energy and matter somewhere in the inconceivable vastness of space. It would seem that our Native Americans were more in touch with nature's plan than we are, for they perceived rocks as the grandfather of all life and considered them to have being and, accordingly, to be honored and revered. It is a humbling lesson to realize that other cultures understand better than we the interrelationships of life and non-life, which we have finally come to respect as the science of ecology.

Hydrogen has played an almost mystical role in the story of the earth, its biosphere and the thin layer of life upon it. It is ironic that the greatest possible release of energy that mankind has been able to develop is derived from the fusion of two hydrogen nuclei. We have reluctantly come to realize that life as we know it could all be terminated by an exchange of hydrogen bombs between so-called civilized societies. Let us pray that our tenure on earth does not end as it was said to have begun; with another brilliant flash of light from the union of protons in the atomic nucleus of hydrogen.

In summary, life has reversed an edict of physics, the Entropy Law, by using energy to organize matter, the common elements available from cosmic events, into units of more and more complex organization. The living bodies formed have cleverly evolved to exploit the extraterrestrial radiation of the sun, largely through the green plants. The green plants, accordingly, have organized themselves to synthesize from several of the most common elements (oxygen, nitrogen, hydrogen, carbon) in earth and air, larger molecules of protein, fats and carbohydrates, which higher animals in turn exploit for the energy to drive an active life of movement and even thought. Essential to the extraction of energy from these three major food sources, both plants and animals make use of other elements or minerals from the primordial cosmic stew, released by weathering from their entombment in the rocks of the earth. It is thus that the search for food becomes a universal quest for that earthly force that powers the

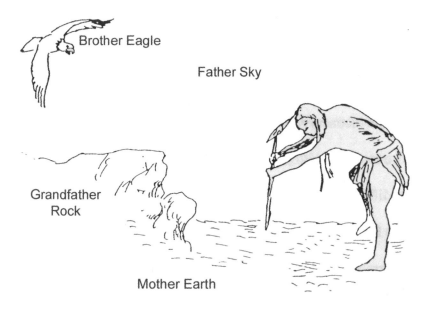

Brother Eagle

Father Sky

Grandfather Rock

Mother Earth

Figure 1. Like ecologists to follow, Native Americans felt that nature was a continuum. They revered the relationship of all things animate and inanimate. They probably knew that without the soil, and its source, the rocks, under the action of rains from the sky and the growing plants, there could be no energy flow that they could intercept and use. To North American Indians, the four great powers (rock, earth, sky, sun) comprised the Wakan Tanka. Mankind's original religion was apparently our relationship with nature.

bodies and brains of ourselves and all the other creatures whose world we share.

Gary Snyder (La Chapelle, 1988) made this remarkable statement about the deeper relationship we have with our foods: "If you think of eating and killing plants or animals to eat, as an unfortunate quirk in the nature of the universe, then you cut yourself off from connecting with the sacramental energy exchange . . . which takes place by that sharing of energies, passing it back and forth, which is done by literally eating each other. And that's what communion is. And that's what the shamanist world foresees . . . one of the healthiest things about the primitive world-view is that it solved one of the critical problems of life and death. It understands how you relate to your food. 'You sing to it. You pray to it. Then you enjoy it.' "

There is no better or more humbling way to appreciate the wonders of life than to understand how we cannot separate ourselves from our fundamental kinship with the universe and all its awesome forms of matter and energy. Although a rock is not a sentient being, it is a participant in our life, for from it come the nutrients that enable us to extract energy and thus to be able to thrill to the wonders of the world, and this is worthy of our respect, if not our reverence.

CHAPTER TWO

Our Primate Heritage

It is revealing to put human anatomy and physiology in perspective with the family of mammals to which we belong, the primates. It helps us to understand how types of foods have made our bodies and brains. Recognizing how powerfully foodstuffs can mold the structure of the body and brain makes us pay more attention to what we eat today and why we eat it.

Let us look at one example of how the type of food eaten may have profoundly altered the bodies and brains of some of the "lower" primates in whose family tree we dwell. For three years, often working alone in the humid rainforests of Panama, Katherine Milton made some significant discoveries. The two kinds of primates she followed through the forest from dawn to dusk were roughly the same size and weight but had entirely different lifestyles. The placid, slow-moving howler monkeys ate primarily leaves (folivores), had longer and larger colons and took twenty hours to digest their meals. The active, fast-moving spider monkeys, on the other hand, ate primarily fruit (frugivores), had smaller guts and took only four hours to digest a meal. Milton found an even more remarkable difference in the size of their brains.

Spider monkeys had brains over twice as heavy as howler monkeys. Her field data told her that, compared with howlers, spiders matured more slowly (had more to learn as youngsters), were much more vocal and ate widely dispersed, high-energy foods growing over several thousand acres. Furthermore, individual spiders had to learn and remember the exact ripening time of at least 100 kinds of fruits. This is especially difficult because, unlike temperate forests, tree species in tropical forests are widely scattered, making long treks necessary to find each tree. Individual spider monkeys could learn and use this information, but howler monkeys, while they had a similar diversity

9

of food trees to visit, had to rely on an extraordinary *collective* memory depending on large social groups.

An interesting side note to this was the reaction of each of two monkeys to Milton when she ate lunch in full view. The dull and placid howlers paid no attention to her while the active spiders came down threatening and teasing, apparently recognizing that a peanut butter sandwich was food.

Milton knew that our small-brained australopithecine ancestral apes had massive grinding jaws and heavy molar teeth, suggesting a diet of tough, low-quality plant materials. She also knew that early humans had smaller jaws and teeth (and increasingly larger brains), indicating that their diet has become less fibrous and higher in quality, with more concentrated nutrients. (Radetsky, 1995.) That our brains grew along with our adoption of a different diet is a fact. What is new is Milton's theory that our changing diet may have been a strong causal factor in the phenomenal growth of human cranial capacity. Milton sees strong parallels between spider monkeys, chimpanzees and early humans: similar diets, aggressiveness, individualistic bent, long-term rearing of young, social systems and large brains. She concluded that: "The behaviors and physiology that define us are the consequences of dietary-driven evolution." She implies that our behavior in modern society translates ultimately into the wisdom of our treks down the aisles of our favorite supermarkets. In view of this, we will later examine *our* current hunting and gathering techniques among the grocery shelves.

Much of what we know about the chimpanzee, in particular, is due to the dedication of the premier field primatologist of our time, Jane Goodall, who has inspired so many to expand our knowledge of our primate background.

Most primates are basically plant eaters. Gorillas get almost all of their food from plants, primarily the green parts, and have enormous paunches for the digestion of all this bulk. Chimpanzees get the bulk of their diet from fruit with some vegetation augmented with animal proteins and fats. Although chimps (and gorillas) branched off some 5 million years ago from human lineage, they still exist in what is considered to be the typical primate home, the tropical forest, with its high diversity of vines and trees.

Unlike orangutans, chimps are not arboreal but travel on the jungle floor along trails, seldom "bushwhacking." Chimps, with a relatively larger brain, are not only more active than gorillas or orangutans, but also have a much more varied diet, cracking

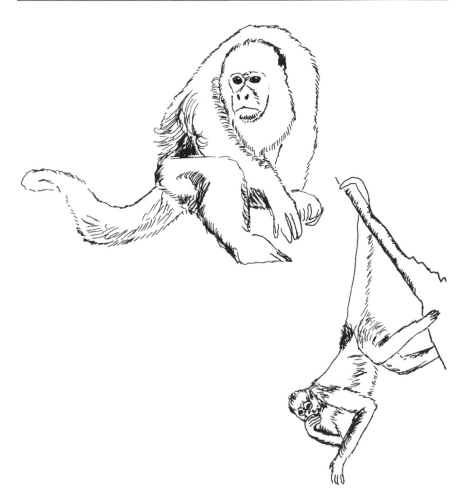

Figure 2. Two monkeys of the Panamanian rainforest, of equivalent weight but with different habits and foods. The fruit-eating spider monkey (below) has a brain twice as heavy as the leaf-eating howler monkey. Such evidence from the lower primates may help us understand how large brains evolved in early humans.

nuts, "fishing" for termites and, by the group effort of a hunting party, capturing and killing monkeys and a few small forest antelopes. It is said that they have made game-killing into a ritual, on the basis that the meat is often traded for copulation with females who rush in with extended hands to get a portion of the kill. Milton (1995) felt that the social implications here were more important than the nutritional ones.

Among primarily vegetarian apes and monkeys, food-getting is not a particularly cooperative effort except that knowledge of adults get the group to the vicinity of the food; then it's every monkey for itself. Cooperation within groups is important in defense of territory or against predators. In the procurement of food, the cooperation of a number of individuals is essential if animals are to be eaten instead of plants. The cooperation of male chimps on their occasional hunting trips demonstrates this. Cooperation is important even in omnivores to catch fish and small game—it is imperative in herding and killing large prey. Cooperation in group hunting goes so far as to involve division of labor, as George Schaller pointed out with packs of African hunting dogs. Some adults stay home and guard the pups, and share food equally, traits not often seen in non-human primates. Speech makes cooperation much more effective. "Lion coming fast on your right" is much more timely than a danger call or even the word "lion."

We can thank our stars that there are no large non-human carnivorous primates. In the forests of the southern Philippines, I was fortunate to be able to study the only totally carnivorous primate, the tarsier. This fist-sized little creature is adapted for leaping like a frog and can jump six feet in the flash of an eye. As I watched these little monsters crunch and swallow a lizard, I couldn't help but shudder to envision tarsiers the size of a chimpanzee, or even a ten-pound monkey. The agility and smarts of such a predator, which operates at night by sound and huge, light gathering eyes, would rival the dinosaurian velociraptor and make it an absolute terror.

The anatomy of the gastrointestinal tract of primates reflects that they are what they eat, as you might suspect. Humans differ markedly from the apes in gut proportions. More than half the total gut volume (56 percent) of humans is in the small intestine, while apes have more volume (45 percent) in the colon. (Milton, 1986.) One monkey, the New World capuchin, has gut proportions similar to humans and, like we once did, eats a high-quality diet of unusually rich, wild foods, including proteins from oil-rich seeds, insect grubs, insects and small vertebrates. This similarity of human gut proportions with those of capuchins and perhaps savanna baboons is an apparent adaptation to high-quality diets that are "digested and absorbed primarily in the small intestine." (Milton, 1987.)

A large colon and caecum (a pouch where the small intestine joins the colon) allows for microbial-aided digestion of plant materials by fermentation. Gorillas, chimps and howler monkeys get as much as 31 percent of their daily energy from microbial fermentation, although it is a relatively slow and inefficient way to produce energy. It is, nevertheless, important in these relatively slow-moving anthropoids. The protruding abdomen of the gorilla is evidence that it can handle large quantities of high-fiber foods.

Because most primates and ancestral humans could handle vegetation in their diets, even modern humans show a surprising ability to digest dietary fiber and possess microorganisms in the colon capable of degrading the structural carbohydrates of plants, especially the relatively unlignified hemicelluloses and celluloses and pectins of vegetables like cabbage and carrots.

Cellulose is the main carbohydrate that gives firmness to plant cells walls forms "wood" and is extremely difficult to break down. Even termites have to depend on bacteria in their gut. Human subjects tested at Cornell University were found to be able to digest 82 percent of cabbage cellulose and "were also notable efficient at degrading bran fiber which has been considerable lignified." (Milton, 1986.) Lignin is the real tough part of "wood." Oddly, a few of the Cornell students could actually digest wood cellulose owing to housing special bacteria others did not have.

We hear a lot about fiber these days. There are two kinds, insoluble fiber like wheat bran and soluble fiber such as psyllium seed husks and oat bran. Both types are good, although some people have problems with wheat bran. Both increase fecal "bulk" and, just as importantly, speed up the time it takes food to go from mouth to anus, called "transit time." Rapid transit is to be desired, since it prevents buildup of toxic compounds that are cancer causing. Both chimps and humans decrease food transit time through the gut with increased dietary fiber, identical hindgut "turnover time" and a high capacity to digest the hemicellulose fraction of wheat bran fiber. (Milton, 1986.) Western societies generally consume less than ten grams of fiber daily per person, while some rural Africans take in more than 170 grams, with transit times two to five times as rapid as that of British navy personnel on refined Western diets—and producing four or five times more fecal matter (and probably defecating as often as three or four times daily). (Burkitt *et al.*, 1972.)

Among our pre-human hominoid ancestors, the "robust" australopithecines, with their large teeth and massive skulls, may have concentrated on tough, fibrous and hard plant foods. As they moved out to forage and scavenge into the mosaic of more varied habitats offered by the African savanna, the lighter ("gracile") australopithecines, although possessing thick molar enamel and large cheek teeth, might have specialized in higher-quality (less fiber) foods. Neither had brain sizes markedly larger than apes. We are presumed to have descended from the more slender form that ate the higher quality foods.

The genus *Homo,* however, with thinner enamel and smaller cheek teeth but with much larger brains, apparently made some sort of dramatic dietary breakthrough beyond an increase in foraging efficiency and ingestion of high-quality foods. This breakthrough, according to Milton (1987), could have been in ways to make low-quality foods higher in quality, such as by separating the nutrients from the fibrous parts of plants or from social innovation, such as cooperative hunting and food sharing, the latter being rudimentary in apes such as chimpanzees. This suggests that both animal protein and fat could then become more important dietary resources for early humans and easier to come by if you have a group of hunters cooperating together. Even chimps, using body language, calls and other sounds, are able to team up sufficiently to successfully hunt. It remained for early humans, however, with their cooperative teamwork and weaponry, to become truly efficient hunters and scavengers, with animal protein playing an important role in their nutrition.

As we might suspect, different lifestyles and foods require different gastrointestinal tracts. We can see the most dramatic differences by comparing the cat, a total carnivore, with the rabbit, a strict herbivore. The cat's digestive tract is short, with 70 percent of the gut volume in the stomach. On examining a rabbit, one is impressed with the long and thin small intestines and well-developed colon and caecum. In the cat, meat not only is stored in their stomach, but also protein digestion begins there. Only the ruminant herbivores like cattle temporarily store large amounts of vegetable matter in the anterior part of the digestive tract. (Birds use an enlarged portion of the esophagus (crop) for temporary storage.)

The human digestive tract is more unspecialized but has a well-developed small intestine and a sacculated colon of fair volume and only a vestigial caecum to which the appendix is affixed.

Treves (1885) found, by actual measurements of the GI tract of human cadavers, that some individuals had colons and small intestines twice as long as others—small intestines between 15.5 and 31.10 feet in males and colons between 3.3 and 6.5 feet in males and females, independent of age, height or weight.

Underhill (1955) who repeated Treves' techniques on 100 individuals, also found that small intestine lengths varied as much as 100 percent with females having the most variation (colons

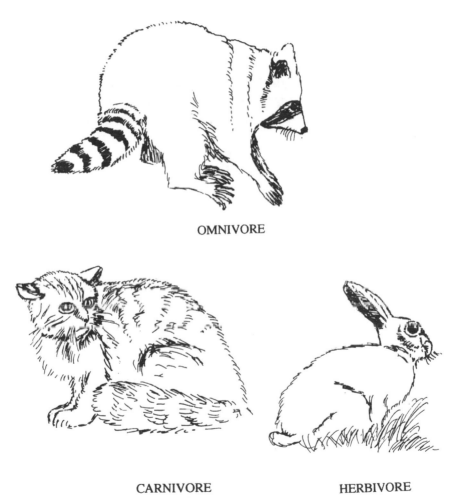

OMNIVORE

CARNIVORE   HERBIVORE

Figure 3.   Cats, with short intestines, live in the wild on other animals exclusively. Rabbits (and some primates) subsist on plant life and tend to have long, specialized gut tracts. Bears, raccoon and many primates, can eat from both animal and plant sources, and have digestive tracts usually intermediate between the other two specialists.

were less variable). She cites Lamb (1893) that there are racial differences in intestinal length, more pronounced in India than in Europe and higher still in American Negroes "in whom lengths of forty feet (12.2 m) are not unknown." (Average length by four researchers from 454 Caucasian individuals was about twenty feet.) This makes one wonder whether this is genetic by reason of our ancestors having adapted to certain types of foods. To confuse this issue it has been discovered that, in certain animals, gut dimensions can be changed somewhat by what an *individual* consistently eats. There is evidence that metabolically active organs such as liver, pancreas and spleen may increase in size with energy needs in swine. (Koong *et al.*, 1983.) Increases in mass of up to 100 percent of the digestive tract have been noted in small mammals (Gross *et al.*, 1985), and many organs, including heart, lungs and adrenal glands were on average 20 percent heavier in lactating cattle over those not yielding milk. (Smith and Baldwin, 1973.) Because of these data, Milton suggests that we sorely need information on human populations on different diets, such as the Africans and Europeans described above.

CHAPTER THREE

Early Man

"We may prefer to think of ourselves as fallen angels, but in reality we are risen apes."

—Desmond Morris

I knelt reverently on a round layer of rock that had formed a floor of rounded boulders. In my hand I held one of the first tools of upright hominids, a palm-sized sharpened stone or "hand axe." Mary Leakey left me there at the *Zinjanthropus*[1] site surrounded by the eroding, naked slopes of Olduvai Gorge. At the bottom of the gorge I could see the volcanic beds of black basalt with some acacia trees, and a few aloes and climbing *Euphorbias*. As Mrs. Leakey left, accompanied by her Dalmatians, she said to keep an eye out for rhinos. There were no trees to climb, and every little dik-dik antelope that I flushed gave me a start. I spent some very pleasant, in fact thrilling, hours looking for and collecting hoof bones of ancient horses, teeth of hippos and bones of catfish, terrapins and birds. I tried to picture how early man must have felt, camped there by some nearby water source. It was eerily quiet in this vast unpopulated corner of Tanzania. Almost everyone who goes to east Africa is profoundly moved by the experience, as if some memory of our ancestral homeland is still with us. It felt doubly so for me at Olduvai at the *Zinj* site or by the little monument erected where *Homo habilis* died approximately two million years ago.

---

[1] Now *Australopithecus boisei*—The hand axes were later identified as belonging to the more "gracile" *Homo habilis.*

Our interest in discussing early man is to get a feel for how humans, given their primate heritage, have eaten and lived for the past several million years. We will see that we would do well to emulate the food habits of our ancestors even today, for our organ systems and major biochemistry have changed little, if at all, since those early times on the savannas of Africa. We have seen that our original niche was that of an omnivore descended from more or less omnivorous primates. Our digestive tracts apparently worked well for at least three million years in African environments which, while near the equator, offered a mosaic of habitats from 5,000 feet upward on the slopes of peaks like mount Kenya. Volcanic activity along the Great Rift Valley yielded mineral-rich soils, along with limy layers (caliche) sought by the large diversity of grazing mammals. No matter how great climatic changes were in the last couple of million years, some parts of Africa were favorable.

In Africa, between five and six million years ago (mya), the gorilla and chimpanzee split off from some ape-like ancestor that led eventually to us. Anthropologists are beginning to believe that "we" (*Homo sapiens),* are not the crowning glory of a line of evolution but merely one terminal twig on a family tree that has twenty or so hominid species that once roamed Africa and Eurasia. To date, our oldest ape-like ancestors are the 4.4 mya *Ardipithecus ramidus* from Ethiopia, followed by several australopithecines, led by *Australopithecus anamesis* (Kenya, 4.2 mya) and including at least four African species (*A. afarenis, A. bahrelghazali, A. africanus and A. garhi*) ranging from 3.5 to 2.5 mya.

Our genus *Homo* split off from the australopithecines some 2 mya. Evidence is mounting that a group of three *Homo* species (*ergaster, rudolfensis, habilis*) along with another hominid (*Paranthropus aethiopicus*) may have foraged the same savannah environments around Lake Turkana in East Africa about 1.8 mya. (Tattersall, 2000.) Their food habits, however, may have differed. *Paranthropus* appears to have been a vegetarian, but our more immediate ancestor *H. ergaster,* clearly ate meat and was the first hominid with modern body form. Ian Tattersall believes that successive waves of humans (genus *Homo*) may have left Africa. Close to the beginning of the ice ages of the Pleistocene, at least by 1.7 mya, *H. ergaster* spread into Europe, and Asia and as far as Java where it is known as *H. erectus.* Of these early waves of migrating humans, *H. antecessor* is the oldest known European form, dating 800,000 years ago and perhaps ancestral to the widespread *H. heidelbergensis.* It turns out that this *Homo* (*antecessor*) was not using the elegant, symmetrical hand axes that its ancestors made in Africa but flaking pebbles and flint and using the core as a hand axe, much as did the people at Olduvai. They ate deer, bison, some elephant and rhino, and human bones were found broken and peeled for their nutritious marrow. (Kunzig, 1997.)

The oldest known "architecture" are crude huts on sandbars at the 400,000 year old Terra Amata site in Greece, where *erectus* ate (in order of fossil abundance) red deer, elephant, wild boar, ibex, two-horned rhino and wild ox, along with seafood and fish. Apparently a successful spear-hunter, he drove now-extinct wild cattle and elephants into bogs. Recently, *H. erectus,* using hand axes and cleavers fashioned from volcanic basalt, was dated to have lived along the Jordan River in Northern Israel 780,000 years ago.

First found in Africa 600,000 years ago, *H. heidelbergensis* became widespread in Africa, Europe and Asia and may have given rise to the Neanderthals, as well as *Homo sapiens.* The first records of *H. sapiens* appears in Africa between 200,000 and 150,000 years ago. (Tattersall, 2000.) They subsequently spread worldwide but apart from the Palestinean corridor (Levantine) "we" (*H. sapiens*) never reached the cold, Pleistocene environments of Europe until 40,000 years ago. When *sapiens* did, their superior technology enabled them to rapidly adapt to the haunts of the relatively unsophisticated Neanderthal hunters.

The stocky, cold-adapted Neanderthals dominated Europe between 230,000 and 30,000 years ago, as far as northern Germany and Kiev. They were hunter-gatherers and Ice Age Europe held many large beasts. It has been said that humans were relatively ineffective hunters between 500,000 and 100,000 years ago. Nevertheless, it is thought that Neanderthals organized group hunts armed with thrusting (not thrown) spears and were able to kill large mammals. Their diet would be dominantly carnivorous. Young wild cattle (aurochs) were taken and adults driven into bogs. Unlike the Cro-Magnon, they are thought to have lacked sewn clothing and warm shelters. There is evidence that Neanderthals harvested reindeer in the Dordogne region on their migrations between summer and winter feeding grounds. The glaciers descended again 180,000 years ago. Evidence from a Croatian cave indicates that by 125,000 years ago they still hunted but also gathered plants, shellfish and small reptiles.

They also practiced cannibalism and used fires to keep warm. It is thought that they were driven south into the Middle East, where they encountered the Cro-Magnon in northern Israel and may have lived with them side by side without interbreeding.

About 40,000 years ago it is thought that technological innovation, clothing, shelters, weapons and more articulate speech enabled a wave of Cro-Magnon to dominate, and the Neanderthals died out. (Gore, 1996.) Jared Diamond's theory is that the elimination of the Neanderthals is the story of a numerous people (Cro-Magnon) well advanced in technology, invading the territory of a less-numerous people with a less-advanced technology. As Cortes proved in his destruction of the Aztec Empire, all you really need is a very small band, technologically advanced.

Cro-Magnon people used needles, awls, mortar and pestle, fishhooks, nets and ropes, spear throwers, and bows and arrows, and indulged in artwork in the caves of southern Europe. Archeologists have found the bones of large animals such as bison, elk, reindeer, horse and ibex, suggesting skilled communal hunting. The Cro-Magnon seemed to have had highly organized animal drives. Near Pavlov, Czechoslovakia, over 100 mammoths were found in one heap of bones, and near Solutre, France, the bones of 10,000 wild horses lay at the bottom of a cliff over which they had been driven. Twenty-thousand years ago the Cro-Magnon migrated into northern Russia and Siberia, where they built elaborate houses, often of mammoth bones, used stone lamps and conducted long distance trade. They may even have been responsible for the extinction of the wooly mammoth and wooly rhinoceros. In fact, Abrams (1987) states that game was the driving force that led Cro-Magnon to occupy all the world's continents.

According to Diamond (1997) anatomically modern humans appeared in Australia before they did in Europe, between 40,000 and 60,000 years ago, in the earliest sea crossings ever made. Diamond claims further that the first Australians and New Guineans, at that time, led the world in technology and art "and that progress could have trickled back to their poorer cousins in Eurasia and Africa."

Scientists have recently found (Dawn of Man Series—The Learning Channel) evidence of anatomically modern people along the South African coast around 100,000 years ago. Apparently shellfish and fish played a significant role in their nutrition. Because such resources are worldwide, theory has it that

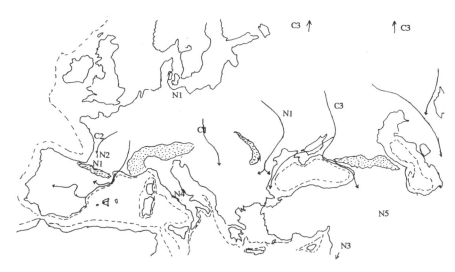

Figure 4. Sites of two sub-species of early man *(Homo sapiens)*, the Neanderthals (N) and Cro-Magnons (C). The Neanderthals and their forebears, *H. erectus,* survived 75,000 years of cold during the Riss glaciation. Between 35,000 and 40,000 years ago the Neanderthals survived the early stages of the Würm glacial period. These cold-adapted people died out between 40,000 and 30,000 years ago, being succeeded by the technologically superior Cro-Magnon peoples who, unlike the Neanderthals, were able to invade northern Russia and Siberia and eventually cross over into North America via the dry land exposed by lowered sea levels, or along coastal routes by boat. The last glacial period ended about 10,000 years ago. Lowered sea levels may have enabled the large herd mammals to pass more easily around the Pyrenees and Caucasus mountains (mountains are stippled) and the Black Sea. Lower sea levels indicated with a dashed line. Hypothetical migration routes indicated by arrows.

Neanderthal sites: (N1) *Homo erectus*/Neanderthal, 230,000 or 30,000 Before Present (B.P.); (N2) Fontéchevade, France, 110,000 B.P.; (N3) Mt. Carmel, Israel, 50,000 B.P.; (N4) Circeo, Italy, 60,000 B.P.; (N5) Zagros Mountains, Iraq, 60,000 B.P. Cro-Magnon sites: (C1) Pavlov, Czechoslovakia, 25,000 B.P.; (C2) Solutré, France, 25,000 (?); (C3) Don River, Russia, 20,000 B.P. Data from *The Emergence of Man Series,* Time-Life Books.

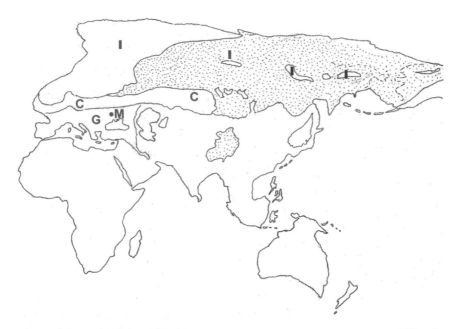

Figure 5.   Map of the important environments in Europe and Northern Asia at the last glacial maximum (21,000 B.P.). Sea levels were lowered during the height of this last Pleistocene glaciation (known as Würm in the Old World). A broad expanse of dry land (Beringia) linked Siberia with Alaska (dashed lines indicate present shorelines). Japan was linked with Asia and the Sunda Shelf connected most of Indo-Malasia out to a narrow but deep trench (Wallace's line), while Australia, New Guinea and Tasmania were joined in a single land mass. Scandanavia and most of the British Isles lay under ice. Cro-Magnon sites occur sparsely in Siberia, Beringia and Alaska, but commonly in Eurasia, Africa, India, Australia and North and South America. The great ice sheet may have protected parts of Europe and Asia from the severest cold. Most of the tundra was not the typical cushion-plant-lichen-moss environment but a mix of four plant communities dominated by low, high and dwarf shrubs along with some grasses, sedges and forbs. Boundaries are approximate. **I,** land ice; tundra (stippled); **C,** cold and cool temperate conifer forest, open woodlands and cold deciduous forest; **G,** mix of grasslands, cold parklands, shrublands and forest (not delineated east of the Caspian Sea); **M,** Mezhirich, Ukraine. Mammoths, either living, or as carcasses or fossils, were so abundant here 15,000 years ago, that Cro-Magnon shelters were constructed of their bones. Data courtesy Jed Kaplan, Max-Planck Institute for Biogeochemistry, Jena, Germany and Patrick Bartlein, Dept. of Geography, University of Oregon, Eugene, Oregon, USA.

these seafood eaters subsequently migrated north along African coasts and east along the coasts of Asia, eventually reaching Australia. Some anthropologists think that these fishing and hunting skills were due to the emergence of symbolic and analytic thought, or there's the possibility that, prior to 60,000 years ago, food was so plentiful they did not have risk encounters with dangerous animals. (Gore, 1997.)

For perspective, some generalities may be useful. From the earliest hominids, man has been highly opportunistic and adaptable, eating what is most readily available, plant or animal. It is logical to assume that evolution would have favored modifying the omnivore gut if people lived long enough in areas offering predominantly either plants or animals. Animal matter, especially if fatty, is our most energy-rich food. (Hamilton, 1989.) Also protein needs are more easily met with animal products, since it takes four medium potatoes to furnish the amount of protein in one ounce of lean meat or one large egg. (Lieberman, 1987.) In the temperate zone, wild game is often available the year around, while, for hunter-gatherers, plant foods are seasonably limited. In some areas man followed the game, as Lapps follow reindeer herds (Abrams, 1987), or he awaited the arrival of migrating mammals (and fish).

Recent research (Pringle, 1998) has refined our knowledge of upper Paleolithic[2] life, between 25,000 and 30,000 years ago in and around Czechoslovakia. It was concluded that while the men

---

[2] To understand the use of archeological terms, let me summarize Cohen's excellent footnotes. Paleolithic refers to Stone Age hunters and gatherers older than 12,000 years who foraged in Pleistocene environments with abundant large game animals (megafauna). Mesolithic (middle Stone Age) peoples were hunter-gatherers in game-depleted environments following the waning of the last Ice Age 15,000 to 10,000 years ago and foraging on a broad spectrum of small animals, plants, fish and shellfish. Neolithic (new Stone Age) refers to farmers of the past 10,000 to 8,000 years. Bronze Age (beginning 5,000 to 6,000 years ago) and Iron Age (beginning 3,000 years ago) coincide with the spread of metal technology, the rise of large urban communities and bounded political states. North American archeologists refer to Paleo-Indian groups prior to 9000 as Archaic (pre-pottery). Early Woodland (9000-1000) peoples were foragers and incipient farmers. Agriculture appeared by 7000 (Mexico-Peru) and crop agriculture began in eastern North America by 3,000-4,000 years ago and full scale maize agriculture around 1,000 years ago.

occasionally killed a mammoth, few were taken prior to the advent of the last Ice Age. Bands had pitched camps next to ancient salt licks and waterholes and simply scavenged the many juvenile and some female mammoths that died there from drought or from miring down in their quest for water. Furthermore, hares and foxes accounted for 46 percent of the individual animals recovered in some sites. Lind Owen and Sarah Mason found that these people had used the fleshy roots of the daisy/aster family. If Ice Age females collected plants, bird eggs, shellfish, insects and trapped small game and also participated in hunting larger game, the conclusion was that women may have contributed 70 percent of the calories consumed by these prehistoric societies, calling into question the typical picture of the female as simply a child-tending, hearth-bound follower.

Recent genetic research on mitochondrial DNA reveals that most Europeans date back to the hunter-gatherers of the late Upper Paleolithic, 11,000 to 14,000 years before present (B.P.), (before the advent of agriculture). (Shreeve, 1999.) Ten per cent go back as far as 50,000 years ago. These two groups would be suspect of needing more protein than the one in five of our ancestors derived from the early (after 8,000 B.P.) farmers that originated in the Near East and who spread through central Europe and along the Mediterranean coast, to eventually reach Britain. While grain farmers and associated villages may have originated in the Near East, in the more northerly parts of Europe other subsistence pursuits may have also led to sedentary village life, but based on animals and possibly different plant foods. Permanent villages have now been found in Turkey dated 10,000 years ago. In these more forested areas no fossil grains were found. Instead pigs were prominent dietary components and other animals such as birds and oxen may have been involved in the local cuisine.

As an overview, Harris (1987) suggests that when populations were small (bands and small villages), people were better off eating high on the food chain (deer instead of seeds, pigs instead of acorns) but that either hard times or denser populations required eating a broader spectrum of plants and animals, setting the stage for cultivation and domestication.

Careful field studies by many anthropologists have revealed that the few existing groups of living hunter-gatherers such as the bushmen of the Kalahari desert and the aboriginal tribes of Australia, with a nomadic life about their only option, are actual relic Stone Age cultures with life styles and diets fairly closely resembling those of Paleolithic man. Some of the investigators lived with the tribes for considerable periods of time. Of special concern are their references to quantity and quality of food killed, gathered and consumed. Some researchers have even drawn up recommendations for modern human diets based upon analysis of things eaten by modern hunter-gatherers, mindful of the fact that for the last two million years cultural man has spent 99 percent of his time as a hunter-gatherer.

Based upon data from living hunter-gatherers today, two anthropologists, Marjorie Shostake and Melvin Konner, and a physician, Boyd Eaton, have formulated what they consider the Paleolithic diet to have been—the ratio was carbohydrate 60 percent, protein and fat each 20 percent. (Eaton *et al.*, 1998.) They also give ratios for the plant and animal foods eaten by contemporary hunter-gatherers, ranging from the savanna-dwelling Hadza of Tanzania (80:25) to the Eskimo of the North American arctic (10:90). In between are the desert dwelling Australian aborigines (90:10), their coastal counterparts (25:75) and two groups in which wild game figures roughly half of the diet, the Aché of Paraguay (50:50) and the Agta of tropical montane forest in the Philippines (40:60). Desert and savanna dwellers eat more plant products than coastal or forest peoples.

In hunting, we generally think of the protein-rich muscle meat as the most sought after portion, but in the context of total nutrition we must consider the sources of vitamins and minerals in the animal body. By instinct or trial and error, our hunter-gatherers had to do this. Organs such as the liver, replete with oil-soluble vitamins, were much sought after. Even the glands were considered. After killing a moose, Canadian Indians divided up the vitamin-rich adrenal gland, which is extremely rich in vitamin C, giving a slice to each member of the family. Fat from around the internal organs, under the skin (blubber) or in the bone marrow was also of paramount importance. Wild animals usually don't have much fat unless they are building it up for survival during the winter. Whereas meat from our domestic stock may have 30 percent fat, the average of wild game is low, about 4.3 percent. According to Eaton *et al.*, the fat of wild game, unlike that of our domestic livestock, contains 2.5 percent EPA (eicosapentenoic acid), one of the Omega 3 family of essential fatty acids derived from alpha-linolenic acid which wild animals get from grazing a diversity of plants. Incidentally, EPA is most abundant in marine fish like sardines and mackerel and sea-run salmon and was presumably not available to Stone Agers living away from rivers draining into northern oceans. Since larval wood beetles are almost little packages of fat, the quest for fat explains why they are so sought after by today's hunter-gatherers. Chimpanzees commonly fish for termites (which are 44 percent fat).

Fat is essential to metabolize protein, for synthesizing the lipoproteins that carry fat soluble nutrients in the bloodstream (such as vitamin A) and, of course, it can substitute for sugar and starch as a source of energy, especially important for Ice Age hunters in northern Europe and Asia and for the Eskimos. For hunter-gatherers fat storage in their own bodies was the key to getting through periods when the pickings were lean. Our own fat stores seem to be designed for intermittent starvation or fasts beyond our control.

Fat is so crucial to hunter-gatherers that they have been known to discard prey animals that had no fat around their entrails. During lean periods, hunter-gatherers in eastern North America killed and ate large numbers of rabbits, which had little or no fat. According to Hayden (1981), these men came close to starvation's door because of the lack of fat in spite of full bellies. Living among the Eskimos, Stefansson (1962) found a similar situation where the natives became ill from gorging on caribou that were fat-free, even down to their tongues and bone marrow. Stefansson said, "one by one the six Eskimos of the party were taken with diarrhea." Brian Hayden (1981) was astounded to see the Australian aborigines of the western desert "kill a kangaroo, examine the intestines for fat, and abandon the carcass where it lay because it was too lean." You may recall the book (or movie) *Never Cry Wolf* when Farley Mowat (1963), having watched the wolves eating the abundant mouse-like arctic voles, decided he too would try to live on them. He could not because he had disemboweled them. He was forced to eat them whole or not at all. There are, of course, other than fat, important nutrients in an animal's organs as well as minerals in the skeleton. After all, we do eat the whole sardine minus the head. Ancient man invariably cracked the bones for their fatty marrow and skulls for their fatty brains. I was raised on scrambled brains and eggs at least weekly, but when I broach this topic with my friends I can watch the gums receding from their teeth in disgust. How far we have come from the hunting-gathering life! Hayden (1981) lists the many cultural groups that place a high value on the fat content of their foods. And you can't be squeamish. The source could be the huge grubs of wood-eating beetles or larval bees in a honeycomb. The aboriginal of the tropical rain forests of northeastern Australia value the fat from pythons as "the greatest delicacy." (Hayden, 1981.)

Protein, of course, is another necessity. The difficulty of getting enough of it in forms to supply the nine essential amino acids urged hunter-gatherers to hunt. Meat readily supplies a balanced intake of amino acids. Vegetable sources like beans, corn and rice have their shortcomings. Hunter-gatherers today are quite protein consumptive, nine groups averaging 80 grams eaten per person per day,[3] comparing favorably with the daily per capita intake of affluent (70 to100 grams) and non-affluent (40 grams) nations. The chimpanzee averages only 6.7 grams of protein per individual per day, but it also gets it from other sources such as termites, which are, by one report (Brothwell, 1969), 36 percent protein. Physiologically, it has been noted that a high protein to carbohydrate ratio lowers blood serotonin levels (you don't feel as good) and elevates the desire for carbohydrates, while one low in protein and higher in carbohydrates increases serotonin and induces a craving for protein. (Wurtman and Wurtman, 1983.)

Regarding total caloric intake, eleven groups of hunter-gatherers from four continents averaged 2,522 kilocalories (KC) daily, which can be compared with the intake of affluent (2,500 to 4,000) and non-affluent (1,600 to 2,100) nations. If I have analyzed Cohen's figures correctly, four groups from Africa, Australia and South America were able to average 6,962 KC per hour of effort hunting large game animals. Gathering (five groups, mainly plant products) generated an average of 2,233 KC per hour of effort. This last figure can be compared with swidden rice agriculture in the Philippines (3,000 to 5,000 KC per hour of effort), irrigated rice (3,500 to 10,500) and horticulture (17,000). Obviously, effort expended on agricultural crops is more rewarding.

Thus we see that ancient man, represented by hunter-gatherer groups living today, had much the same dietary needs as we

---

[3] This assumes that game has 25% protein per 100 grams of meat.

do. By taking a close look at surviving hunting gathering groups, we can conclude with reasonable certainty that man's biological and biochemical needs have changed hardly at all in the last several million years. The lesson is this: today's hunter-gatherers live in natural environments of many different kinds, from desert to rainforest. Wherever they live, it is in intimate balance with the plants and animals around them. Whether by centuries of trial and error or not, they have come to know they must eat certain things and do so without question. They cannot satisfy whims of appetite but can only eat what nature provides and when she provides it. They are, in general, superbly healthy and do not need dentists. They know where it all comes from and respect and revere the natural world that gives them life. Colin Turnbull recounts the story of the Ituri forest pygmies, who, each evening, gather and sing praises to the spirit of the forest, thanking the powers that be for what they are allowed to hunt and gather from the forest's productivity. To live their lifestyle requires that they learn to identify and know the characteristics of a staggering number of life forms with which they must share their world.

The following, quoted by Price (1941), was written by the distinguished anatomist and anthropologist, M.F. Ashley-Montagu, in the Scientific Monthly under the title *The Socio-biology of Man*.

"In spite of our enormous technological advances we spiritually and as human beings are not the equal of the average Australian Aboriginal or the average Eskimo—we are very definitely their inferiors. We lisp noble ideals and noble sentiments—the Australians and the Eskimos practice them—they neither write books or lecture about them. Theirs are the only true democracies, where every individual finds his happiness in catering to the happiness of the group, and where any one who in any way threatens the welfare of the group is dealt with as an abnormality."

There is a paucity of data about the actual efficiency of gathering plant foods in the Northern Hemisphere, as done, say, by Native Americans. A highly suggestive experiment was conducted with students collecting acorns in an oak forest (red oak, white oak, chestnut oak) in central Pennsylvania. It took five times less energy to collect acorns than it would with conventional grain cultivation. Their data suggested that 160 hectares of forest could provide the total energy requirements of a forty-person clan for five months. (Gerwing *et al.,* 1999.)

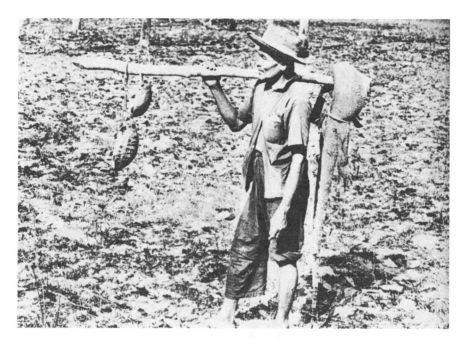

Figure 6. In the monsoon forests of northern Cambodia, local people revert to hunting and gathering during the dry season in particular, setting fires to facilitate visibility. Here, a Cambodian returns to camp after a successful afternoon, having captured a large monitor lizard (*Varanus salvator*) and some terrestrial terrapins. The arid savanna forest has been newly burned. (Wharton, 1966.)

Jared Diamond has taken many expeditions to the highlands of New Guinea, primarily to study bird life. He found that hunters of the local tribes knew well over a thousand plants and animals and knew the rock types as well. They were, as he put it "walking encyclopedias of natural history." This intimate acquaintance began with the primate need to recognize the many forms, shapes and colors of leaves, flowers, seeds and fruits of the tropical forest. Chimpanzees are reported to eat 200 plants and even use some for medicinal purposes. They also consume forty animals, including ten primates and four hoofed mammals. Kung bushmen of the Kalahari Desert of Africa use 100 plants and 144 species of insects, reptiles, birds and mammals. Queensland Aborigines 240 plants and 120 animals. This is only what they use, not the number they can identify. The Philippine Hanunoo use over 2,000 species (Hayden, 1981), including 108 insects and

461 vertebrates. Common sense tells us that native peoples have a much broader knowledge of their total environment, since their very survival has depended on not just in knowing things (taxonomy) but in knowing how things relate (ecology), including weather, soil types and natural cycles. Contrast this with the modern urban citizen, while street-wise in his artificial surroundings, probably doesn't know the original home of tomatoes, carrots or pistachio nuts, or even chickens for that matter. If we were plunked down in some natural environment somewhere and forced to live off the land for a week or two, I can guarantee that, in addition to a weight loss, we would acquire an admiration, and even a reverence for, the knowledge and wisdom of early man and the living groups of hunter-gatherers whom we are fast pushing into oblivion.

From ape through australopithecine to *Homo habilis* and *erectus* and, eventually, to us, *sapiens,* there came a genetic and, later a cultural endowment. The heirs of this profound knowledge of how man is supposed to live are the hunter-gatherers. In the provocative book "Ishmael," Daniel Quinn (1992) calls the hunter-gatherers the "leavers" and the rest of us the "takers." The hunter-gatherers, developed by principles of natural selection "in the hands of the gods," were an integral part of the community of life in earth's diverse environments, their populations controlled by the same inexorable laws that apply to all animals, i.e., you must not override the carrying capacity of the land in which you live, or, in other words, the ability of its soils and life forms to sustain only a certain number of animals parasitic upon its productive largesse. The last trick of the gods, Quinn says, was "that they did not exempt man from the law that governs the life of grubs and ticks and shrimps and rabbits and mollusks and deer and lions and jellyfish . . . any more than they were exempted from the law of gravity." About 10,000 years ago, with the inception of the agricultural revolution, we began to erode our reservoir of knowledge of how to live sustainably with the world.

That we are not divinely appointed to modify the world to suit our needs, that we are not the apex of creation and that we cannot overcome nature's rules with our technological genius, has been a hard pill to swallow. With no certain knowledge of how to successfully live with nature, the peoples who followed the hunter-gatherers came to depend on prophets for guidance. Unfortunately, most of the wisdom they dispensed seldom included how we should relate to the rocks, soils, waters, air, plants and fellow animals. Nor did they address the inescapable fact that earthly health and happiness is vitally dependent on how they treat and respect the acreage that sustains them. In the opinion of many, we have cut the ground out from under the feet of our youth by denying them the knowledge of how man has been able to live happily and healthily without the trappings of civilization or the myth of the god-like status of humans. Quinn's wise gorilla asks his human friend, since we can't seem to stop screwing up paradise (ultimately when all the fish and forests are gone and the air and waters are dead) and enacting a wretched story without anchorage in the fundamental truths and laws of nature, why we wonder that so many of our young people live lives stoned on drugs, booze or television. They are, as many have said, looking for meaning in a life bereft of the laws of nature, the solid foundation leading to the grandest of all visions, the spiritual awareness of the unity of all life and non-life throughout the universe.

I once stood in a Guarani village near the Pilcomayo River. I saw in the fire before me a dozen little armadillos, their feet sticking up in the air, getting roasted, entrails and all. I realized that ancestral man must have always been an opportunist making the best of wherever he lived and exercising his greatest advantage over the other animals, his incredible adaptability. My Argentinean friends had adapted to the great thorn forest of the Gran Chaco with many species of armadillos ranging from tiny, mole-like forms to giants that could out-pull a horse (so I was told). Adaptability allowed early man to scrounge anything edible. Later, individual cultures adapted to predominantly meat or predominantly vegetable diets, dependent on their environments. Subsequent chapters address how modern man, with all his mobility, mixed up the dietary bloodlines so that some of us may now have to pay a price to eat like everyone else. While we're still extremely adaptable, our physiology just cannot adapt that swiftly to the speed of our technological progress.

According to Morris (1994), going to work is a major substitute for hunting and we still "bring home the bacon." Even collecting things like rocks, stamps and art work, he says, can be symbolic of hunting, with the careful plans, prolonged searching, stealth tactics (bargaining) and the joy of the final "kill" of acquisition. Our sports and games, hikes and travels and even our celebratory feasts that recreate the "primal tribal sharing of the hunter's kill," all may bear the hallmarks of our hunting past. Our love of gardening may titillate some atavistic urge. It has been said that our preoccupation with semi-open terrain around our homes and especially grassy lawns may be an attempt to satisfy some innate longing for the savannas of the African plains where we spent those millions of years. Edward O. Wilson, the Harvard biologist who has popularized the word "biodiversity," thinks that man is innately a lover of nature, a biophile. He offers the evidence in a book devoted to and named *"Biophilia."* Both this emotional approach and our intellectual grasp of ecology may be needed for our very survival.

We wish we knew more about the environments of early man. We know that humans lived with much of the Pleistocene megafauna such as the huge wooly mammoths and reindeer herds that could survive the harsh winters of northern Eurasia. Perhaps early humans followed or intercepted their migrations around the flanks of the Alps, Carpathians, Caucasus and Pyrenees, or waited for their annual return to the warmer regions nearer the Mediterranean. It is hard to see how the massive mammoths, requiring up to 600 pounds of vegetation daily, could have survived the winters of northern Europe and Asia without some migration.

It so happens that the most revealing evidence of what the conditions of life must have been like back then comes from the ice frozen in place for tens of thousands of years, and from ocean sediments at the bottom of the sea. Figure 7 shows climatic fluctuations over the past 100,000 years, based upon ice cores from the Greenland ice cap and from ocean sediments. Based upon these ice cores drilled to great depth, Alley and Bender (1998) have been able to identify major and minor fluctuations of ancient temperatures that affected both hemispheres. During the past 100,000 years, there were five major warm periods, the last one roughly 10,000 years ago. They were apparently caused by a wobble (precession) in the tilt of the earth's axis relative to the sun. These warm-ups fitted a 20,000-year cyclic wobble, predicted by the Serbian astronomer Milutin Milankovitch.

The Greenland ice cores, however, in addition to those predicted by the Milankovitch cycles, showed a remarkable number of smaller-warming cycles, 24 in fact, for the past 100.000 years. These shorter cycles lasted from "a few hundred to a few thousand years." They were abrupt, changing climates 5 to 10 degrees Celsius or more, sometimes in as little as a few years. The ice

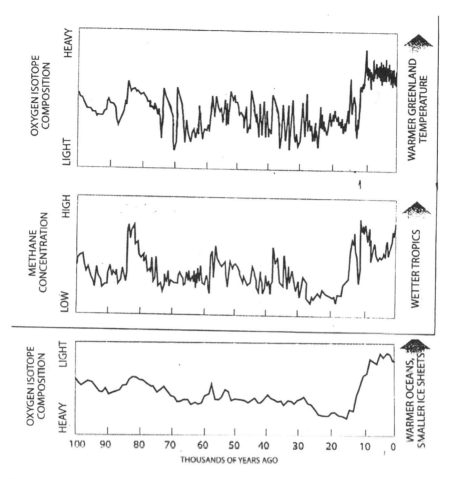

Figure 7. Climatic fluctuations from the Greenland Ice Cores (upper two graphs) and ocean sediments (lower graph). Note the abrupt shift about 10,000 years ago to a new average temperature much higher than the average levels of the preceding 90,000 years. This coincides with the rapid spread of man in North America, the demise of the great Ice Age mammals and the advent of agriculture. (Graph after Alley and Bender, 1998.)

"thermometers" used by the scientist also recorded the coldest periods. The severest periods of the last Ice Age (roughly 30,000-15,000 years ago) found Greenland 20 degrees Celsius colder on an average than it is today.

To me, the startling conclusion of this science is that, between 12,000 and 10,000 years ago there was a dramatic, rapid and substantial shift to a warmer average temperature in the Northern

Hemisphere, as visible in the graphs of Figure 7. The climate suddenly got quite a bit warmer and stayed warm. Gone were the approximately 24 large fluctuations between cold and warm of the previously 90,000 years, which presumably were adapted to by both the great Ice Age mammals and a scattering of Neanderthal clans. The first waves of Cro-Magnon man apparently also endured the end of this long period of changing climates and especially the last great glaciation, presumably with the aid of caves, fires and animal skins as clothing. Their advanced culture may have left the Neanderthals literally "out in the cold."

The effects of the abrupt climate change about 11,000 years ago can be seen in North America as well. Certain environments in the southern Appalachians such as boulder fields are obviously peri-glacial features in our higher mountains. (Wharton, 1978.) Other studies had shown that about 10,000 to 9,000 years ago freeze-thaw phenomena such as rock cleaving ceased and was supplanted by the emergence of erosion as a dominant theme controlling certain environments. Heavier rains may have also been implicated.

Recently, while watching the NOVA program "Warnings from the Ice" I was stunned to see the upper graph of Figure 7 on television, depicting the sudden shift in the earth's temperature regime beginning about 11,000 years ago. What was so startling was a possible relationship of this climate change with three other post-Pleistocene events: the rapid spread of man in North America, the demise of the great Ice Age mammals and the advent of agriculture in the northern hemisphere. It just seemed too much of a coincidence.

When the glaciers covered Poland and the British Isles (Figure 5), the tundra in France and Germany was apparently warmer and provided more grazing than later when it withdrew to the Arctic Circle. (Claiborne, 1970.) The extensive prairie-like steppes south of the tundra also grew an herbaceous flora that supported many large mammals. As the climate warmed and the glaciers withdrew far to the north, neither the cold strips of tundra that remained or the conifer forests of the taiga that closely followed it, yielded sufficient summer refuge or forage for the great herds of Pleistocene herbivores that fed early man in Europe and Asia.

In the Northern Hemisphere, at least, as the glaciers retreated, the width of the temperate zone expanded, and the grassy and game-rich prairies of the steppes were replaced by the less hospitable forests of the taiga. (Claiborne, 1970.) With the demise of the Pleistocene megafauna, humans began to eat a wider variety of terrestrial faunas and, in coastal areas, marine resources became more important, such as the spring biomass peak in oysters. (Yesner, 1987.)

In any event, mankind, north of the Tropic of Cancer, suddenly had less meat to eat and perhaps, for whatever reasons, ceased to be a follower of the great beasts, soon discovering that the proteins of grains and domesticated animals could substitute for the former wealth of the wild game. Obligatory or not, the shift to sedentary agriculture began the long goodbye with the natural world that had nurtured us for countless millennia. We are still groping for the recovery of some of that physical, mental and spiritual kinship with the world we tried to leave behind.

CHAPTER FOUR

Agriculture

"Ceres . . . (from which the word 'cereal' is derived) . . . took him in her chariot, drawn by winged dragons, through all the countries of the earth, imparting to mankind valuable grains, and the knowledge of agriculture."

The Age of Fable—Thomas Bulfinch

"Demeter (Ceres) rewarded Triptolemus by giving him a bag of barley seed and a plough. At her orders, he went all over the world teaching mankind how to plough the fields, sow barley seed and reap the harvest."

Greek Gods and Heroes—Robert Graves

From early man on, there were places on earth where animals did best and places where plants did best, and some places where both flourished. Being opportunistic omnivores, humans evolved to exploit all these environments. Those who could not adapt to the local diet did not reproduce. As theory goes, their food supply forced them to genetically adapt.

Unlike plant-based cultures, animal-based cultures and mixed-base ones (hunter-gatherers), had little permanent effect on their environment. Imitating the movements of the great assemblages of Ice Age beasts, pastoralist herders moved or followed their herds. Early horticultural gardens in small forest clearings and aquaculture with marsh plants such as rice, began to change things somewhat. Plantings in large areas cleared of forest, coupled with the use of fire, could seriously modify the forest environment.

Apart from its environmental impact, tilling the soil began a new social concept: that one could own or permanently possess a part of the earth, heretofore available to all that could use its resources.

Agriculture has been called the greatest tragedy ever to befall the human race. This shocking news must be viewed objectively within the context of historical, ecological and medical perspectives. Most of the problems facing the world today are a direct result of overpopulation, which is largely due to agriculture. Anthropologists would say that, given such a large brain, it was inevitable that man would domesticate plants and animals, thus making it possible for them to dominate the ecosystems of earth.

The transition from hunting and gathering to agriculture has enabled man to achieve two characteristics of modern civilization: a stable food supply and leisure time. Carefully examined, this transition suggests to Jared Diamond another conclusion: "For most people, it meant infectious diseases, chronic malnutrition and a shorter life span. It brought a class-based inequality, worsened the lot of women and represented a halfway station between noble traits such as art and language, and unmitigated vices such as genocide and destruction of the environment." (Diamond, 1992.) This is not based on conjecture. As Diamond says, " . . . the archeological evidence shows the introduction of agriculture to have been a mixed blessing, seriously harming many people while benefiting others." Nesse and Williams (1994) state: "How ironic that humanity worked for centuries to create environments that are almost literally flowing with milk and honey, only to see our success responsible for much modern disease and untimely death."

Until about 12,000 years ago, man was just another biped creature playing out his role as a social omnivore. Oblivious to his primate heritage and his forthcoming role as de facto ruler of the earth, he was nourished by the largesse of the biosphere, living from the surplus production of plants and fellow animals.

Many of us will agree that, in the short space of 10,000 years, as worldwide populations explode, the Amazon burns, ethnic and religious struggles show no sign of abating, and while we are preoccupied with sickness rather than health, humans appear to have violated natural laws that have successfully controlled the welfare of the earth and all its life. It has to do with agriculture. The mindset of those early cultivators in the Fertile Crescent appeared to change from a working relationship with the entire network of the natural world to one in which man began to feel that he was some sort of special organism that could mold nature to his needs. Accordingly, he gradually began to exempt himself from natural laws that exempt nothing or no one, and in 500 generations has brought the world to the point of both natural and artificial apocalypse.

Plants live on the constant flow of energy from the sun. The cycles of water and weather linked to this energy flow release minerals from rocks and atmosphere. Drawing on a small increment of minerals from the rocks, plants can continuously recycle their principle nutrients while maintaining other elements in the atmosphere consistent with life, in accordance with the Gaia theory.

Plants always produce a few more leaves, flowers and fruits than are actually necessary, in order to survive sporadic environmental events such as droughts and outbreaks of insects. In addition to being able to lose a certain percentage of their leaves, buds, and fruits to worms, birds or mammals without damage, plants have another technique for survival. They store extra food in their stems and root systems. Some trees can be entirely defoliated for two or even three years before they succumb, and grasses can be grazed, harvested or burned yearly and will regrow from the energy stored in the rootstock. Thus plants, with their built-in energy storage, evolved to cope with the vagaries of environments, provide a huge biomass of food to support plant-eating animals from insects to elephants. Furthermore, the carbon compounds in their cast-off leaves provide energy to fuel a host of bacteria, worms and insects and millipedes, which decompose the tons of organic matter that fall to the ground, releasing from it nutrients that are in a reusable form.

Actually, many plants, by color, flavor, or nutrient content advertise their edibility and invite all kinds of animals to assist them in their reproduction. It is a mutual and highly satisfactory arrangement. Because plants have "learned" to "cooperate" and even depend upon plant-eating animals, herbivores, including fructivores and granivores have flourished, their life cycles beautifully integrated with those of the plants, all existing on the legacy of those first tiny free-floating cells that acquired an incredible internal chemistry to harness the energy of the sun.

Wouldn't you know it, with all that plant-generated flesh running around some vertebrate animals would evolve to live on the surplus production of meat, just as the herbivores evolved to live on the surplus production of plant tissues. Indeed birds of prey and various predators adjust their reproduction to the fluctuations of the numbers of rodents they prey upon. Some scavenging and killing may benefit an ecosystem. The dinosaurian reptiles established a herbivore-carnivore balance similar to the mammals today and it worked very well for them, for they dominated the earth for 50 million years.

So, for millions of years, animals and plants evolved in balance with each other, both dependent on the nutrient reservoir of a fertile soil and a supply of pure water and air. Then along came some adventurous primates with their insatiable curiosity, intelligence and social cooperation and spread all over the world. They didn't really upset nature's apple cart until about 12,000 years ago when, after sampling anything that looked or tasted at all edible, they discovered that munching the large seeds of certain grasses would give them energy. They probably watched the birds eating them and found the storage caches of rodents—this may have given them the idea initially. For two million years at least, early man had participated in the grand plan of nature as just another animal, weird as he looked, with his body hair and big head, stalking around on two legs, babbling and shouting strange sounds. Waving his arms and throwing sticks and stones, he was even harder to deal with than the troops of long-fanged baboons that hunted and gathered on the African plains.

We have already seen that human hunting and gathering societies had developed a life style that well satisfied their quest for energy and balanced intake of protein, fat and carbohydrate. The daily levels compared favorably with those of modern civilized humans, didn't take all that much more effort, and left them with an enviable amount of leisure time. The Kung Bushmen of Africa's Kalahari Desert area have a diet which is 60 to 80 percent vegetable, including the protein-rich Mongongo nut. The Anthropologist Richard Lee estimated that a Kung woman could gather enough food in one six-hour day to feed her family for three days. The studies of Eaton *et al.* have shown that in many ways hunter-gatherers ate better than we do at, least health-wise, and we would be prudent to emulate their recipe for success. As intimated above, however, about 12,000 years ago hunter-gatherers began to depart their time-honored ways. In certain parts of the world, such as the Fertile Crescent of the Near East, they discovered that the seeds of wild grains, ancestral wheats and barley, were not only good energy sources but, unlike wild game, roots and tubers, could be stored for long periods. They were far enough north where "laying by" for the winter was a fact of life with most animals. Other animals had to store fat, hibernate or migrate or otherwise adapt to slim pickings in the season of cold. So it was that in the land of grasslands and oak-pistachio woodlands lying between the Zagros Mountains and the Mediterranean (now largely Iraq, Syria and Jordan), the first agricultural economies emerged between 10,000 and 8,000 years ago. Herbert Wright (1977) stated that pollen studies in Iran, Syria, Greece, Italy and Spain showed that, between 35,000 and 11,000 years ago, the entire northern Mediterranean region had a cool, dry, steppe climate, dominated by composites of the genus *Artemisia*. About 11,000 years ago, these steppes withdrew to southern Asia, leaving a dry, summer climate to which cereal grains were adapted. This dramatic climatic change is precisely recorded by evidence from the Greenland Ice Cores (see chapter on Early Man). In the area of southwest Asia, ancestral grasses with their large seeds grew in patches almost as thickly as cultivated fields are today. One researcher of wild wheats, Jack Harlan, using a stone sickle, proved that in only three weeks a family could gather enough grain to last them an entire year. Wild einkorn wheat grew in the ecotone or edge-zone where scrub oak woodlands met the open savanna grasslands. It did not take our large-brained ancestors very long to figure out that you could sow those seeds in disturbed places conveniently close to their camps. The necessity for wandering around became less and less. And of course what you needed to complete this picture were some animals always close by which you could butcher as needed.

By a remarkable coincidence, this same part of the Fertile Crescent was also the original home of four of our major domestic animals, goats, sheep, pigs and cattle. These were domesticated around 8,700 to 8,000 years ago. Some eight plants were

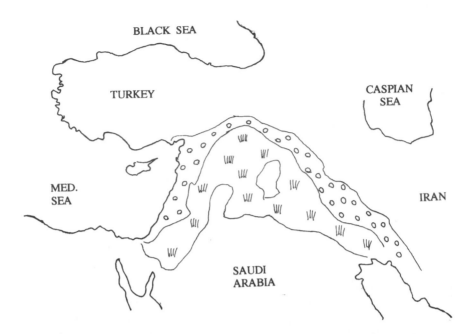

Figure 8.   Ecological zones of the Fertile Crescent where eight species of plants including wheat, barley, peas, lentils and flax were first domesticated between 10,000 and 8,000 years ago, principally in sub-tropical woodland (round symbols) and steppe grassland (grass symbols). In this same area four important animals were domesticated; goats (9,000 B.P.), and sheep, cattle and pigs between 8,700 and 8,000 B.P., mostly in present-day Iraq and Syria. (Smith, 1995.)

also domesticated in the Fertile Crescent between 10, 000 and 9,700 years ago: lentils, peas, and chickpeas, bitter vetch, flax, emmer, einkorn wheat and barley. The exact area has been pinpointed as a 10-40 kilometer wide strip from the Damascus Basin to the lower Jordan Valley, called the Levantine Corridor.

It has been suggested that we invented a mythology to explain why we had to work so hard, often "against" nature it seemed, while other less "advanced" cultures fitted themselves more or less harmlessly into the natural world and were emotionally and spiritually thankful to be the recipient of God's generosity and compassion.

It seems that the Garden of Eden was a metaphor for the pre-agricultural life. Adam and Eve apparently represented, at first, the hunter-gatherer and herder cultures that had developed modestly for three million years without destroying their rivers, soils, prairies, forests or oceans.[4]

These prior cultures, now just scattered remnants, unlike agriculturists that followed, did not assume that they had a god's prerogative of what and who should live and what and who should die. When Adam and Eve ate the fruit of the tree of the knowledge of good and evil, these first biblical humans assumed that they no longer had to depend on the bounty of nature and they could reproduce without limit, for they now had god-like power. But, as the story goes, they were found out and banished from the Garden of Eden, to be forever condemned to wrest their livelihood from the soil by the sweat of their brow.

The story of Cain and Abel is revealing. The ancestral Hebrews were the original agriculturists in the Fertile Crescent between and close to the Tigris and Euphrates Rivers. Their uncontrolled population expansion led to desire for more land and they encroached on the domain of and destroyed the pre-agriculture herders, the Semites. By 4500 the southern expansion of the tillers of the soil was blocked by the nomadic Semite herders (called respectively the "takers" and the "leavers" by Quinn (1992)). Quinn claims that the Cain-Abel story is itself a metaphor for the confrontation between the agriculturist and the herders, and that the story where God accepted Abel (a herder) and rejected Cain (a tiller, and killer, of herders) actually originated among the Semite herders. It was apparently difficult for the herders, who had controlled their population for so long, to understand why the "new" people, the soil tillers, could be so murderous. (Don't forget how we tillers destroyed the Native American culture, which were both tillers and hunter-gatherers.) Unlike many "primitive" cultures, which out of respect or fear honored the territorial boundaries of other peoples, this new culture of tillers that spread from the Mid-east recognized few boundaries. We can now understand why Ritchie Calder wrote about "the age-old struggle between the nomads, the Sons of Abel, and the tillers, the Sons of Cain . . . " and how this enmity was exaggerated by the "metal-working barbarians" and the refined

---

[4] With the exception of certain islands they apparently did not seriously impact the great mega-faunal assemblages on the southern continents. There is still controversy over their exact role in the demise of the great boreal megafauna of the Northern Hemisphere during the waning of the last Ice Age.

armaments which made more devastating the wars, eventually setting tiller against tiller as well as tiller against nomad.

The manipulation of nature was not unique to the Near East. In Australia, where hunter-gatherers have lived for many millennia without agriculture, the natives manipulated habitats by burning to encourage some species of grasses. They would also intervene in the life cycle of plants such as wild yams, the tops of which they replanted after cutting off most of the tuber, much as we plant potatoes today by leaving an "eye" or bud in a small

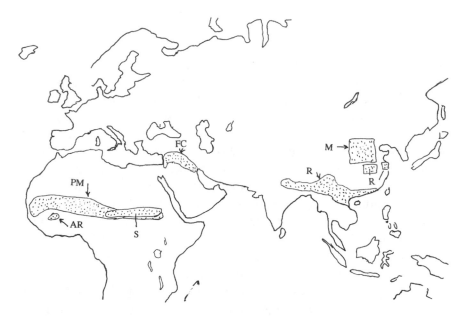

Figure 9.   Areas of origin for the domestication of food plants in the Old World (stippled). The African zone of pearl millet (PM) and sorghum (S) lies in a rainfall zone of 4 to 24 inches. The center for African rice (AR) is in a zone of higher rainfall. The Fertile Crescent (FC) in the Mid-East was the source of many important food plants such as wheat and barley as well as four important animal species. In East Asia, the center of rice origin (R) (about 8000 B.C.) is thought to be in China's Yangtze Valley, and by 5,000 to 3,000 years ago was established in broad areas of India and southeast Asia. Millet (M) (which feeds nearly a third of the world) was cultivated along the Yellow River. Broomcorn and fox-tail millet (M) was cultivated along the Yellow River by hunter-gatherers as early as 9,000 to 7,500 years ago. The jungle fowl (our chicken) was thought domesticated in China 7,000 to 7,200 B.P., along with pigs. Water buffalo came later (3,500 B.P.). (Data from Smith, 1995.)

piece that we put back into the ground. A pre-agricultural stage might be called a horticulture where you just move plants around but don't mess with their genetic traits, such as seeds that don't shatter off the stalk when harvested.

The Kumeyaay Indians of the California coast as late as 1769 were still creating groves of oaks and nut-bearing pines and planting and transplanting agave, grapes, desert palms and cacti to end up with a complex mosaic of manipulated wild plants. (Smith, 1995.)

Domestication of plants led to the formation of compact easily gathered seed heads preferably at the top of the stem. Our common cultivar, sorghum, a source of molasses, has such a compact terminal package of seeds. How this human selection came about is exemplified by a common garden "weed," lamb's quarters (genus *Chaenopodium*), the leaves of which make a tasty and calcium-rich pot green if picked young. It would be difficult to harvest the seeds of lamb's quarters as they are borne loosely all over the plant. Caves in Arkansas and eastern Kentucky reveal that Native Americans were eating and storing the seed of a domesticated lamb's quarters *(Chaenopodium berlindieri)* by 3500 B.C. In the 1720s this "grain" plant was still being grown by the Natchez Indians along the Mississippi River. At the same time, a close relative, quinoa, was being domesticated in the Peruvian Andes. Its very nutritious seeds are now available in most health food stores.[5]

Present day hunter-gatherers have little need for agriculture. When Bushmen were asked why they didn't plant things they replied that why should they, with all those Mongongo nuts out there for the gathering.

In any event, agriculture seemed to set the stage for the haves and have-nots, and the acquisition of wealth by some individuals over that of others. The earliest villages, as with many societies today, were communal, with little personal property and often based on an extended family, with the sexes sometimes

---

[5] Experimentation with plants led to seven areas where wild species were independently domesticated and distinctive economies emerged. They are as follows with the approximate dates B.P. (before present): Near East (Fertile Crescent) (10,000); South China (Yangtze Corridor) (8,500); North China (Yellow River) (7,800); sub-Saharan African (4,000); South Central Andes (4,500); Central Mexico (4,700); and eastern United States (4,500). (Cohen, 1977.)

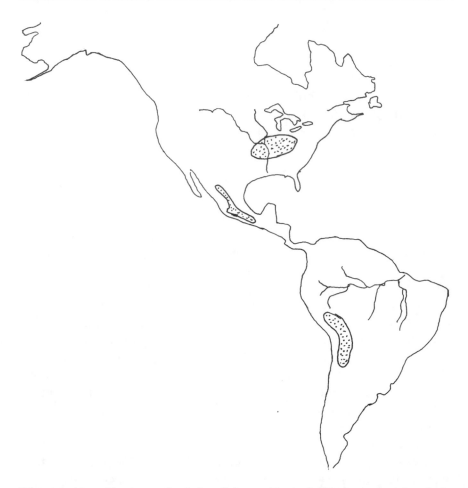

Figure 10.   Centers of origin of domesticated plants and animals in the New World (stippled). The U.S. site saw the cultivation for their seeds, principally, of lamb's Quarters *(Chaenopodium),* marsh elder *(Iva),* sunflower *(Helianthus)* and wild gourd *(Curcubita sp.)* as far back as 4500 B.C. By 500 B.C. other plants appeared (erect knotweed, may-grass and little barley). Beans, corn and squash were late arrivals (A.D. 1 to 200). The Mexican center is the site of origin of corn about 5000 B.C., which arrived in the U.S. by 3200 B.C. Five high elevation Andean species were important domesticates: llama, alpaca, guinea pig, white potato and quinoa *(Chaenopodium quinoa),* domesticated about 4,500 years ago. (Data from Smith, 1995.)

sleeping apart. Later, with agriculture, these egalitarian villages gave way to structures housing a single family, which could proceed to accumulate things like grindstones and livestock, possessed by the family instead of by the group.

What caused certain hunting gathering societies to turn to agriculture? It has been theorized that when hunter-gatherer groups had expanded into all available ecological zones and territory, population growth became the driving force. (Cohen, 1977.) It has been stated that, ordinarily, hunter-gatherers have a low population density of one person per square mile. You need this space, especially in rainforests poor in larger mammals or in deserts. These environments seem to be exactly where hunter-gatherers survive today. Some, like the African Bushmen, have been driven to these marginally productive areas by agricultural peoples such as the Bantu. Hunting and gathering groups were forced to limit their populations to the amount of energy that could be extracted within a given territory. Other tribes had adjacent territories and, like most other animals, survival depended on having just the right number of square miles to feed the number in their camp, and no more. No extra mouths were possible because the territory could not be expanded. They had to practice birth control with herbs, infanticide, sexual abstinence, or lactational amenorrhea, or expel adults from the group, as do most wild creatures. You can move camp to a limited extent, eventually making a circuit of your tribal territory. Monkeys and apes are almost constantly on the move through their group's territory.

In the Fertile Crescent, unlike the rainforest or desert, the living was apparently so easy that hunter-gatherers there did not have to move camp but could live in year round settlements. One ancient site (Netu Hagdud) was a settled hunting-gathering group transitional to farming, with the first domestication of cereal grains. In addition to gathering the wild grasses, including three species of wild oats, wild emmer and wild barley, they ate everything else in sight: mollusks of all sorts, crabs, frogs, ducks, eels, fish, chameleons and other lizards, rodents, fallow deer, wild pigs and gazelles. They collected over fifty wild grasses. At the same time, they had learned to plant and harvest two-rowed barley, the first domesticated cereal. At the same time another group on the eastern edge of the Fertile Crescent found life determined by the necessity of moving up and down the Zagros Mountain slopes to harvest wild grasses and to hunt wild sheep and goats. In any event, following the waning of the last great glacial period in Europe, there came a time when the hunter-gatherers succumbed to the lure of "easy food," the abundant wild cereals that could be stored for the winter and yielded more energy per unit of work than did foraging and hunting. The relatively sudden warming of post-glacial temperatures, coupled with the diminished large animal populations, may have been crucial factors. Low-density hunter-gatherer populations could now afford to increase their densities.

I suppose it was what would become a vicious circle, the more food, the more new additions to the tribal group you could support and the more labor you had to grow additional food. If every community tried to have more pistachio trees and range more sheep, a build-up of population pressure might occur. Be that as it may, agriculture spread across Europe at a snail's pace, barely 1,000 yards per year. This, according to Jared Diamond, is "hardly a wave of enthusiasm." But nonetheless, emmer wheat had spread to Greece by 6500 B.C. and to Germany by 5000 B.C.

Elsewhere, agriculture took other forms. In equatorial zones based on tubers and things like starchy bananas (plantains), gardens were prepared in clearings and visited periodically. A worldwide favorite, and probably very ancient technique, is called slash and burn, or shifting cultivation (Figure 11). Trees were ringed and allowed to die or chopped down and burned, the ash making a temporary fertilizer. A few plants are cultivated for two or three years, then the villagers move on, basically because the soil is so poor in organics and with the heavy rainfall, unable to maintain fertility. Because of this rainfall plants do not build up a nutrient-rich soil as in temperate forests, but suck the nutrients back up from their fallen leaves and twigs about as fast as they can to conserve them. The slash and burn agriculturists may return after eight or ten years and reclaim what little fertility has accumulated in their absence. If forced to do this too often, the soil degenerates to the point where only a grass such as the dread "cogon" can grow. With low population densities, slash and burn can be a reasonable way to exploit tropical environments, maintaining the original diversity of the forest.

As might be expected, the domestication of herding animals such as cattle, horses, camels and reindeer, enabled other people to take advantage of fundamental ecology, especially where ex-

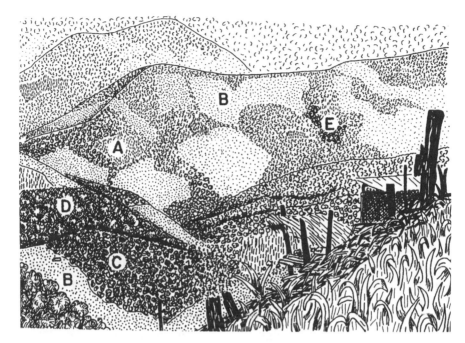

Figure 11. Shifting cultivation in Sabah, Borneo. From a photo looking at the southwest flank of Mount Kina Balu. Generations of Dusuns have removed nearly all the original vegetation up to the 3,000 foot level (about the top of the figure). When the field is in use the shelter is occupied to warn off hungry birds and mammals. The entire field of view is a mosaic of secondary succession in various seral stages: **A.** Recently cut and burned (bamboo stage); **B.** Shrub-height fallow, following abandonment; **C.** Older fallow (mixed shrub young tree stage); **D.** Old fallow approaching a closed canopy; **E.** relict mature trees, probably a ravine or rocky terrain. (Wharton, 1968.)

tensive areas of grasses dominated, such as the Asiatic steppe or the African savanna. The herbivore eats the grass that you can't use and you eat the herbivore or drink its fluids. This is a contemporary model of those hardy early Neanderthals and Cro-Magnon, who may have followed or intercepted the massive herds of gregarious mammals across the grasslands and tundras of the upper Pleistocene, killing when they could. Over 100,000 horses are reported to have been killed at one site in the Rhone Valley. Reindeer were preferred prey in western Europe, mammoths in central Europe, reindeer and horse in central Russia and bison in southern Russia. (Cohen, 1977.) Later, with the pronounced climate changes that followed the retreat of the last ice sheets, herds were forced to migrate seasonally and the hunters could intercept them as they passed, going and coming. The logical next step for our intelligent forebears was to domesticate some of these herding animals and then to move them at will, either up and down mountains or relocate them to better grazing in response to alternating wet and dry seasons. Large herds of herbivores must be moved from time to time today, but misguided outsiders, by digging wells or whatever, have today forced the natives to overgraze their herds instead of moving them. This has resulted in the abandonment of large areas of sub-Saharan Africa, where the grazing was marginal at best.

Some Asiatic peoples developed the novel and deadly technique of riding their "herd" animals, armed to the teeth, on devastating long forays into the territories of others. While they may have had victuals aboard wheeled ox carts creaking along behind in their support, the warriors of Genghis Khan each herded eighteen horses and would live on their blood by opening a vein of a different horse every ten days so it could recover. (Harris, 1985.) Wouldn't it be great to have a history book that told how everybody really lived?

And then there were the flies. It was one of the most vivid memories of my visits with the Masai, those dozens of flies ringed around each child's eyes like they were drinking from a trough. Everything was cattle. The huts were plastered with cow dung. The Masai drink milk and eat some blood and meat. Rather than being nomads following herds, they don't move all that often, but do move their herds about. Each night, the cattle have to be driven behind a thorny fence to protect them from lions. And yet I have never met a healthier looking people with beautiful white teeth, standing tall and fiercely proud, never stooping to ride a bicycle or adopt any custom from the outside. They are pretty much left alone. As you gaze out across the ten-mile wide crater of Ngorongoro, you don't see the villages of the Masai, nor can you see the lions, wildebeest or rhinos. Humans there are just another unobtrusive member of the ecosystem. They have developed a sustainable way of life that does not permanently damage the ecosystem, albeit at the cost of a few less herds of hoofed wild animals. They seem to know instinctively that agriculture-oriented Kikuyu would permanently change an economy based upon grasses inedible to humans and permanently alter one of nature's most workable scenarios for life in that climatic zone.

Eating the products of domesticated plants is probably not the first choice of most people. Mark Cohen says that people worldwide eat meat and fruit when they can and cereals and tubers when they must. Agriculture has one great economic benefit: more food per unit space per unit time. Any animal that can eat from the lowest trophic level (green plants) can theoretically have a population ten times that of one living solely on meat. A cow must convert ten times the amount of low energy grass in order to concentrate it into one pound of meat. Eating from both plants and animals is like the best of both worlds and, though labor intensive, the combination of domesticated plants and animals has worked very well for mankind so far. There are costs, especially in eating a plant-based diet. One is reduced dietary quality, another a less reliable harvest potential and equal or greater labor than with hunting and gathering. Add onto this the difficulty in getting certain essential fatty acids and the epidemic diseases bought about by the close proximity of many people. A genetic result is often a reduction in skeletal size and "robustness." (Cohen, 1987.) And, on a plant-based diet, you have to face up to a protein shortage. There's no getting around the fact that manioc and plantain (that maintain the Amazonian Yanomami) yield only 1.0 percent protein. (Good, 1987.) On the other hand, fish ranges from 17 to 25 percent (dogfish, flounder), while whale meat averages 23.3 percent protein. Shellfish run as high as 24.6 percent. (Yosnor, 1987.) Normal lean meat has about 21 percent protein. The worse short-range impact of agriculture is that it allows an almost unlimited population expansion. The long-range effect is an equal disaster, for it breaks the bond between plants and the soil that nourishes them. Soil was not designed to have its fertility used up quickly by fast growing plants that are toted away from it. Soil has evolved as part of nature's machinery to establish and maintain a steady state, cooperative homeostasis of soil, plant and animal, that would survive the toughest conditions that the climatic cycles could throw at it. Earth once resembled the surface of the moon. Life changed all that and the natural systems are programmed not to allow it to look that way again. Vast areas of the earth's surface have, largely by the action of mankind, become deserts. Closer to home, you should try to visit the copper basin of Tennessee or see how this devastation brought about by acid fumes from copper smelting shows up on a satellite (Landsat Band 5) image.

The effect of steel plows pulled by domestic animals can hardly be overestimated. According to Diamond (1997) the first prehistoric farmers appeared in central Europe about 5000 B.C., where soils were light enough to be tilled with digging sticks. With the ox-drawn plow 1,000 years later, farmers could tear up the tough sods and heavy soils that occupied the grasslands of Asia. Native Americans farmed the river valleys. Only much later (nineteenth century) did our animal-drawn plows begin to cut the great grassland sods of the American Plains.

Because of high rainfall, the soils beneath tropical rainforest have little residual fertility and can support crops only briefly, perhaps three years. This has led to the demise of rainforests that are planted for several years then, when fertility wanes, sold to ranchers for grazing beef cattle. Temperate forest soils are somewhat more enduring but are relatively thin. In the southern Appalachians, most Native Americans and early settlers confined their farming to the bottomlands where flooding had accumulated fertility for centuries. They farmed upland forest soils in mountain coves or on broad flat areas where nutrients were able to accumulate and form deep, organic soils. Here, mostly potatoes were raised. Grasslands, on the other hand, with their low, non-leaching rainfall, become fertile to great depths, owing to the considerable root-death of grasses and the upward concentration of nutrients, where evaporation exceeds precipitation. It was when man obtained the power to break the dense grassland root systems and replace the native grasses with more energy-rich domestic grasses that the stage was set for a truly big population explosion. Unfortunately, such farming has a finite life span.

Instead of allowing the time-honored and balanced cycle of alternating growth and decomposition, most commercial agriculture mines the soil of centuries of accumulated nutrients, depriving it of any way to restore itself. In a later section, we'll see that there is a glimmer of hope. Some human societies have found a way to sustain a farming lifestyle without major damage to the ecosystem. This is reflected in their physical and mental health in the midst of an industrialized and technological world that appears to ignore the fact that its roots must remain forever

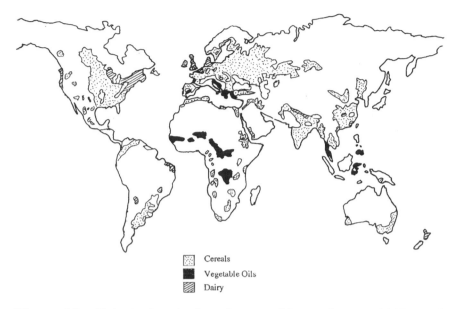

Cereals
Vegetable Oils
Dairy

Figure 12. Principal agricultural areas of the modern world. Tea, coffee, cocoa and vines, sugar crops and fruit growing areas not shown. (After Goldsmith *et al.,* 1990.)

deep in natural processes acquired during millions of years of our prehistoric past.

In the meantime, we can take a lesson from the fate of the birthplace of agriculture, the Fertile Crescent. Originally clothed with forests, it was transformed from fertile woodland to eroded scrubland and desert, overgrazed by sheep and goats. Erosion silted up the valleys and almost finished the job. The final blow, in this area, where evaporation exceeds or is close to precipitation during much of the year, salt accumulates when the bottom-lands are irrigated, and crops can no longer grow. As Jared Diamond says: "Thus, Fertile Crescent and eastern Mediterranean societies had the misfortune to arise in an ecologically fragile environment. They committed ecological suicide by destroying their own resource base." From the domestication of animals, agriculture and metallurgy Diamond says, "it was then but a short further step to those monuments of civilization that distinguish humans from animals across what used to seem an unbridgeable gulf—monuments such as the Mona Lisa and

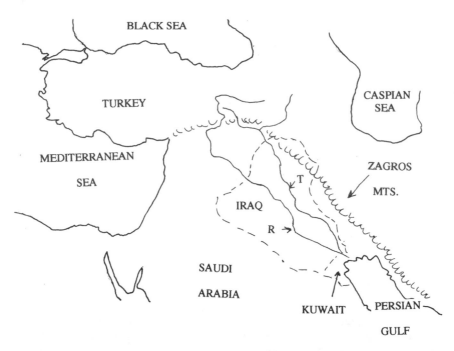

Figure 13. The relationship of the formerly fertile valleys of the Tigris and Euphrates Rivers to the Fertile Crescent (See Fig. 8) and the mountains that surround it to the east and north. Approximate boundaries of Iraq and Kuwait (dashed line) are indicated. The original Eden was supposedly located about where the Tigris (T) and Euphrates (R) Rivers join the Persian Gulf.

Eroica Symphony, the Eiffel Tower and Sputnik, Dachau's ovens and the bombing of Dresden."

In conclusion, please note that the production of food by cultivating the soil is essential to feed a burgeoning world population. This book is not intended to be critical of those who nurture their soil with love and respect. Rather it is to honor those individuals and cultures who seek to learn how to live more closely with nature by reducing dependence on commercial fertilizers and pesticides and by using traditional methods to assure a sustainable agriculture.

CHAPTER FIVE

The Staffs of Life

" . . . In the sweat of thy face shall thou eat bread, till thou return unto the ground; for out of it wast thou taken . . . "

—Genesis 17:19

Reay Tannahill (1988), in her delightful book *Food in History,* from which much of what follows is derived, recounts human diets from ancient Greece to modern day. Especially interesting is the common food of the common man. Most of us know whether our ancestors came from Africa, South America, India, the Middle East, or from specific areas in Europe or elsewhere. It seems important to know what our own ancestors were adapted to eat for hundreds of years prior to their immigration to the New World. Presumably, if they couldn't handle the foods available to them, they did poorly and either died or did not reproduce. Our Paleolithic inheritance must have been subject to rapid Darwinian selection at crucial times such as brought about by the Industrial Revolution, the adoption of agriculture and urbanization, and swapping the home garden for supermarket shelves. Earlier, our flexible genotype had enabled us as omnivores to take advantage of diverse life styles such as the carnivore niche of the Eskimo or the herding nomads of the Asiatic steppes and African savanna, or the near-vegetarian dietary niches of India, the high Andes and parts of China.

Perhaps the majority of people ate, and still eat, close to their primate heritage as omnivores. Save for those with certain religious convictions, few of us would reject protein, whether it came from fish, fowl or mammal, or disguised as egg white or dairy products. Some of us omnivores lean heavily towards carnivory, some more heavily because of faster metabolisms, others less so because of slower metabolisms, or we lean towards herbivory, again in degrees that vary with our metabolic needs.

The gestation period of modern civilization is said to be the 7,000 years prior to 3000 B.C. As we have seen in a previous chapter, during the course of his Neolithic "revolution," European man changed from a hunter-gatherer to a settled farmer and stockbreeder, and much of humanity, in Europe at least, went from predominantly meat-eaters to predominantly grain-eaters.

Conditions in parts of Southern Europe favored fast growing plants that could set seed before either the intense winter cold or the hot, dry summer. Grasses, with their large starchy seeds, were a natural growth over areas of the Middle East. Neolithic tribes found it easier to move and settle near these wild grain patches than to harvest and carry grain from long distances away, as did the hunter-gatherers. Wheat, rye, oat and barley, and their offshoot, bread, were to play a dominant role in nourishing Europe, the Near East and northern Africa. Other grasses, such as millet and rice, would feed other areas of Africa and Asia.

While grains and, later, breads were the staff of life, wouldn't you know that we would come up with a way to feel really good from all this carbohydrate that we worked so hard in the fields to produce. While the Egyptians had fifteen kinds of bread made with natural yeast (the sourdough method), barley beer was the national drink, and was carried to the fields in clay jugs. Perhaps beer and bread built the pyramids. The Egyptians also occupied themselves with making ale from crumbled bread made from sprouted grain. As early as 1750 B.C., the Sumerians made eight kinds of ale from barley, eight from wheat and three from mixed grains. A staggering 40 percent of Sumerian grain went into ale. So the corn patch and vats of fermenting corn meal of the Appalachian settlers, was not just a modern innovation to ease the monotony of subsistence agriculture. Early on, grains were made into alcoholic beverages and most of us have a very long heritage of drinking grain-based spirits.

In fact, ale making may have contributed mightily to the raised breads we enjoy today. It is thought that the leavening of bread may have been accidentally discovered when someone used ale instead of water to mix the dough. Prior to this, leavening was achieved only by letting the dough sour. Sourdough bread is delicious but to make it is time-consuming. Leavened bread, in which yeast expands the gluten-forming proteins of wheat (barley, millet and oats are unresponsive to leavening), became common in Greece in the fourth century B.C. Bread was a later development in grain use. Archeologists say that Neolithic peoples probably first started cooking grains as porridges or gruel around 5000 B.C., along with the pit boiling of meat. The toasting of grains and then pounding them up on rocks to make a grain-paste with water is another step (still in use in twentieth century Tibet).

About 8,000 years ago bread wheat appeared, a hybrid between emmer and goat-faced grass (with forty-two instead of twenty-eight chromosomes). What made it especially valuable was that it could tolerate cold winters and rainy summers and did not require the Mediterranean climate (mild rainy winters and hot, dry summers). It had more gluten and would rise well with the natural yeast in the air. Barley also later developed tolerance to a broad range of climates.

Barley pastes, gruels and flatbreads were Grecian staples until 500 B.C. Wheat, however, was preferred in central Italy and the Roman Legions are said to have carried a quern (a circular two-part grindstone) for each ten men on the march. In addition to bread and porridges of millet or lentils, they carried a fermented fish oil or *liquamen,* full of vitamins and minerals. (Fallon *et al.,* 1995.)

Coarse ground flatbreads, probably first cooked by being plastered on a hot rock, have been dietary staples of humanity for thousands of years. Many are still enjoyed worldwide and include the Mexican *tortilla,* the Scotch oakcake, the Indian *chapatti,* the Amerindian johnnycake and the Ethiopian *injera.* By 500 A.D., dark, whole-grain breads of rye and other grains nourished northern Europe and Russia. In addition there were whole-grain porridges as well as dried legumes.

Because whole-grain bread was such a basic food throughout history, it might be helpful to consider some fundamentals about the use of grain. We eat bread for the energy value of the starchy endosperm, but also (ideally) for the vitamins and minerals in the outer layer (bran) and in the embryo (germ) (Figure 15). There are also drawbacks: all grains and many seeds such as beans contain phytic acid which, for the plant's advantage, ties up nutrient minerals as an insoluble phytate molecule. Seeds did not evolve for our benefit, so our intestinal tracts lack the enzyme

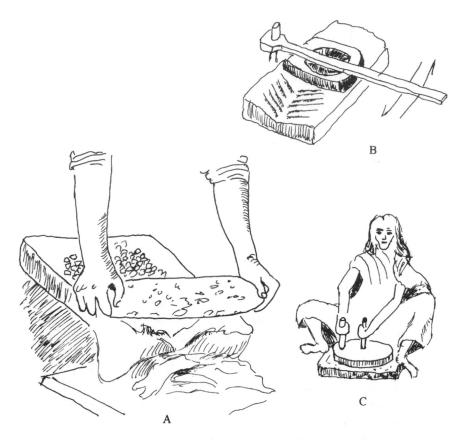

Figure 14.   Grinding grain by hand on millstones. **(A)** The "saddle stone," used for grinding corn for tortillas in Guatemala, dates back to Egyptian carvings 2700 B.C.; **(B)** Side-to-side rubbing stone with a hopper top; **(C)** a portable version of this rotary quern was carried by the Roman Legions. It was still in use in nineteenth century India. Donkeys turned larger versions, as waterwheels do today in the southern Appalachians. Grindstones first appeared on the Island of Cypress, 10,000 years ago. (Partly from Tannahill, 1988.)

(phytase) to release the minerals from the phytate of grains and legumes. The good news is that seeds also contain the enzyme to unlock the minerals that are mostly found in the outside covering of the grain. All it takes is water. You can either soak the grains and germinate them and then grind up the sprouts and make bread or you can grind the grains to flour first and add water to make a dough. It is a matter of time. In ordinary dough 75 percent of the phytate is broken up within ten hours. Yeast speeds up the action because it also has the phytase enzyme, but the longer the bread-making process, the more phytate can be broken down. If you soak oatmeal, you should use the soak water as it contains valuable minerals. If you soak legumes such as beans, you need to throw away the soak water two or three times.[6] Unfortunately, baking powder allows a fast rise and if immediately baked denies us some minerals in the grain. Neither will you get much minerals from pita bread if the dough is promptly cooked after mixing. In fact, some Near East peoples (and health nuts elsewhere) may get mineral deficiencies by insisting on unleavened breads such as pita. The best rule is to let whole grain dough stand over night or with a long fermentation process, as the old "sourdough" prospectors out West learned to do. If you use white flour, it doesn't matter, since there are few or no minerals left after the millers have gotten rid of the bran and germ of the original grain. So, simply enjoy your hot biscuits, pancakes or cornbread for the good taste, use the starch as an energy source, but get the missing vitamins and minerals from other foods or supplements. The value of the "old style" traditional ways of making bread is immediately apparent. Areas of the world that cannot afford to buy supplements must get their nutrients from their foods the old fashioned way and, frankly, they'll be better off.

While bread was a cornerstone of diet for many people, other foods were important to sustain health. During most of medieval times a large stew pot or kettle called a "cauldron" hung constantly over the hearth fire in every house. It contained a stew or soup constantly replenished by whatever meat and vegetables were available. It remained an essential feature of the northern European kitchen until the eighteenth century. Common vegetables were cabbage, kale, spinach, sprouts, nettles, onions and, later, potatoes. On the other hand, the mobile nomads of the Asiatic steppes had an entirely different and bread-free diet based largely on meat and milk. They had little fuel for fires anyhow. Milk came from a variety of herd animals; horse, cattle, camel, sheep, goat or yak. A clarified butter, ghee, would keep for weeks even at high temperatures. Diets based on herd animals required a high degree of human mobility since herd animals

---

[6] No need to soak rice, barley or millet.

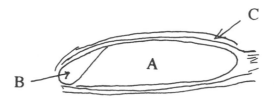

Figure 15. Wheat seed or "berry." **(A)** Starchy endosperm, the principal ingredient of refined flour; **(B)** the germ contains protein and oil-soluble vitamins; **(C)** the bran adheres fairly tightly and covers both endosperm and germ. It contains fiber and water-soluble vitamins. The germ is removed to prevent flour from becoming rancid and bran is removed so that the flour will be white. It is sold as a livestock supplement.

must be moved periodically. The ancient Sumerians learned this the hard way by following sheep and goats up and down the mountains of the Near East on their annual migrations to greener pastures. Until recently, even Western Europe was heavily involved in moving livestock around. In France, tens of thousands of sheep were moved from the mountains of Provence to the winter pastures of Arles and pigs were driven each fall to harvest the acorns of Vancluse.[7]

Each Mongol warrior, the quintessential nomad, would drive eighteen head of horses on a campaign of conquest. He could live on horse blood, withdrawing one-half pint from each of his eighteen horses on rotation, each horse being bled every ten days. Along with dried milk invented by the nomads, such ration enabled the armies of the great Khans to dominate most of Asia.

Other pastoralists to invade were the Aryans from around Iran who penetrated into northern India in 1750 and contributed the Vedas or Aryan bible. Further south in India, the Hindus adopted aspects of the Aryan Veda and came to equate meritorious living with vegetarianism. Most of India couldn't be herders and they needed cattle for draft and dung. Eating them became a threat and the cow became sacred. The other two principal reli-

---

[7] It is interesting to note that, from around the tenth and eleventh centuries, the 90,000 people of the city of Florence annually ate 4,000 oxen and calves, 60,000 sheep, 20,000 goats and 30,000 pigs.

gions, Buddhism and Jainism, were also advocates of a vegetarian diet because they sanctified all life. For their carbohydrates, Indians in the south ate rice and in the north, wheat.

Most North Americans are of European origin. In Europe, the vital relationship between soils and food shaped our civilization. Early Neolithic man apparently ate well, his crops withdrawing nutrients from the organic-rich virgin soils. He did not need to replenish the nutrients and organics that he used up, or so it seemed at the time. Even the scratch-plow did not markedly alter the fertility. It was the introduction of the horse and oxen-drawn moldboard (turning) plow between 1000 and 1492 that made the conquest of huge expanses of virgin soils possible. The deep, fertile soils beneath the grasslands of Eurasia could now be reached and elsewhere the forests were stripped away and their relatively thin topsoil exploited. Erosion by water and wind has ever since robbed us of much of the principal wealth of nature's bank. Long term agriculture with or without the plow modified entire biomes. Its forests and fertile soils gone, much of Greece was left with rocky slopes best adapted to things like goats and grapes.

Following the voyage of Columbus, New World crops had a profound impact on European diets, especially the potato. Originally, many varieties of potatoes were the principal carbohydrate source (along with grains like quinoa) for Andean natives above 11,000 feet where corn will not grow. The potato, introduced in 1580 to Ireland, became an essential dietary component. A potato patch could not only support a family but livestock as well. The cow was essential to the health of the potato farmer. The middle class could be carnivores but the poorest classes had to make do with potatoes. Like the Indians, you couldn't afford to kill your cow and lose all that milk, curds, whey, cheese, butter and manure. As in our own formerly rural culture, it was the pig that provided the occasional taste of meat. Chickens were more valuable as egg layers than as pot birds.

Another great dietary impact was liquid. As in the case of earlier Sumerian and Egyptian cultures, there was not much choice in the beverage line. Again, it was either dangerously polluted water or milk and alcoholic drinks, at least until the introduction of coffee from Ethiopia, tea from the Orient, and chocolate from Central America. Is it any wonder that many Europeans, Poles, Germans, Dutch, Russian and English became heavy drinkers?

Lest we feel too superior, rum was the great lubricant in early American society.

It appears that most European communities were self-supporting through medieval times. They could even support local monasteries that, in the ninth century, demanded of them, in addition to bread, a staple ration of sixty gallons of ale daily. Societies, however, in addition to depleting their limited store of topsoil, are vulnerable to the risks of placing all their eggs in one basket, depending on only one or two species of plants grown in what is called a monoculture. It is a formula for disaster. The ninth and tenth centuries were a black age for northern Europe when outbreaks of the ergot fungus attacked the wheat crops. This led to twenty "grievous famines," some lasting three or four years. Southern Europe saw fifteen waves of plague when the Arabs introduced the barberry bush along with a rust fungus that ravaged wheat monocultures. Great famines also swept Spain in 915 and 929 A.D. It got so bad that killer gangs waylaid travelers, cooked and sold their flesh. Cannibalism persisted in areas (Bohemia, Silesia, Poland) until the end of the Middle Ages. This was a foretaste of another disaster to a monoculture, the utter destruction of the Irish potato crop in 1845.

Traditional foods, derived from a quasi-sustainable agriculture where the family and livestock contributed to the maintenance of soil fertility, could support only limited numbers of people. International trade brought not only new kinds of foods, but could supply energy-rich foods like grains in quantity. This led to an increased population, which in turn needed more food, beginning a vicious cycle from which the world has never recovered. The first major decline in health can be attributed to the change from a hunter-gatherer way of life to a sedentary, agricultural one. It is a toss-up whether the second great health decline came from the disruption of the one family plot of ground with a large diversity of edible products, or from the Industrial Revolution that led to urbanization. Both events set the stage for malnutrition.

In the early eighteenth to mid-nineteenth centuries, the Chinese population jumped from 150 to 450 million, made possible by the "new" foods: maize, potatoes, sweet potatoes, and peanuts, that could grow on land never before farmed. Previous agriculture was largely centered in the large river floodplains. The period 1800 to 1900 saw a huge population increase in Europe due to the importation of large quantities of grain from abroad. In the United States alone, 400 million acres were put under the plow. At the same time, people were leaving their farms and backyard gardens to produce machines, not food, for the Industrial Revolution. The impact on human health is attested to by the fact that 41 percent of 2.5 million English men were rejected as unfit for service in World War I. That there was no more damage than this was due to a realization that man had to participate in natural processes, not continuously exploit nature, especially the finite fertility of soils subject to continuous crops each year.

What we eat has been and probably always will be the result of the interaction of solar energy with a fertile substrate, through the courtesy of a green plant or the animals that eat them. Man, with his intelligence and incredible adaptability, attempted to improve his relationship with the topsoil, arguably the most precious resource in the world. He realized that, year after year, you couldn't continue to get a good crop yield from the same field without somehow cooperating with nature.

Holland, it appears, led Europe in adopting an ambitious seven-course crop rotation plus a thriving dairy industry. Most of Europe became a four crop variant, allowing each field to pass sequentially through wheat or barley, clover, a root cover crop like turnips, and then to remain fallow for a year. Even this could not relieve massive urban poverty with its bad housing, bad food and bad sanitation. In an English manufacturing town around 1850, a semi-skilled worker fed his family weekly on: five four-pound loaves of bread; five pounds of meat; forty pounds of potatoes; seven pints of beer; three ounces of tea; one pound of sugar; and one pound of butter. In bad years there was no meat, beer or butter.

Then came the evils of tinkering with our staple foods. The second half of the nineteenth century saw new methods of processing milk, such as into the condensed form. New methods of milling resulted in whiter bread, lacking both the embryo germ with its oil-soluble vitamins and the bran with its water-soluble ones. These changes increased the incidence of malnutrition.

In the late 1960s, we began to play around with the plants themselves, seeking high yield genetic varieties to feed a burgeoning population. While the first "Green Revolution" increased crop yield 250 percent in some cases, it required an unusual amount of water and fertilizers and often proved a magnet for pests. The bottom line was that in the 1970s the wealthiest families (who could afford fertilizer) prospered, while poorer farmers were driven out of business. The specter of cash crops that could be sold abroad began to dominate the third world, forcing people to need money to buy things rather than to depend on the former subsistence agriculture that had been well adapted to the local ecology. Paddy fields in the Philippines once grew fish as well as rice. Artificial fertilizers eliminated the fish and reduced the protein intake. Pests and disease took an enormous toll of the huge fields needed for mass production of the "new" crops sent to the Third World, leading to the use of more expensive herbicides and pesticides. All this showed that it was much easier to destroy ecological balance than to restore it. By 1981 countries where agriculture had been revolutionized by the first Green Revolution were once more reduced to importing grains from exporting nations, notably the United States, "where three million acres of land a year was being lost to erosion to cultivation by erosion and urban development." The question now before us is, where will the second Green Revolution, based upon gene juggling by genetic engineers, lead? Meanwhile, thousands of native food plants have been lost—it is only by last minute efforts that we have saved a small percentage of the fifty or more kinds of potatoes originally grown in the high Andes.

Society's concern with human health had to surface. While a health food store opened in Orlando, Florida in the 1950s, it took a long time, prompted by lonely voices like Adele Davis, to realize that something was wrong in the land of plenty. Serious concern began in the 1960s with the "flower children," influenced by the vegetarian edicts of Indian gurus. "Health foods" and new ways of eating came into being. The 1980s saw the rise of militant "health evangelists" who sought every scrap of scientific evidence available to support their dietary choices.

Meanwhile, in the 1970s, eighteen African nations experienced serious food shortages. Fourteen million people in Ethiopia and Bangladesh were starving. By 1985 United States citizens had sent aid but also spent six billion dollars trying to lose weight. Sedentary workers ate half again as much as their active predecessors at the end of the 1800s. Twentieth century diseases became the result of twentieth century diets.

Long gone were the nutritious dark, slow rising breads, the fermented cabbage and the kettle on the hearth with its nourishing broths and stews. Gone the mineral-rich curds and the protein-rich whey and the butterfat of milk. Seldom seen were the thick barley soups, the lentils, meals of game and fish, the yogurts, in short, most of the traditional foods that had maintained the health of much of the northern hemisphere for centuries. Formerly, man had been forced to come to grips with how to subsist sustainably on local soils, for which he developed a modicum of respect and even love. All this changed when we were able to buy anything we wanted to eat, much as did the wealthiest Romans who, from a graceful reclining position, indulged their most exotic tastes and feasted on dishes of flamingo tongues.

Now that we are able to afford to eat almost anything our heart or appetite desires whenever we want it, our survival seems to demand that we make sense out of that enormous smorgasbord of foods presented to us by the marketing skills of agribusiness and the commercialization of our daily bread. To thread our way along this perilous path should occupy every intelligent being. The alternative of being the victim of degenerative disease is not a pleasant choice. Our judgments on how to eat and live must be based upon knowledge of our individual bodies and how we came to be that way. Discovering your own nutritional type may be the end result of an evolution that began with the first large primates millions of years ago in the forests and savannas of Africa.

CHAPTER SIX

Traditional (Sustainable) Agriculture

*"Traditional agriculture in the Third World is fre-
quently dismissed as primitive and unproductive. In
fact it offers the best hope for the future."*

—Edward Goldsmith

While we decry the negative aspects of agriculture, it has been
an incredibly successful means to support billions, for better or
for worse. After all, it is an imitation of one phase of ecosystem
resilience—the freezing in time of a stage of vegetation from a
sequence of steps by which natural plant communities recover
from a total wipe-out by fire, landslide or other calamity ("ecological succession"). In forested areas of the world it means a
stage naturally dominated by either herbaceous ground cover
plants (substitutes: root crops, legumes, vines), shrubs (substitutes: cultivated shrubs like blueberries) or trees (substitutes:
cultivated orchards of nut or fruit trees). In prairie or steppe
areas of the world, as in the western United States, rather than
an arrested stage back towards climax forest, it is a more
natural substitution—that of non-native, single species grasses
(wheat, corn) for native grasses of many species. Pastoral
peoples, living off livestock that graze native grasslands are exploiting a more natural relationship which, as Eugene Odum
says, is ecologically sound.

It is not so much this intervention in nature's plan that raises
concern, but the way agriculture is conducted. Improperly done,
it can ultimately bring disaster to both the environment and the
people using it, as the demise of the original Fertile Crescent and

the deterioration of soils worldwide attest. Its intelligent use, however, can be a credit to the highest human attributes, including ingenuity, humility, affection for life and respect for both life and non-life. All over the world, people have proved that they can evolve an agriculture that will yield energy and essential nutrients for plants and animals almost indefinitely. This is what we mean by sustainable agriculture.

It enables us to stay in one place and use the same soil. It is accomplished by imitating natural processes, fertilizing the soil by the recycling of organic materials, enriching it by adding fertile sediments, or by using skillful use of irrigation to exploit soils that were either already extremely fertile but had insufficient natural water, or were renewed annually by silt deposition from flooding.

Most of the human cultures reported by Weston Price (Chapter 8) were living healthily, supported by the sustained productivity of natural environments and using nutritious foods harvested from them, either sea, forest or prairie steppes. Others, like the pastoral peoples of Africa, took advantage of immense natural grasslands for their livestock. Some, such as the Australian aborigines, living in the more arid regions, had to move about a good deal. Others, such as the Peruvian Indians of the coastal zone, were able to adopt an intensive agriculture in one environment, namely the fertile soils along rivers draining the Andes.

The largest of the sedentary, most of which were sustainable, agricultures have been called the great "hydraulic civilizations," based upon the human management of water. One of the oldest of these was under the Han Dynasty when, 2,000 years ago, the main population of China was based on irrigation in river valleys. (La Chapelle, 1988.) Other examples are the Nile Delta, the Khmer Empire of Southeast Asia, the fertile valleys of coastal Peru, and areas of Sumeria, Babylonia and Sri Lanka. One of the most ingenious was the use of underground aquifers. Ancient Iran had 170,000 miles of underground channels that made gardens of uninhabitable deserts. These and those of Iraq were destroyed by Mongol invaders. One of the most sophisticated examples of this type of irrigation were channels constructed by the Chagga people of Tanzania's Mount Kilimanjaro. (Goldsmith, 1998.) Almost all of these huge irrigation projects were communal in nature and required the unity provided by powerful rulers who could command the labor of enormous numbers of workers.

Cleverly, the Cambodian Khmer Empire used the natural annual water cycle to irrigate their rice fields, built in low-lying wetlands surrounding the great Tonle Sap lake which, during the dry season, feeds into the Mekong River and occupies about 1,800 square miles (Figure 16). During the monsoon rains, the Mekong reverses the outflow in the river flowing out of the lake and floods some 6,200 square miles, much of which is wetland terrain. Thus, by using this natural phenomenon, the Khmer were able to feed their large population. One city, Angkor, covered 100 square miles and contained an estimated one million people (about 1000 A.D.).

The small reservoirs or "tanks" of Sri Lanka, like the "quanta" aquifers of Iran and the furrows of the Chagga, provided villages with only the amount of water that the ecosystem made available. This is an important lesson from sustainable agriculture—

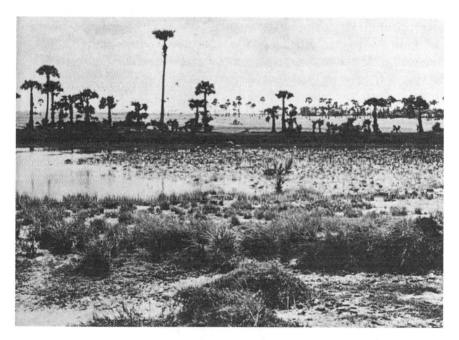

Figure 16. Without expensive irrigation systems, sustainable rice production cultivation is largely confined to the moist, flat terrain surrounding Cambodia's great lake (Tonle Sap) and the Mekong Delta. Ducks are also raised in this natural hydrophytic plant community, with its heavy annual monsoon rains. The skyline is dominated by the sugar palm (*Borassus*). (Wharton, 1966.)

do not depend on assistance from outside the area in which you live. Depend only on your soils, the local climate and energy of the local labor, human or animal. Such systems are functional only if the slopes of the watershed remain forested. Forests provide water steadily and in perpetuity. Scientists at the Coweeta, North Carolina, Forest Service Experiment Station filled a large wooden trough with enough forest soil and tilted it at a slope matching the surrounding terrain and saturated it with water that then oozed steadily out of the lower end for seventy days. Watershed water is thus provided in perpetuity, with no social or economic costs. Perennial irrigation schemes based on huge dams and reservoirs lead to a myriad of environmental problems, including raising the water table and increasing salinization. The secret of sustainable irrigation is that this type of water management be devised and controlled by the local farmers familiar with the geology, hydrology and biology of their area, not by distant bureaucracies with self-perpetuating officials often in pursuit of short-term political gains.

There are biological perils from the attempt to provide perennial water to an ecosystem such as the Nile Delta that was adapted to annual flooding with yearly deposits of fertile silt from as far away as the Ethiopian highlands. Now salinization, the dread disease schistosomiasis, the loss of annual silt deposits and the death of the delta fisheries have been the result of the Aswan Dam.

The most important feature of traditional sustainable agriculture is that it is "geared to producing food for local consumption rather than for export to some distant land." (Goldsmith, 1988.) Cash crops for export have converted vast areas of the world away from local sustainable agriculture. Half of the prime agricultural lands in the Philippines and Central America and half of the wet zone land of Sri Lanka are now used to grow cash crops. (Goldsmith, 1982, 1988.) Since large dams are expensive, the water-retaining forests are sacrificed to finance them. A further violation of ecological principles (nature's laws) was the attempt to impose a system of agriculture on the prairie soils of the southern plains of the United States, leading to the great dustbowls of the 1890s and 1930s where we indeed trampled out the vintage where the grapes of wrath were stored, a story of nature's retribution so eloquently told by Steinbeck.

One of the earliest methods of sustainable agriculture was the step-like terracing of land in mountainous regions, thought to have originated some 4,000 years ago. In the Western world, it was probably first practiced in Lebanon by the Phoenicians and eventually covered 55 percent of the Judean Mountains. Whether by Canaanites, Israelites or Arabs, traditional cultures well understood how nature worked in the Mediterranean climate of the Near East. (Bunyard, 1980.) The great terrace systems in the mountains of Luzon (Philippines) cover an area of 250 square miles. They were reportedly built by immigrant Chinese about 2000 B.C. and are still productive 4,000 years later. Just as impressive are the famed rice terraces of Borobudur, Java, where fingerling fish are introduced to feed among the growing rice stems. (Calder, 1961.)

Terracing reached perhaps its highest development on the western flank of the Peruvian and Bolivian Andes. Constructed by the Pre-Incan peoples, they were studied and described by

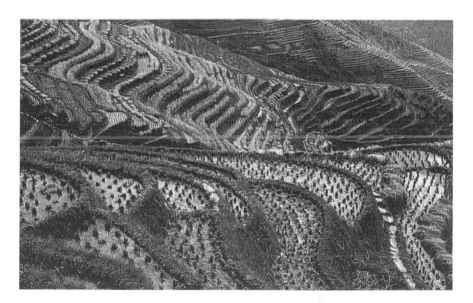

Figure 17. In steep, mountainous terrain, man has evolved a traditional agriculture, with step-like terraces. These rice terraces are near Guilin, China. In the Andes, these "staircase farms" reached nearly to the snowline. Courtesy, Reinhart Wolf/Bilderberg and W.H. Freeman. (From Smith, 1995.)

O. F. Cook (1916). Cook described four early stages of agriculture: nomadic clearings, tillage, fertilization with natural organic substances and irrigation. The crowning achievement was terrace farming by a pre-Incan megalithic culture of Peru. Terraces were made of rocks, sometimes huge, and fitted so astoundingly that the joints "are in many places too fine to be seen by the naked eye." Behind these walls, an artificial soil profile was constructed with a subsoil layer of stones and clay supporting a three-foot layer of topsoil. Even the rocky floodplains were terraced and leveled and the river channeled.

Even forty-five degree slopes were farmed, the terraces often wide enough for only one row of potatoes. Bands of fifty terraces, each being ten feet high, would rise up the steep slopes as high as the Washington monument. These hanging gardens rose almost to the snowline and in grandeur and height exceeded the world wonder at Babylon. They were irrigated by incredible aqueducts that brought in silt-rich, glacial water from as far away as 100 miles, as reported by the Spaniards.

The ancient Peruvian cultures had three crop zones: a low tropical belt up to 6,000 feet (for cassava, etc.); an intermediate zone up to 11,000 feet for things like maize; and above that a zone for potatoes. Cook documented sixteen varieties of potatoes in one field. Michael Palin (Full Circle, PBS) reported 360 varieties near Cuzco. Hardy potato varieties grew up to 14,000 feet. More plants were domesticated in this section of Peru than in any other part of the world, including "white" potatoes, sweet potatoes, tomatoes, maize, beans, pineapple, peanuts, and quinoa. The reason was the range of altitudes from the tropics to the arctic. As Cook said, standing in the valley of the Urubamba and gazing up at the Andes was like "looking from Jamaica to Alaska."

The terraced fields of the Pakistani Hunzas were likewise narrow fields of staircase gardens on steep slopes, the down slope edge being a strong stone wall. Individual fields averaged as many as twenty per acre, occupying an estimated five square miles (Wrench, 1938) and were fed mineral-rich water from the Ultar Glacier. In addition, the Hunzas returned organic wastes and inorganic silts to their fields and used both animal and human manure, fallen leaves, ashes and alkaline earth.

Large populations in the Far East would not have been possible without traditional wetland, rice paddy agriculture. The smaller, labor intensive plots that nourished family and village have been in sustainable production for hundreds of years. Again, this is an imitation of natural processes by using the slow decomposition of natural materials. For at least 4,000 years the Chinese have made manuring and composting an essential feature of their sustainable cultivation of plants. In pits they compost mud from canals, clover from fields, stubble roughage, manure and ashes. Whenever possible, enormous volumes of river silt are evenly spread over the fields, imitating natural flooding. The Japanese follow much the same procedures. Both treasure the fertility of human excrement. I recall each morning in the Japanese cities where I was quartered, the passing by of the "night soil" collectors, with their wooden pails or "honey buckets" swinging from a shoulder stick.

With some rice farming, the relationships with nature are indeed complex. Figure 18 depicts sustainable rice paddy agriculture in Sri Lanka, following descriptions by Goldsmith (1982), Senanayake (1983) and Pereira (1991) (Figure 18). The ecology is fascinating. No expensive fertilizers or pesticides are required. Nitrogen is supplied by leguminous weeds, algae, floating ferns, tree leaves and the excreta of bats, ducks, buffalo and people. Birds, which can be positive or negative, are "trained" to use their own little paddy planted just for them. Large monitor lizards, living on the adjacent high ground, feast on fresh water crabs whose holes make leaks in the retaining walls of the paddy. Top minnows, which control the malaria-carrying mosquito, are kept alive during dry weather by a buffalo wallow refuge. Rice was once grown with 280 varieties.

Masanobu Fukuoka (1978) described an advanced type of traditional agriculture called "natural" farming in his book, *The One-Straw Revolution*. He used a summer crop of rice alternating with a winter crop of rye and barley, essentially a "no-till" system using clover and controlling weeds naturally rather than destroying them with manual labor or poison. Fukuoka, however, unlike traditional farmers in his area, used no compost pits but simply returned the straw to the fields with a little manure. No artificial fertilizer, herbicides or tilling was ever used. The wiser Japanese farmers had apparently discovered early that chemical fertilizer quickly destroyed the natural humus content of their soils. Fukuoka also stated that the standard daily diet of Japanese farmers which "gave long life, a strong constitution, and good health . . . consisted of rice and barley with *miso* and pickled vegetables."

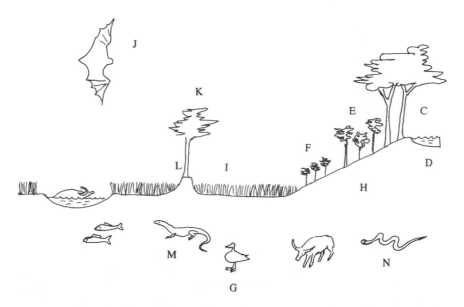

Figure 18. Traditional rice paddy agriculture in Sri Lanka. This quasi-natural marsh and the surrounding terrain exhibits a remarkable ecology, involving the cooperation of a variety of plants and animals. **(C)** Mature forest with wild fruits (jackfruit, avocado, wood apple, etc.); **(D)** Reservoir "tank" (lotus seeds, *kaketi* roots, fish); **(E)** Wild areas ("pillawas") (source of leguminous seeds grown in paddy between harvests); **(F)** Fruit gardens; **(G)** Ducks eat snails/insects and provide fertile droppings; **(H)** Rest area provides buffalo and human droppings; **(I)** Rice paddy contains fish when flooded and nitrogen-fixing algae, pond fern and duckweed; **(J)** Bat feeds on Mee tree fruits, droppings fertilize paddy; **(K)** Mee tree grows on dikes; **(L)** Dikes (levees); **(M)** Monitor lizard eats crabs that damage dikes; **(N)** Snakes control rodents. (Goldsmith, 1982; Senanayake, 1983; Pereira, 1991.)

There is a new, fascinating, sustainable rice paddy agriculture called the "Aigamo method," developed ten years ago in Japan, by the Furuno family. It is rapidly spreading throughout Southeast Asia, increasing the income of Third World farmers from 20 to 50 percent. It might be called the "One Bird Revolution" since ducks are the keys. Twenty ducklings released per tenth of a hectare eat insect pests, golden snails and weed seeds and save 240 hours per hectare of manual weeding. Ducks remain on the paddy twenty-four hours a day until the rice forms ears of grain. Then they are penned. Nitrogen-fixing *Azolla* fern and duckweed cover the water surface, feeding the ducks and providing cover for edible fish (roach) which feed on duck feces and organisms fertilized by the ducks. The only external input is a little waste grain fed the penned ducks. The output is a nutritious harvest of organic rice, duck and fish. The productivity is remarkable—1.4 hectares yields seven tons of rice, 300 ducks, 4,000 ducklings and an adjacent 0.6 hectare supplies organic vegetables for 100 people. It was calculated that, by using the Aigamo method, no more than 2 percent of Japanese farmers could feed the nation and make it self-sufficient. (Ho, 1999.)

When you think about it, the fast-growing technique of organic farming in the United States, which eliminates chemicals and uses natural decomposition, is a return to traditional agriculture. It differs but little from the traditional Oriental agriculture practiced in China, Korea and Japan for many centuries. This system emphasizes the fundamental importance of recycling animal wastes, composting, crop rotation, and green manuring (use of cover crops of clover, vetch and alfalfa). It is a cooperative venture between animals, plants and man.

Some of the most ingenious approaches to sustainable agriculture involve alternating narrow platforms of soil with water-filled ditches. In the Peruvian Andes, present day peoples are restoring a system of raised fields that the Incas evolved about 3,000 years ago on the Altiplano. Here, platforms were made of soil dug from adjacent ditches, which filled with water. They produced bumper crops in the face of floods, droughts and killing frosts at altitudes of 4,000 meters. The one-meter-high platforms were fertilized with nutrient-rich muck from sediment and vegetation in the canals alongside the raised beds. The nearby water also ameliorated the extreme temperatures. No modern tools or fertilizers were used.

A similar type of agriculture is the famed *chinampa,* originated by the Xochimilca and Chelmeca Indians, in shallow lakes in the wetland basin where Mexico City is now centered. In certain shallow lakes, large masses of aquatic plants and mud from the lake bottom were formed into platforms up to ten meters wide (Figure 19). Held together with posts and branches, they projected about thirty centimeters above the water. Willows planted around the edge provided shade and, eventually, anchorage of the platforms to the lake bottom. Rich organic lake bottom mud, aquatic plants, bat guano and human wastes were also used, as well as crop rotation. Chinampa agriculture reached its zenith during the Aztec reign and helped support a huge population of from one half to two million souls. As late as 1986, remnants of these ancient structures in Lake Xochimilco produced 25 percent of the vegetable demand of Mexico City. (Outerbridge, 1987.) Today this technique, nearly destroyed by neglect and development, is now being reconstructed in Vera Cruz and Tabasco.

Most environmental authorities and ecologists view sustainability as the key to the survival of life as we know it. In spite of hundreds of organizations in the U.S. dealing with this topic, there needs to be a social movement fueled by powerful forces within each individual to counter the growing power of transnational industry. Ecosystem destruction is an assault on creation. Defense must invoke the spirit within us and the religious community and provoke a worldview that captures "the emotional imagination of a public so removed from the natural world that it doesn't take physical reality as seriously as abstractions like the economy." (Bill McKibben, Sierra, 2000.)

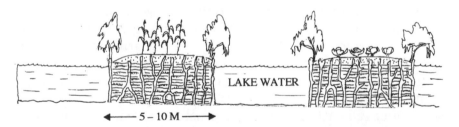

LAKE WATER

◄——— 5 – 10 M ———►

Figure 19.   Mesoamerican swamp agriculture. Cross-section of Chinampa plots. Platforms were built up of dense mats of emergent and floating aquatic vegetation from the lake shore and towed by boats. The compacted mats of vegetation were capped with organic-rich mud from the lake bottom until the garden surface was 30 cm above the water level. Height of the beds was between three and four meters. Willows planted around the edge eventually anchored the giant rafts to the bottom. This was one of mankind's most ingenious plans to utilize shallow lakes and wetlands, by a sustainable agriculture capable of supporting a large population. As late as 1950 the "Chinamperia" produced the greater part of Mexico City's fresh vegetables. (Modified from Outerbridge, 1987.)

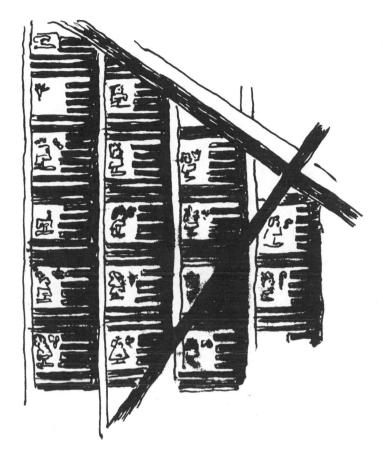

Figure 20. A small section (plan view) of a gigantic island garden *Chinampa* system of Mexico. Water is dark, footpaths (running north and south) and garden strips (some 300 feet long) are clear. Major irrigation canals conducted spring water from the mainland. Each owner was identified by a symbol and a name. Sketched from an Aztec map by a Spanish scribe. The chinampas supplied food for the 300,000 inhabitants of the Aztec capital Tenochtitlan, now Mexico City. Replete with flowers, a few of these "Floating Gardens of Xochimilco" that still exist are a popular tourist attraction. (From Leonard *et al.,* 1973.)

CHAPTER SEVEN

Gardens

"Agriculture is a way of life. It cannot be maintained by reluctant farmers or by slave labor. It is essentially the identity of the peasant with his soil. . . . Neglected, it becomes sickly and dies. That was the fate of the granaries of the Roman Empire."

—Richie Calder

A final type of traditional agriculture involves gardens. It is here that man has his most intimate relationship with the soil. Any changes in fertility are vividly apparent and threaten the immediate nutrition of a family. To most of us, gardens are small areas of soil close to our dwellings that we work lovingly from spring to fall in the Temperate Zone.

Gardens often contain a variety of plants and may serve but a single family. Mostly, they are devoted to herbs and do not contain shrubs or trees. They do not therefore imitate the structure and diversity of a natural ecosystem such as a forest, but may represent the "weed stage," the frozen-in-time counterpart of the primary stages of plant succession.

In rainforest areas such as the Amazon, villagers practice a small-scale replica of the widespread shifting cultivation used on quickly exhaustible tropical soils. These communal "gardens," with manioc and bananas, are used until productivity wanes or the nearby forest is depleted of game (Figure 21). Then the village is moved to another site.

A few cultures, however, do attempt to mimic the structure of a forest. An example is the Javanese multi-story garden as described by Freeman and Fricke (1984). While the Javanese traditionally practiced shifting cultivation on upland areas not

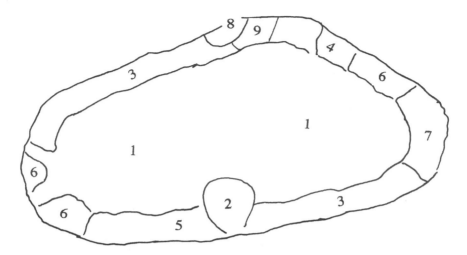

Figure 21. Generalized plan of shifting garden cultivation, where the rain forest is felled and burned and the opening is planted for about three years, then abandoned. The Yekuana Indians of southern Venezuela are said to use over seventy different food plants, depending on soil conditions. Manioc and maize **(1)**; sometimes with squash **(2)**; plantain and maize **(3)**; plantain and bottle gourd **(4)**; plantain and tobacco **(5)**; sugar cane **(6)**; *fa'ada,* papaya, *tania, tupiro* **(7)**; sugar cane **(8)**; chili peppers **(9)**. (From Goldsmith *et al.,* 1990.)

suited for paddy rice culture, they have discovered a highly productive, stable system for their volcanic soils in a tropical setting (up to 160 inches of rain yearly) in west and central Java. This is a type of home garden called a *pekarangan.* Tall fruiting trees such as cinnamon and jackfruit substitute for the top canopy of the forest. There is a middle story of tall and fast-growing plants such as coffee, banana and papaya, and then a herbaceous ground layer of corn, upland rice, cassava, peanuts, and cumin. Vines (pepper, vanilla, etc.) climb the woody stems. This type of stable, man-designed ecosystem is said to equal the rice paddy (*sawah*) in carbohydrate production. It provides regular harvests of food, fuel, fodder, fiber and medicinal products for the cash and subsistence needs of rural people.

A more common sustainable form of agricultural support is the "doorway garden," seen but not recognized by many travelers in the tropics (Figure 22). It is a collection of plants and animals more or less fitting the modern concept of "permaculture." Pigs and chickens may run free, feeding from and fertilizing a host of fruit-bearing trees and shrubs. Commonly, an outside carbohydrate source is necessary, usually rice. It is not too far from what many dwellers in sub-tropical parts of Florida pridefully attempt. It is a horticultural effort; a planting around the house of citrus, guava, mango, banana, papaya, coconut and other species.

If you are ever in Miami at the Fairchild Tropical Garden you can see the components of a skillfully planned doorway garden that emulates nature. Here, in the Mayan Garden, developed by Richard Campbell, you can see the fruit, vegetable, medicinal and ornamental plants of a traditional Central American garden (minus pigs, chickens and dogs) adapted to the ecology of the Mayan Region (Yucatan, Guatemala, El Salvador, Belize and Honduras) with its shallow, calcareous soils and seasonally dry climate. There is a shade canopy of Mayan breadnut, Spanish cedar, Guiana chestnut, tamarind, cashew and *Inga,* the latter

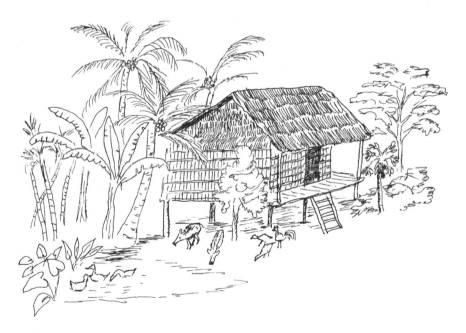

Figure 22. Typical "doorway garden" in Indomalaysia, surrounded by coconut palms, papaya, banana, mango, bamboo, breadfruit, tamarind and fruiting shrubs with emergent aquatics such as taro (edible rootstocks). Chickens, ducks and pigs provide eggs, meat and fertilizer and contribute sanitation and insect control. The horticultural and animal mix bears similarities with the modern concept of permaculture.

adding nitrogen to the soil and providing livestock forage. Underneath is a sub canopy of coffee, papaya, custard apple, siricote, star apple, cacao, sapote, avocado, Spanish lime and banana. Canopies are regularly thinned and pruned. In wetter locations, palms are grown for roof thatching. Ground level plants may include pineapple, cotton, pomegranate, prickly pear, corn, beans, melons, herbs and spices. A type of tall corn is used for fencing and construction.

There was a time in the United States when gardens were an essential part of life for a large rural population who still lived on the land. In the late 1800s, for most folks distant from the cities, if it wasn't grown locally, you just didn't eat it. My father said that, as a child, the greatest treat they could look forward to was the once a year orange in their Christmas stocking. A close look at early American traditional agriculture can tell us about when the health of many of our people began its downward slide. It is a story of soil and society. An example was the Anglo-Saxon settlers of the southern Appalachians whose way of life persisted until roughly the 1950s in isolated areas. They set up their small subsistence farms and large gardens on fertile soils in narrow, mountain valleys. Here they practiced a type of permaculture. Until the 1960s in north Georgia, they ranged their hogs and belled cattle free, providing them with salt and some grain. In the fall, the livestock fattened on acorns and, before their demise in the 1930s, chestnuts. I got to know intimately the life of some mountain families, one in particular in an isolated mountain valley in Towns County, in Georgia (Figure 23). This family lived in a 120-year-old log structure with a clay-chinked stone chimney. There was a cow for milk and butter. Pigs (in pens) provided most of the cured and smoked meat and bacon fat needed in cooking. Yard-run chickens laid eggs with almost orange yolks. Ducks dabbled in the branch over which was suspended an outhouse. (Pigs, chickens and ducks are notorious for pursuing the "dung factor" perhaps for vitamin B-12 in mammal droppings). Nothing was wasted. The corn crop provided cornbread and fed the hogs and for a while, a horse for ploughing. There was no running water in the house. Refrigeration was unnecessary since saturated fats in butter rarely turns rancid and unpasteurized milk keeps very well if kept cool (unlike pasteurized milk) in a spring box. Root cellars kept vegetables fresh for long periods. The ceiling beams supporting the cabin loft sagged dangerously from the weight of canned vegetables from the garden. Hot peppers and beans were threaded on strings and hung on the walls. The garden, of course was the key. Forest and streams provided fish, game, nuts, berries and medicinal plants. Furs and ginseng provided "spending money." A dose of ramps (a wild garlic) acted as a spring tonic and vermifuge. There were apple and cherry trees. Young sprouts of cornflower *(Rudbeckia laciniata)* and certain wild mustards were relished as greens. Alcohol was locally available. In spite of purchases from the "outside" world such as tobacco, salt and white flour (for cathead biscuits) the people were remarkably strong and healthy. Occasional comments about "rheumatiz" or "the swimhead" were the only medical complaints that I heard. This way of life, however, was not as sustainable as one based on composting and careful recycling, as done in the Orient.

In the valleys of the southern Appalachians a productive environment and the lack of convenient stores allowed a large population to develop a good, life-sustaining diet, and after 300 years, we were on the path to developing a traditional United States diet. The exodus from the little mountain homesteads to the towns was more or less when the larger fabric mills or other industry came into the area. At the same time most of the virgin timber had been logged out and the mining of mica, corundum and gold had terminated. A few relict farms persisted into the early 1970s.

It is important to realize that these subsistence farmers with their productive gardens had evolved a diet that sustained them in reasonable health. When they moved into town and started buying their food it was the beginning of the end. They lost their relationship with the soil and the natural environments in which they lived. Now, instead of eating the balanced diet that had sustained them for many years, suddenly convenience, seductive tastes, whimsy and economics determined their choice of food at the local stores. Chain stores and later supermarket chains began to purchase foods from everywhere and anywhere. Neither the buyers for the grocery chains nor the consumer public had the slightest idea which soils grew their foods or what fertilizers or poisons were used in their production. When the profit motive reigned supreme, food quality took a back seat. It was not deliberate: the buyers and store managers just didn't recognize that quality foods could only come from quality soils. The saving grace

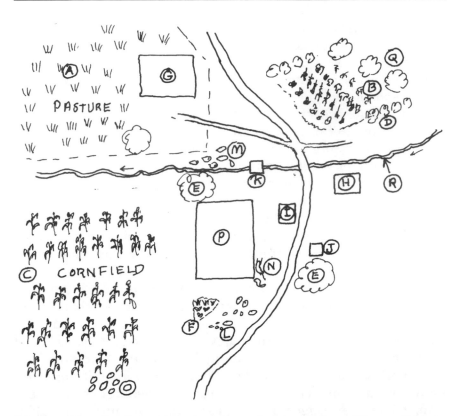

Figure 23. Southern Appalachian subsistence farm (Towns County, Georgia 1900–1965): (A) Pasture with one cow, one horse; (B) Garden; (C) Cornfield; (D) Berry bushes; (E) Black Walnut trees; (F) Herb garden; (G) Barn (for stock, hay and farming implements); (H) Pigsty; (I) Smokehouse; (J) Springhouse; (K) Outhouse; (L) Chickens; (M) Ducks; (N) Dog(s) and Cat(s) (hunting and mice control); (O) Guinea fowl (optional); (P) Main house (log cabin); (Q) Fruit trees; (R) Small creek.

was that, if you selected a wide variety of foods, you'd get the necessary spectrum of vitamins and minerals and other essentials.

In most restaurants in this country, the main course is almost invariably a meat dish. The vegetables seem to come as an afterthought and are conspicuously absent from the menu of the evening meal. Eyeing the list of luncheon vegetables, one generally searches in vain for those that rank high in nutrition: greens such as kale, sweet potatoes and pinto beans. The "soul food" restaurants maintained by Afro-American citizens may have sustained the closest thing to a traditional nourishing cuisine in the

South. In them you could be fairly sure of finding cornbread, collards and buttermilk, at least in Atlanta in the 1970s. Even a dish of regular slow-cooked oatmeal is hard to find on the morning menu of many restaurants. Oatmeal porridge appears to be one of the last "holdouts" of traditional foods. The point is: with a national cuisine in tatters and, apart from some food group pyramids, how in the world do we know what to eat? With no collective diet to depart from, each of us must chart his or her own course through the restaurants and down the supermarket aisles.

If you travel abroad and stay for any length of time in one area, at least for some, the wisest course appears to be one that tries to eat as close to the native or local diet as possible. The French are not drinking that red "vin ordinaire" just to get high. This lesson was vividly brought home to me in a little village in Paraguay's Gran Chaco, miles from anywhere. I had studied parasitology and medical entomology at Cornell and my symptoms did not seem to fit any endemic diseases. I reasoned that it must have something to do with food or drink. I had been eating the basic bread and beef local diet that everyone else ate. But, I had noticed that the local people all drank copious quantities of Yerba Maté tea, starting with hot tea in the morning and sipping a cold infusion all day long through a special metal filtering straw. I thought that this might be the missing ingredient that made an acidifying diet, almost completely lacking in fruits and vegetables, possible. I sent a boy to the market for the special flask, straw and tea. Within hours, I was up and ready to set off into one of the largest and most remote thorn forests on the planet.

Following the period when we grew most of our own food, there was a time when locally-grown food was locally sold in towns by bakers, green-grocers and butchers and when local nutrition was still tied to local soils. This was followed by "farmers' markets" and most of those were some distance away and served as regional centers for distribution. A farmer in Union County, Georgia, would get up at 2 a.m. to deliver a truckload of fresh collards to a farmers' market near Atlanta by 6 a.m. Comparatively few Americans can shop at this type of market. The freshness of some vegetables is questionable as some, like tomatoes, are picked green. Then, of course, came food "processing" with a host of additives and preservatives. Freezing has been a partial solution. The point is that local health was no longer tied to local soils and gardens and products were grown, sometimes in foreign countries on non-local soils of unknown nutrient content and with unknown treatment by pesticides and herbicides. Most supermarket managers have no earthly idea where their products were grown or how they were treated. The death of many cultures and even some empires attests that it is dangerous to break man's connection with the soil.

Agriculture has become agribusiness and a vast acreage is farmed not for quality of nutrition but for quantity and cosmetic appearance. Who is to blame? After all, it is the outcome of competition in a capitalist society. To be fair, consumers today seem to desire the most unblemished fruits and vegetables, not realizing that this has little relationship to nutrient content. Other regions of the world have developed traditional staple foods that are regularly, if not daily, eaten. In much of the Far East, rice is the main carbohydrate and energy source. In Mexico, corn, beans and peppers are standard daily fare in most rural areas. Corn *tortillas* are dependable energy sources, as are wheat *chapattis* in northern India. Unfortunately, in this country, it we had a traditional cuisine, we seem to have lost it. We have opted for a boundless variety of foods. This is great, but the catch is that it is not accompanied by a collective wisdom about which of those foods will be eaten, nor when and how often.

Since we don't have a national diet standardized through centuries of trial and error, most of us are at the mercy of the agriindustrial complex and the advertising media they so intensively use. The recent massive surge of interest in non-traditional medicine, health foods, organic produce and any and all supplements could be due to the public feeling of vulnerability in having drifted so far from the stable nutrition of the farms and gardens of the past.

CHAPTER EIGHT

Traditional Diets

"In order to believe that our society has 'progressed,' we must believe first that the lives of our ancestors were indeed nasty, brutish and short. But, as study after study has confirmed, the health of traditional peoples was vastly superior, in almost every way, to that of modern industrial man."

—Sally Fallon

In previous chapters, we have seen that man has struggled to adapt to new ways of life completely alien to his prehistoric past. Devastating diseases, famines and wars have apparently forced rapid changes and may have imposed "unnatural selection." The pliable nature of the human genotype has even enabled genetic response against specific diseases such as malaria, where the survivors breed and the unfit do not. Modern medicine, with all of its altruism and compassion seeks to ensure that even the unfit breed and perpetuate defects that normally would have been eliminated. While morally admirable, this unfortunately leads to a weakening of the human body, with ever more dependence on the availability of modern medical technology and its pharmaceutical support, neither of which is readily available to much of the world.

It is said that we spend $900 billion a year on food, surpassed only by the costs of medical care. (Meyerowitz, 1999.) Chronic illness affects at least one third of all Americans and causes three out of four deaths. "It is estimated that by the year 2000, about 50 percent of Americans will be chronically ill." (Marshall, 1998.) Fifty years ago it might have been 5 to10 percent. "One person in three suffers from allergies . . . one in five is mentally ill."

(Fallon, 1999.) The CDC says 25 percent of all Americans will be mentally ill by the year 2025. We've all seen the incredible cost of our national health care, such as $100 billion per year for Alzheimer's disease alone, and $270 billion for menopause-related conditions. The cost of cancer is staggering. This is "disease care," not health care. There are, or at least were, too many healthy people still left in the world to believe that disease is an inevitable and "normal" condition of the human race. Several nutrition pioneers who have studied and lived among peoples and cultures eating traditional diets adjusted by centuries of trial and error have ably documented this.

The most important documentation was the work of a dedicated dentist, Weston Price, who in the 1930s, became concerned with the loss of teeth and deformities in the faces of children especially—not only crowded and crooked teeth but actual changes in the bone structure of the face, causing it to be narrow, pinched, or otherwise abnormal. He also noted associated afflictions, such as arthritis, osteoporosis and diabetes.

For ten years Price, often with his wife, traveled literally to the ends of the earth, seeking societies isolated from civilization and living in a stable and sustainable relationship with nature. He visited at least fourteen groups, including natives of Alaska, the Pacific Islands, Australian aborigines, and Indians of the Peruvian Andes and the Amazon basin. In these isolated groups, tooth decay was rare to nonexistent; neither could he find cancer, heart disease or tuberculosis. Not only were the teeth beautiful, but the faces were strikingly similar in appearance, totally unlike the enormous variation we see in the streets of a civilized nation, even apart from the effects of ethnic mixing. Price found no toothbrushes, dental floss, braces, water piks, or dentists.

His epic book, *Nutrition and Physical Degeneration,* should be the bible of every nutrition-minded person in the world. It is replete with photographs of healthy and apparently happy natives, with perfect teeth and broad dental arches who lived on their native foods. A facing page often shows vivid photographs of the deformed dental arches and faulty facial bones characteristic of the first generation after their parents had adopted the foods of modern commerce (white flour, sugar, etc.). These children could hardly be recognized as belonging to the same racial type as their parents.

Price also arranged to analyze foods of the isolated societies for vitamin and mineral content. He tested salivas. He began his work in the Loetschental Valley of Switzerland which, in 1931, had just been opened by railroad to the outside world. The Swiss children between seven and sixteen years of age had only 0.3 cavities per individual on a diet that "consists largely of a slice of whole rye bread and a piece of summer-made cheese (about as large as the slice of bread), which are eaten with fresh milk of goats or cows. Meat is eaten about once a week."

Of the other cultures Price observed, some were modern hunter-gatherers in Canada, Amazonia, Africa, and Australia. They consumed available prey animals and ate the blood, bone marrow, glands (especially the vitamin-C rich adrenals) and organ meats as well as vegetables, tubers, grains and fruits, depending on their local environment. Others ate a great deal of seafood along with pig meat and fat, with available plant foods. Widespread geographically, such cultures naturally did not eat the same foods, but all had found, through centuries if not millennia of trial and error, the foods that kept them in perfect health and teeth. Price found six cattle-herding carnivorous African tribes (living largely on blood, milk and meat) to be entirely free of dental decay, while the more vegetarian Bantu tribes had five to six percent decayed teeth.

Price was forced to conclude that, while many "primitive" types continued to thrive on the same soils through thousands of years, American human stock has declined rapidly within a few centuries and, in some localities, within a few decades. No era, he says, "in the long journey of mankind, reveals in the skeletal remains such a terrible degeneration of teeth and bones as this brief modern period records." "And," he asks, "must nature reject our vaunted culture and call back the more obedient primitives?" The alternative is a complete readjustment in accordance, as he puts it, with the controlling forces of Nature. The controlling forces of nature are, of course, obedience to the laws of sustainable use of fertile soil, the non pollution of air and water, and the acknowledgement that our present life places demands and restraints upon the nervous system, glands and organs of each of us as individuals. As a collective population we are manipulated by the economic goals of commercialization, or, as Dolores LaChapelle puts it, the IGS or "Industrial Growth Society."

To further confirm that such dental-facial changes are not hereditary Price (1941) experimented with pigs, demonstrating that if you deprive female pigs of vitamin A for some weeks before mating and for thirty days afterwards, but then add vitamin

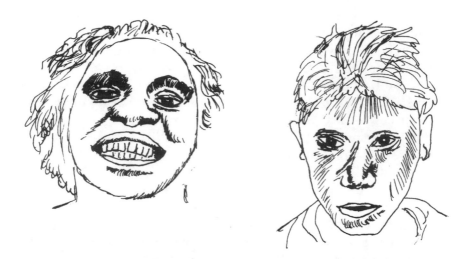

Figure 24. Comparison of the faces of Australian Aborigines on a traditional diet (left) and on "white man's food." The "modernized" young boy (right) shows some of the typical facial deformities such as the narrow face, pinched nostrils, narrow dental arch and undershot mandible. Where the middle third of the face is undeveloped like this, mouth breathing is common. (From photographs by Weston Price, 1939, 1948.)

A liberally to the sow's food, serious defects have already been established. Fifty-nine young from six sows so treated were all born without eyeballs or optic nerves and had cleft palate, harelip, club feet and spinal bifida. He also found cleft palate and harelip in puppies when both mother and sire were deficient in fat-soluble vitamins. He goes on to cite human studies that palatal deformities were present in 82 percent of mental defectives, 76 percent of epileptics and 80 percent of the insane.

Another pioneer in nutrition was Sir Robert McCarrison (M.D.). Most of his work was in India in the 1920s. He compared the diets of healthy Punjabis in northern India who ate fresh-ground whole wheat *chappatis,* milk, butter, curds, varied vegetables and fresh meat with bone and fat once a week. This contrasted vividly with the diet of the unhealthy Madrassis of southern India who ate polished rice, some vegetables, pulses, coconut, vegetable oils and coffee. McCarrison fed rats on the Madrassi diet. They fell ill, but those on the Punjabi diet throve. In another famous experiment, he fed his rats on a healthy Indian diet, others on a poor English diet composed of white bread, boiled vegetables, margarine, canned meat, jam and sugar. The rats on the English diet had double the mortality of those on the healthy Indian diet and were "ill-grown, poor-coated, weakly and listless." McCarrison went on to do classic deficiency disease studies of the effects of cooking on rice and other foods given to pigeons, guinea pigs and monkeys. His report is complete with visual comparisons of internal organs, glands and images of microscopic slides of tissues. (McCarrison, 1921.) His work is not only an indictment of the damage caused by eating milled grain such as polished rice, but of the deleterious effects of heat on grains and dairy products.

James Mount (1975) discussed McCarrison's work but also added other research documenting the value of experiments and cultures that declare the value of "whole food." He records an interesting experiment on dental health. Children fed whole-meal bread and porridge, wheat germ, fresh and dried fruits, cooked and uncooked vegetables, butter, cheese, eggs, milk, nuts and vitamins, were almost immune from tooth decay (0.58 cavities per child) with sixty-three out of eighty-one children completely free of cavities for five years.

Another very relevant nutritional pioneer is Francis Pottenger, Jr. (M.D.). He conducted famous and oft-cited experiments with over 900 cats on various diets for a period of ten years. He found that changes in facial structure and the onset of degenerative disease in cats paralleled the human degeneration that Price discovered in tribes and cultures that had abandoned traditional foods for the refined flour, sugar and other processed foods of the so-called "modern" diet.

Why would anyone select cats, strict carnivores, to compare with omnivorous humans? Being strict carnivores, cats vividly mirror any changes in their diet involving protein foods. This cleverly eliminates the confusion of testing an omnivore. Even dogs would not do for they apparently can digest and use carbohydrates. I recall being amused at our coonhounds gobbling up ripe persimmons; and, of course, commercial dog foods are mostly derived from grains.

If you've watched a cat eat a mouse, it usually begins with the head, its shearing carnassial teeth mincing up the skull and bones for calcium while organs such as the liver yield essential fatty acids and so forth—making a mouse a complete diet in one little package. Pottenger kept cats healthy by substituting a diet of meat, milk and cod liver oil. He discovered, and this was his stunning conclusion, that either cooking the meat or pasteurizing the milk utterly destroyed the cats over time, so that the third generation died within six months of birth and, in the interim, suffered skin diseases, allergies, parasites, soft bones, and personality changes, many females becoming vicious jezebels and males becoming spineless wimps. The cooked-meat cats had heart problems and were short or near-sighted; abortion was common (25 percent in first-year, 70 percent in second-year litters). There were structural changes in the cat skull bones leading to narrow, pinched faces, as Price had found in humans. Interestingly, studies in prisons, reformatories and homes for the retarded have revealed that a large majority (nearly 100 percent) of inmates had marked abnormalities of the dental arch, often with changes in the shape of the skull. (Schmid, 1994.)

Pottenger postulated that the heat of cooking or pasteurization adversely affected the proteins, changing the physiological utilization of certain albuminoids and globulin's, as well as reducing or destroying vitamins and enzymes. A resume of his research was presented in a classic paper (Pottenger, 1946), complete with X-ray images and photographs. Francis Pottenger, Jr. was probably influenced by an early study of the autonomic nervous system done by his father, also an M.D., prior to 1919 (Pottenger, 1944) who emphasized that much of our disease is the result of altered nerve and endocrine activity of physical or psychic origin. This work has inspired investigators who use the autonomic system in their assessment of metabolic typing.

Weston Price not only studied and analyzed the foods of contemporary human groups but also examined thousands of skulls of ancient peoples. (He looked at 1,276 skulls of fossil Peruvians alone). His and Pottenger's data must be taken as incontrovertible evidence of the physical and mental changes "that have accompanied the abandonment of humanity's traditional native foods and the adoption of the refined foods of modern industrial society." (Schmid, 1994.)

In addition to the studies reported above, there have been other studies pinpointing cultures that have lived with nature long enough to find sustainable health and freedom from degenerative disease.

McCarrison (1921) himself spent some seven years (1904-1911) among the fabled Hunzas of Pakistan. Here he found long-

RAW MILK

PASTEURIZED MILK

EVAPORATED MILK

SWEETENED, CONDENSED MILK

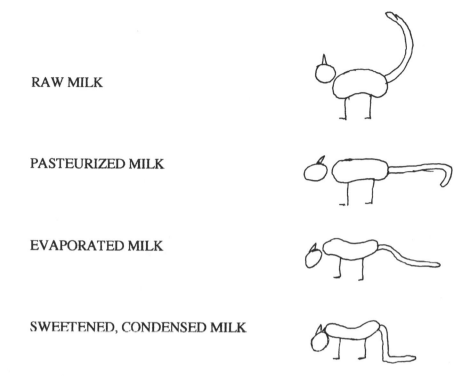

Figure 25. The health of adult cats fed raw milk versus processed milks. Raw milk produced healthy litters, homogenous in size and skeleton. Pasteurized milk produced changes in skeleton and reproduction, and kittens showed the same progressive body and respiratory problems as did cats on cooked meat. All diets were two-thirds milk, one-third raw meat, plus cod-liver oil. (Data from Pottenger, 1946, 1983.)

lived people with "continued vigor and perfect physique." Their maladies, he concluded, were not connected with the food supply. The Hunzakuts had somewhat of a restricted food supply, particularly relating to domestic animals, and seldom kept dogs. They mostly ate whole-grain wheat, barley and abundant apricots, according to McCarrison. Later (1950 to 1951), a geologist, John Clark (Ph.D. 1956) spent twenty months in Hunza and treated fifty or sixty people a day at a medical dispensary. At that time he found the Hunzas desperately poor. Some were malnourished. The problem may have been with food quantity, not quality. During Clark's stay the main foods were wheat, barley, buckwheat or millet, freshly ground along with some vegetables and fruit. Meat was rarely available and some soured goat milk products were taken. It is difficult to get the facts about the Hunzas since something of a mythology has since developed, following these two early and reliable reports.

People of the village of Vilcabamba in Ecuador were studied by a gerontologist, David Davies (M.D. 1975) between 1971 and 1973. The Vilcabambans have also been touted as healthy and long-lived, subsisting on small mountain farms at an altitude of 5,000 feet and growing grains and vegetables, harvesting yucca and wild potatoes and raising chickens, cows and goats. Cottage cheese and eggs were common foods. These villagers were also free of cancer and other chronic diseases as reported by a cancer specialist, Dr. Jorge Santiana. (Schmid, 1994.)

A third group reportedly replete with centenarians was the people of Georgian Russia investigated by the physician Alexander Leaf (1973). He examined 15,000 people over eighty, a number of which were centenarians. The older people were active, revered and had an active sex life into their nineties. They derived about 70 percent of their calories from vegetables and 30 percent from meat, dairy and eggs. Some raw milk and raw milk cheese were used at nearly all meals. Protein intake averaged seventy to ninety grams per day. Several glasses of wine were routinely taken daily and many people enjoyed homemade grape vodka.

All three of these social groups apparently live in or close to valleys supplied with trace-element-enriched, silty waters. Hunza water is of glacial origin.

The isolated communities of healthy beings described above can also be labeled "traditional societies" eating traditional foods. From some of the practices of the traditional lifestyle, we can hope to derive important information for our own dietary program, regardless of which metabolic type we find ourselves to be. We need to know what traditional diets can tell us about the broad categories of carnivory, omnivory and herbivory. It turns out that certain habits of traditional societies such as soaking grains and beans, fermenting grains and pickling vegetables, have been found essential to nurture sustainable health, vitality and longevity. In our own culture, we can see that the abandonment of these practices has gone hand in hand with the deterioration of our health. It will then be easier for us to see why leaving the land or local soils for the ease and convenience of city life can, for many of us, have disastrous consequences, as it has had for other civilizations with populous cities, now relegated to crumbling ruins.

Once adapted, these cultures find it very difficult to change their standard diet or substitute foods from other cultures. Most immigrants, coming from a different food niche such as the Orient, soon suffer the same incidence of the same diseases as their new host country. I'll never forget the problems endured by the Mennonites who immigrated to eastern Paraguay from Canada in the 1940s. My daily meals with them consisted basically of cassava roots and peanuts. In the sub-tropical forest, they were unable to grow their familiar crops. Disillusioned, many returned to Canada. It is an expensive problem for our military forced to live in exotic places. Some of our troops are not adapted to local foods and must be supplied with the costly fare of their homeland. Opposing them is often a population well adapted to an inexpensive and highly portable traditional diet, such as rice and dried fish.

The leadership in documenting traditional diets appears to be Sally Fallon (M.A.) and her collaborator and scientist Mary Enig (Ph.D.). Fallon has an extensive background in both nutrition and in the culinary arts and has devoted many years to the study of traditional methods of food preparation. Enig is an internationally recognized expert in lipid chemistry and is the leading authority on the dangerous trans-fatty acids such as are created by the partial hydrogenation of vegetable oils. Their Human Diet Series, published by the Price-Pottenger Nutrition Foundation (now retitled Health and Healing Wisdom), addresses details of what traditional peoples really eat and covers Australian aborigines, Merrie Old England, Sub-Saharan Africa, China, Cavemen and Americans (then and now).

Since we are concerned with the ratio of proteins, fat and carbohydrate in individualizing our own diets, we need to briefly review the conclusions of these talented authors as presented in the human diet series and in the book *Nourishing Traditions* (Fallon *et al.*, 1995), which is highly recommended. Furthermore, as these authors emphasize, the *type* of nutrient is extremely important as well as the way in which it is prepared. For example, they offer data that clearly refute the concept that cancer and heart disease are caused by the increased consumption of saturated fats and cholesterol from butter, cream, eggs and meat.

They analyzed cook books from the 1895-1896 period and discovered that Americans at the turn of the century consumed an estimated 2,900 calories per day with 40 percent derived from fats, with a ratio of saturated to unsaturated fat at least 1 to 1. (Fallon and Enig, 1996.) Here are ratios of carbohydrate, protein and fat based upon the 1896 *Boston Cook Book* in percents: Breakfast 42-23-35 (632 calories); lunch 52-17-31 (1,043 calories); dinner 41-18-41 (1,143 calories). It is well established that heart disease and cancer were relatively rare before the turn of the century. To quote the authors, "this rich diet of cream, butter, eggs, meat, vegetables, grains and fruit produced a generation of healthy, hearty, intelligent Americans, in spite of the fact that they consumed substantial amounts of sugar and white flour."

We've all heard the nursery rhyme "Jack Sprat could eat no fat, his wife could eat no lean . . . ," perhaps one of the first references to individual nutritional needs or the coupling of a carnivore with a vegetarian. We recognize that, in cold climates or in temperate climate winters, one desires and needs more fatty foods. A surgeon in the Royal Navy, T. L. Cleave (1973) wrote that in northern Europe, 40 percent of the calories are derived from fat against 20 percent in southern Spain and Italy. He further indicated that in England, where the population is of mixed descent due to past invasions from both the north and south of Europe, and in the heterogeneous United States, you would find both Jack Sprats and their herbivore opposites in a mixture.

Let's look a little further into the current confusion about fats. The case against polyunsaturated fats or vegetable oils is strong. They have been highly touted as being "better" for you than saturated animal fats such as lard and butter. According to Fallon and Enig (1996) a high intake of polyunsaturated oils invokes a host of problems: they "increase cholesterol levels in tissues, increase fat cell synthesis in growing animals, alter the response of the immune system, increase peroxidation products such as ceroid pigment, increase gallstone formation, and of all things, decrease HDL cholesterol in the blood." In addition, it is now recognized that store-bought oils, especially if not refrigerated, rapidly become rancid and carcinogenic. This is arguably a greater danger than heart disease, supposedly prevented by their supposedly cholesterol-lowering effects. Traditional diets relied heavily on fats like butter and lard, neither of which rapidly oxidize or grow rancid and keep well in a cool place. I can remember in the 1960s, living in the mountains of north Georgia with an isolated corn-patch farmer's family for an entire summer. We fished out slices of "fat back" floating in a bowl of hog fat; the delicious "cat-head" biscuits were made with fat rendered from the annual hog killing.

Fallon and Enig (1997) made a strong case that the high-fat proponents "are the most likely winners of the great Paleolithic fat debate." They indicate that Stone Age man and many present day hunter-gatherers prefer fatty portions of their animal prey and actually consume a diet quite high in fat, which, on average from wild game, is at least half-saturated. (Wild boar fat or lard is about 41 percent saturated.) The gut protozoa of ruminants like sheep and cows saturate the oils of plant foods. Also, to keep our perspective, remember that wild game fats contain a proportion of healthy Omega-3 fats while domestic beef contain little. (Eaton *et al.,* 1988.) One frequently reads about the high amount of fat in domestic meats. Fallon and Enig assure us that our practice of breeding and feeding domestic animals, if naturally and humanely done, is not to be disdained, but was a forward step in man's evolution of food. One of the caveats, however, is that we can overdo stock raising by diverting too much land to feed animals instead of using the extra energy we could derive from feeding the grains to people. The other caveat is that because it is delicious and we can afford it, we overeat the juicy, fatty meats and overwhelm our sedentary bodies with too much of a good thing.

Another traditional practice that we have gotten away from, inherited from the omnipresent kettle over the hearth-fire, is gelatin-rich broth made from the bones of chicken or beef, or, in the Orient, largely fish. During my several years in Southeast Asia, I grew quite fond of the inevitable fish stews or soups replete with fish heads. I didn't realize it at the time, but the eyes and the tissues in the eye sockets are a rich source of vitamin A. (Price, 1939.) Back home my friends wrinkled their noses at this sensible approach to good nutrition. To simulate this aspect of traditional diets, ask your supermarket butcher for a tray of chopped up backbone, neck bones or other bones. Not only is the marrow nutritious but the morsels of meat are uncommonly tender. Do not be deterred if they are labeled "dog bones." The gelatin in broth improves the digestion of beans, grains, meats and dairy products and helps normalize a stomach acid deficiency. (Osborne, 1998.)

In the chapter on breads and grains (The Staffs of Life) we discussed the problem of eating grains because of the phytates, which rendered the minerals unavailable, and the enzyme (protease) inhibitors, which prevent protein utilization. Since protease inhibitors are so effective against cancerous growths, it could be that they interfere with or block the cancer's insatiable need for amino acids to appease its rapidly dividing cells. In any event, with no knowledge of the chemistry of enzyme inhibitors or phytates, our ancestors survived by soaking and fermenting grains before eating them. They soaked grains such as oatmeal overnight in warm water or clabbered milk. They made naturally leavened "sourdough" breads and soaked whole meal flour in buttermilk before making pancakes and biscuits, according to Sally Fallon.

Traditional societies also discovered that they had to soak beans at least overnight with changes of water and then cook them long and slowly. "Southern" cooking is often derided because things appear to be over-cooked. Half the critics don't realize that, for many vegetables, cooking well is necessary to release the nutrients from the cells. The beta carotene of cooked carrots is much more available than that from raw ones. The other half of the critics are totally unfamiliar with phytates, enzyme inhibitors, and lectins.

Fortunately, cooking also inactivates lectins, protein-like substances present in many grains, vegetables, fruits, spices and seeds. Lectins apparently can damage intestinal walls. For example, lectins in raw kidney beans (as few as five may cause illness) bind to the microvillae of the small intestine and impair nutrient absorption, thus suppressing growth. (Liener, 1986.)

According to Leiner, proper cooking inactivates most lectins. Beans must be boiled for at least ten minutes. Viscous masses of beans and corn, especially in earthenware vessels, if not consistently and vigorously stirred, still retain lectin activity. Cooking at higher elevations also means longer cooking. Slow cooking, as in crock-pots, without pre-boiling, does not eliminate lectin activity. Detectable levels of blood agglutination remain, even after slow cooking of kidney beans for five hours at ninety-one degrees Celsius, although they are acceptable in texture and palatability. (Liener, 1986.) This is all the more reason to use fermented foods traditionally evolved by various cultures. Some pulses, such as lentils, mung beans, split peas, black eyed peas and *sprouted* beans (sprouting deactivates lectins) have relatively low, non-toxic levels of lectins.

Lectins apparently serve plants as insecticides and are being used by the agricultural industry to alter the genes of edible crop plants. Rodents suffer damaged immune systems and stunted organ growth from eating raw potatoes genetically engineered to contain a lectin from another plant. On the basis of such tests, a British scientist, Arpad Pusztai, accused the industry of using humans as guinea pigs "in a vast experiment with genetically modified (GM) foods." (Firth, 1999.)

There is a highly controversial theory that lectins, if either injected or carried into the blood stream during digestion, cause red blood cells to agglutinate or clump together. (D'Adamo and Whitney, 1996.) These authors claim that each of the four blood types react differently to specific lectins; for example type B's should avoid tomatoes, presumably raw, at all costs. Michael Klaper (M.D., 1999) wrote an extensive critique of the Blood-type Diets of Peter D'Adamo. He feels that D'Adamo failed to provide evidence of his own or other research that would document his theories. To support this criticism, Klaper asserts that modern medical pathology has never documented "lectin reduced red cell agglutination as a cause of disease in any humans." He fears that D'Adamo's claims will cause unnecessary worry and concern for millions of readers attracted to "an evolutionary fairy tale."

A physician, Robert Rowen (M.D., 1999) compared the blood types of his patients with their diets and found almost no accuracy for blood types other than O, and found two individuals with blood types "who should be eating a vegetarian diet more fit for blood type A," according to D'Adamo. Rowen had learned metabolic typing techniques from Harold Kristal. Osborne (1998) indicated that there is evidence that all four blood types existed back in the Paleolithic era. She suggests that the success of D'Adamo's books (see Chapter 26) resulted from his advice to eliminate commercial breads, bagels, muffins, flours, cakes, cookies, pasta and cereals (whole grain or not) which give gluten-sensitive gut linings "a chance to rest and recover." Also, all four blood-type diets improve health by eliminating chips, candy, doughnuts and junk foods containing "sugar, wheat, salt, hydrogenated fats, and other known health destroyers." (Osborne, 1998.)

There is another controversy, to eat or not eat soy products. Unfortunately, according to some, everybody seems to be jumping on the soybean bandwagon these days. Most of southeast Asia and Japan have the wisdom to eat them largely as fermented condiments (tempeh, miso, soy sauce). Besides, unlike ourselves, they have had many years (since the Chou dynasty) to adapt to soy products such as tofu and bean curd.

Some studies have shown that the isoflavones of soy (genistein, diadzein, glycetein) have been effective against breast cancer in post-menopausal women. According to Harold Kristal, there are other studies showing that isoflavones may promote breast cancer in these same women, as well as in pre-menopausal women with a previous history of breast cancer. "Soy protein products, isoflavone supplements and (most disturbingly) soy infant formulas deliver concentrated levels of isoflavones never found in traditional Asian diets." (Kristal, 2000.) For additional information Kristal recommends the web site *www.soyonline.com*.

It so happens that soy phytates are highly resistant to even long, slow cooking and only a period of fermentation will significantly reduce the phytate content of soybeans. (Fallon and Enig, 1995.) The soybean also contains potent enzyme inhibitors which block the action of trypsin needed for protein digestion, and can cause chronic deficiencies in amino acid uptake. While reduced in tofu and bean curd, they are not completely eliminated. When consumed with meat, the effects of phytates are reduced, which means that Asian children might suffer rickets and other problems without adequate meat and fish in their diets. The production of soymilk, while destroying most of the anti-nutrients, also denatures the proteins. The alkaline soaking solution used produces a carcinogen and reduces the cystine content, rendering useless the entire protein complex of the soybean (according to Fallon and Enig). One alarming aspect of this is that soy protein isolates may be principal ingredients in soy-based infant formulas, leaving them with a high phytate content as well as trypsin inhibitors, although the latter can vary as much as five-fold. Neither do soybeans supply the important fat-soluble vitamins such as retinol A and vitamin D, found only in certain animal foods such as organ meats, butter, eggs, fish and shellfish. (Fallon and Enig, 1995.)

A final major contribution of traditional diets concerns the process of lacto-fermentation. Lactic acid is a natural preservative produced by bacteria, usually lactobacilli. The process enabled our forebears to preserve vegetables without freezers or canning. Lactic acid not only enhances the enzyme content of vegetables but also apparently increases vitamin levels and improves digestibility. Examples of lacto-fermented foods are sauerkraut, pickles, cucumbers, beets and turnips, and include our relishes, chutneys and the famed Japanese *umeboshi* plum. Other valuable fermentation products are (apart from alcohol and the rising of bread dough) buttermilk, yogurt, cheeses and various sour beverages made from grains, fruits and nuts. Koumiss, fermented mare's milk, is the principal food of wandering tribes in European Russia and the plains of south, western and southern Asia. The fermentation of milk allows lactose-intolerant people to drink it; and both the vitamin B and C content of milk appear to be increased by the process. Like koumiss, there are a number of less well-known fermentative products. My fieldwork in northern Cambodia in the 1950s and 1960s would not have been possible without the fermented fish sauce *nuoc-mam,* prepared by burying minced, salted fish in earthenware pots in the ground for several months. The resultant oily liquid that rises to the top is drawn off and is rich in amino acids, certain vitamins and minerals. It is quite tasty. I cannot say as much for the other fermented product, a fish paste, *pra-hoc,* ripened in open jars in the sun for about a month. When we unsealed the jars in the backcountry, we had to first scoop out a layer of maggots before we could ladle out the more edible portion. After this anecdote, if you still want to learn more about fermented foods and how to prepare them, I recommend a fascinating book, the "bible" of fermentation, Steinkraus' (1983) *Handbook of Indigenous Fermented Foods.*

Fallon cites Tom Valentine's book (*Search For Health*) about a finding by Soviet researchers concerned with the dramatic increase in cancer following World War II. In the midst of dreadful cancer statistics, two districts in the central western Ural Mountains stood out "like neon lights" having hardly any cancer, even though they were heavily polluted by toxins. Investigators accidentally stumbled on the fact that every home had fermenting crocks of Kvass or Kombucha.[8]

---

[8] The Kombucha fermentation of tea and sugar forms a bacterial "mushroom" that can be propagated. The very pleasant tasting liquid in which it resides is said to boost the immune system and detoxify the body.

In conclusion, man can benefit from the many nutrients in plant foods as long as he takes care in their preparation. It has been said that the methods of preparing plants by primitives, pounding, soaking and fermenting imitates the time-consuming processes that take place in the digestive tracts of ruminant animals such as cows and sheep. The teeth of ruminants do the crushing and special compartments of their stomachs do the soaking and fermentation, the bacteria creating additional protein.

According to Marshall (1998) among civilized nations we rank twenty-seventh in survival yet spend more than twice per capita on health care than any of the others. He also sagely comments that we keep our houses and cars in top shape but ignore the needs of our bodies.

The Oldways Preservation and Exchange Trust has prepared "diet pyramids" (Figure 26) which summarize amounts of what type foods are ingested by much of the world. In these three diets, proteins and fat are largely provided daily by the plant kingdom.

Note that protein-rich beans and other legumes, nuts and seeds are prominent *daily* diet components in all three pyramids. Also note that red meat plays a relatively minor role in these diets. There are good reasons for this and ecology gives us perspective here. While you can generally produce ten times the food energy by growing plants instead of animals, not all nations are created equally in this regard. Countries blessed with a grassland climate and large areas of fertile soil can afford to feed grains to livestock. It is estimated that one pound of American beef requires sixteen pounds of grain and soy, plus one gallon of gasoline (chemicals, transportation and processing). (Rifkin, 1992.) We are talking here about stall-fed, not range-fed, livestock. Stall-fed animals are eating things that could be eaten by humans. Actually, much of the world is unsuited to cultivation and there it is more efficient to let livestock convert what we can't eat (grass, shrubs) to what we can (meat, fat and dairy products). In the days of the old west cattle, like bison before them, efficiently converted grass to protein with no soil depletion. They were not fattened with grains. It was an ecologically sound use for immense areas that were too dry or otherwise unsuitable for agriculture at that time.

Today, unfortunately, to raise those fattening grains and "marble" that beef does deplete organic matter and minerals from the soil where they had been built up for eons by the low rainfall

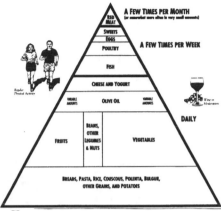

The Traditional Healthy Mediterranean Diet Pyramid

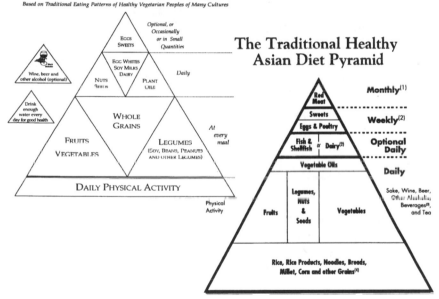

Figure 26. Three traditional "diet pyramids." Note that in all three diets, proteins are largely provided on a daily basis by grains, legumes, nuts, seeds and certain vegetables. Dairy foods are generally not part of Asian diets except in India and areas of nomadic herders to the north. (Courtesy Oldways Preservation and Exchange Trust, 1994, 1995, 1997.)

and root death of the grasses. Our current use of the mid-continent breadbasket is ecologically unsound and unsustainable, compared to the time when cattle ranged like buffalo over immense natural pastures. Only comparatively wealthy nations can afford the luxury of grain-fed livestock. Meat and expensive deep-ocean fish like tuna are beyond the means of much of the world.

Even in nations that are not heavily industrialized, wide gaps between the "haves" and the "have nots" mirror the high-energy costs of expensive foods such as protein. For example, the average Mexican middle-class diet contains 100 grams of animal protein daily and costs 14,000 "agricultural calories" and 500,000 "industrial calories" (fuel, transport, equipment, etc.). Contrast this with a less advantaged family eating predominantly maize, beans and vegetables, whose foods require only 2,000 "agricultural calories" and 8,000 "industrial calories." (Martinez *et al.*, 1976.)

There are, of course, cultures where hunting (Eskimo), herding (nomadic or sedentary herders of Asia, Africa and Scandinavia), or fishing (some island and coastal cultures) has made humans more dependent on animal products, and, by climate or physiology, adapted to them. Because of our genetic heritage in the United States, some of us had ancestors who were more adapted to animal protein and fats. The rest of us enjoy the luxury of red meats, fish and fowl because it tastes so good and we can afford it. The problem is that we may or may not be adapted to such a protein intake, hence the utility of knowing our own metabolism.

One is impressed, even awed, by the almost religious fervor of so-called "vegetarians." Most would seem to be offended if you dared suggest that they might be eating improperly. The vegetarian diet pyramid (Figure 26) seems to apply only to ovo-lacto vegetarians. Let's look briefly at vegetarianism. Remember that most humans are basically omnivorous but that some of us have metabolisms that are adapted towards either carnivore or herbivore (vegetarianism).

The Carnivore-Herbivore Controversy

As discussed elsewhere, if you are on the slow oxidizer side of the typical omnivore you will do better on more plant-based foods. If you are fairly far from the central omnivore position, you can call yourself a vegetarian, in which case you may get some animal protein from things like eggs and dairy products. The general term "vegetarian" also includes a very strict category the "vegan," eating no animal protein at all.

Randall White (M.D.) and Erica Frank (M.D.) have neatly summarized the literature (1994) on vegetarianism. According to these authors, vegetarians generally receive adequate protein *provided* they eat high-protein vegetable sources such as grains, nuts, seeds and beans regularly *every* day. Vitamin intake is usually good except for vitamin D and B12, especially a concern for vegans. Potassium loss seems to be higher in vegetarians. These authors cite a study which indicates that omnivores have a third of the stool bulk of vegetarians, which makes it all the more imperative to eat within your nutritional type. Carnivorous wild animals seldom seem to have colon problems. It would seem that humans with a hereditary carnivorous metabolism shouldn't either. The nearly carnivorous Eskimos seem rarely plagued with colon cancer. The prevalence of colon cancer today suggests that some of us at least are either eating the wrong diet for our presumed metabolic type or consuming too many low-fiber, processed, refined and concentrated "modern" foods. Vegetarians are said to have a lower risk of Type II (adult onset) diabetes. A high fiber intake has been postulated as protecting hunter-gatherers and subsistence agriculturists from excessive post-meal rises in blood sugar as well as increasing bowel transit time.

White and Frank found that vegans and lacto-vegetarians are indeed rare and cite an incidence of 1.5 percent among 605 physicians and lawyers. While most vegetarians seemed to them to be more health conscious, to exercise and to eat fewer calories and less fat, "there were no significant correlations between vegetarianism and morbidity as measured by sick days, clinic, or hospital visits."

Stephen Byrnes (N.D., Ph.D.) has discussed the myths of vegetarianism (1999). He indicates that vegans on their abnormal diet would not have survived 100 years ago without modern supplements and that the largely vegetarian inhabitants of southern India have the shortest life spans in the world. Byrnes reviews the evidence that low cholesterol diets are not healthier and that saturated fats do not cause cancer or heart disease. This ties in with the endorsement of animal fats by Sally Fallon and Mary Enig. Byrnes makes the interesting point that fat must be eaten with beta carotene so that bile salts can convert it to vitamin A.

Apparently many people, including infants and diabetics, make the conversion poorly, if at all.

Klaper's (1999) Institute of Nutrition Education and research is conducting long range studies of the effect of vegan (no animal protein) vegetarian and omnivore diets and will track thousands of individuals. They will attempt to answer questions such as: "Are *Homo sapiens* metabolically required to eat the flesh of other animals for optimum health and function, and can we identify people especially suited (or unsuited) to plant based diets?" Klaper admits that there are "significant metabolic differences between people."

Klaper has an interesting theory: One's metabolic type may be culturally determined by the kind of food eaten in the early years, setting "biochemical patterns that last for a lifetime." If adults had meat-eating childhood, so his theory goes, their enzyme systems might not be able to make the change to a plant-based diet and after months or years on a flesh-free diet, they would understandably feel better when meat was added back. Long-term omnivores who made an abrupt change to a vegan diet may be in the same boat according to Klaper and may need to taper off gradually in an "attenuated weaning process in order to overcome metabolic patterns begun early in life." The field of metabolic typing will clearly benefit by the Institute's research agenda.

In conclusion it might be wise to consider the words of an authority on the eating habits of un-modernized human societies worldwide: "As yet I have not found a single group of primitive racial stock which was building and maintaining excellent bodies by living entirely on plant foods. I have found in many parts of the world most devout representatives of modern ethical systems advocating the restriction of foods to the vegetable products. In every instance where the groups involved had been long under this teaching, I found evidence of degeneration in the form of dental caries, and in the new generation in the form of abnormal dental arches to an extent very much higher than in the primitive groups who were not under this influence." (Price, 1939.)

CHAPTER NINE

When Is a Tomato a Tomato?

"Indeed, the whole of ancient society depends entirely on the soil, and in the final test the history of these times is not written on the temple friezes, the clay tablets, the parchment rolls or the rock writings, or in the conventional history book writings of today. It is written in the soil."

—Ritchie Calder

Nutrient-rich topsoil is perhaps the most precious resource in the world. You can desalinate salt water to make fresh water but you can't make new fertile soil. You can only do agriculture similar to hydroponics and beyond the means of much of the world. And unless taxpayers of the wealthy nations intend to provide huge and perpetual sums of money, either to buy the soil amendments or feed the starving of the less fortunate nations, there is only one solution. It is to help the Third World restore fertility in their depleted soils and conserve what is left of their fertile soils, the forests that help water them, their locally adapted plant varieties and the farming techniques of their past.

Unfortunately, here is where many of the multinational corporations can be indicted. Regrettably, they turn peoples that once supported themselves by subsistence agriculture into purchasers of their products. By raising export crops to sell instead of to eat, former subsistence farmers can earn enough money to buy things, including fertilizer, pesticides, and "modern" refined foods. The local, time-honored relationship of man with his sustainably productive soil is broken. People are driven to exhaust the forests and realize only a transient, temporary gain from the soil bank in which the forest has been depositing nutrients for hundreds of years.

The nutrients in plants that we want come from the soils in which they are grown. As we all know, certain plants have nutrients that other plants lack. The trouble is that the sensory organs of humans cannot, apart from sweets and fats, tell either what nutrients a plant contains or how much. So one of the reasons for our large brains may be to learn, store and pass on our learned and experiential knowledge of what we must eat and to make all the associations that would allow us to thoughtfully invade other new, unknown habitats and to be able to find suitable foods.

Katherine Milton's monkeys certainly knew how to eat a nutritious diet in the jungles of Barro Colorado. Primates have keen vision. Odor and taste may simply inform them of degrees of ripeness or palatability. I have no data that tell how well primates can detect the content of proteins, fatty acids, vitamins and minerals by odor or taste. Perhaps we began as vision-dependent generalist omnivores eating everything that looked edible and rejecting things that tasted bad or made us sick, and our young learned by imitating their parents.

Humans can detect sweet carbohydrates and recognize fats and meat proteins by sight or taste. Beyond that, our ability to analyze foods is limited. We eat what we observe our parents to eat or are given. This is not the case with most wild creatures that "instinctively" know what to eat. Most have a highly developed sense of smell which domestication does not destroy. Total carnivores, like cats and crocodiles, don't need to evaluate the nutrient status of their prey but cows and pigs are recognized as excellent organic "chemists," being able to detect by odor the nutrient quality of their food. It may all look green to a cow but they can readily detect the amount of nitrogen, calcium or other substances.

Albrecht (1947), whose book on soil fertility and animal nutrition is a classic, relates the case in which twenty-five acres of virgin prairie hay were cut and put up in four haystacks. One quarter of the twenty-five acres had been given soil treatments one season and the grass from this area was segregated into one of the four haystacks every year. The cattle ate this one haystack first and, from 1937 on, each year thereafter for eight years. The cows were able to detect a 5 to 7 percent increase in calcium, phosphorus and nitrogen in the grass from the four fertilized

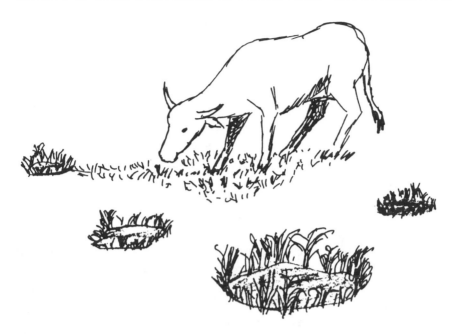

Figure 27. Cows as chemists. Cattle avoid the lush, green grass growing around a cow-pie. The high nitrogen content has lowered the quality of the faster growing grass.

acres even after eight years. In another case, hogs turned out into a forty-acre cornfield to glean corn (accidentally dropped during harvest) each day made a beeline across the entire field to feed in a distant corner where, several years before, the farmer had tried to grow a small patch of alfalfa and had used lime and fertilizer but had forgotten about it until the hogs reminded him. You may have noticed that cows do not eat the fast growing nitrogen grass that grows in and around their droppings. This is not because they are being sanitary or fastidious—the quality of the grass is too poor to eat.

As our omnivorous primate ancestors ventured out into the "new" environments such as the open savanna and had to deal with new foods such as turtles, lizards and all sizes and shapes of game animals and the predators that went along with this new diversity, it must have placed a premium on the brain's ability to adapt. Being a part-time predator and being forced to migrate long distances to find water and shelter and game, either alive or scavenged, were new demands on a brain that was suited to a more stable life in the rainforest. Certainly, tools and speech became more essential for survival. Whatever the cause, increased brain capacity was the hallmark of early man and prepared us for the long epochs of hunting and gathering which occupied 99 percent of our past. The verbal history, as maintained by the "dreamtime" of the highly mobile Australian aborigine hunter-gatherer, was supplanted by the written history of the sedentary farmer. Groups of people in the Swiss Alps and Himalayas, in the rice paddies of Asia and even in the Appalachians had to develop a new wisdom of how to live sustainably, based on empirical observation and trial and error. The Industrial Growth Society of LaChapelle and "progress" changed all that. So, cut off from nature and natural laws, we stand in the produce department of a large supermarket fondling a tomato. At least, it *looks* like a tomato, but we don't have a clue as to how much nutrients it contains, on which soil it was grown, whether or not it was picked green, or what temperatures it has been kept at or how long since it was picked. It is red and looks like a tomato. There is just enough evidence to suggest that all is not well with commercially grown and marketed foods.

Bear *et al.* (1949) collected samples of vegetables from commercial fields in Georgia, South Carolina, Virginia, Maryland, New Jersey, New York, Ohio, Indiana, Illinois and Colorado. Detailed analysis was made of tomatoes and snap beans. Tomatoes showed the greatest variation in calcium, magnesium and copper. Calcium ranged from 4.5 to 23.0 (milliequivalents per 100 grams (me/100g) dry matter); magnesium from 4.5 to 59.2. Tomatoes also varied from 1.0 to 68.0 ppm (parts per million) of manganese and from 0.0 to 53.0 ppm of copper. Spinach showed wide variation: 84.6 to 257.0 (me/100g) in potassium; 46.0 to 203.9 in magnesium; 0.8 to 69.5 in sodium and between 19 and 1,584 ppm of iron.

Soils of the eastern Coastal Plain states have been thoroughly leached and have limited supplies of mineral nutrients. Of soils from the eastern north central states, some were developed from calcareous glacial drift, some were prairie soils. The Colorado soils were high in calcium carbonate and were under irrigation. One can conclude that different vegetables from different soils differ, sometimes drastically, in their nutrient content. In the case of copper and iron, values can range from none, or nearly none, to very high. Trends were noticed. Calcium in-

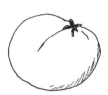 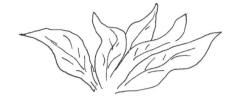

	LOW	HIGH		LOW	HIGH
Calcium	4.5	23.0	Potassium	84.0	257.0
Magnesium	4.5	59.2	Magnesium	46.0	203.0
Manganese	1.0	68.0	Sodium	0.8	69.5
Copper	0.0	53.0	Iron	19.0	1,584.0

Figure 28. The striking variation in mineral content in tomatoes and spinach grown on commercial fields in different states (and thus different soils). In millequivalents per 100 grams. (Data from Bear *et al.*, 1949.

creased and magnesium decreased from south to north; calcium, magnesium, potassium, boron, iron, molybdenum, copper, and cobalt increased from east to west and sodium and manganese values decreased from east to west.

In 1989, a nutrient testing laboratory tested eleven commercially grown vegetables from supermarkets in five states (California, Colorado, Massachusetts, Florida and New York). The tests for thirteen minerals were designed to uncover mineral imbalance in the soils on which the foods were grown. The mineral content in each food tested varied widely from region to region. There was three times more phosphorus in California potatoes than in those from New York. Florida tomatoes had eighteen times more calcium than Massachusetts samples (Florida tomatoes were probably grown near Homestead over a calcareous substrate) but Colorado's spinach had five times more iron than Florida's. Some of the vegetables sampled had zero content of important trace elements such as boron and zinc. (Jensen and Anderson, 1990.)

Comparisons of organic and commercially grown foods are also revealing. Smith (1993), over a two-year period, purchased apples, pears, potatoes, wheat and corn from markets in Chicago. These were analyzed by Doctor's Data Laboratory in west Chicago. The vegetables organically grown had on average, over 90 percent more nutritional elements than similar commercially grown food. Sweet corn had 2.5 times more nutrients.

Factors other than vitamin and mineral content are also important. Lampkin (1990) cites evidence for a longer storage life for organic grown vegetables, less pesticide residues, and less nitrate accumulation (nitrates may convert to carcinogenic nitrites when ingested or cooked). Lairon *et al.* (1986) compared analyses of carrots, lettuces, leeks and potatoes from organic and commercial sources and found that organic fertilizers could reduce roughly by half the nitrate content of vegetables and increase levels of phosphorus and magnesium. There have been pros and cons concerning organic methods. In 1980 there seemed to be insufficient evidence that organically grown produce was superior to that grown with commercial fertilizer. (Hornick, 1992.) In her 1992 paper, however, she indicated that some carrot varieties could provide three times as much beta carotene as commercial types. She cited 1958 data that showed that both the cultivar and the altitude (the latter affecting soil type) affected the protein content of dried beans. She also cited Salunkhe and Desai (1988) who emphasized that both ascorbic acid and carotenoids of different vegetables grown at six geographic locations varied significantly. In another study, increased nitrogen application (as from commercial fertilizer) lowered protein quality in barley, wheat and rye, but not in oats or corn.

Hornick's comments on handling and storage are relevant to supermarket foods. Apples, apricots and peaches contained no ascorbic acid if picked green. By contrast, mangos have much more vitamin C when green (60 mg/100 mg) than when ripe (14 mg). Now I understand why we knocked down green mangos (and ate them with *nuoc mam* sauce) in Cambodia's backcountry. It seemed dumb to me at the time, but the natives knew more than I did about how to survive.

Temperature and humidity can markedly affect vitamin content in the grocer's bins. Kale kept for two days at twenty-one degrees Celsius had 60 percent less ascorbic acid dropping to 89 percent less with low humidity) than when kept moist at 0 percent Celsius. Potatoes can lose 60 to 70 percent of their ascorbic acid in storage, although their B vitamins remain stable up to 240 days. Hornick summarizes a number of studies substantiating the fact that excess nitrogen from commercial NPK fertilizers can diminish taste, lower resistance to insects, reduce the biological value of protein and reduce carbohydrate synthesis, in addition to decreasing ascorbic acid.

Some authors, like Gussow (1996) have suggested that the best argument for organic foods is that they conserve natural resources and their use "solves, rather than creates, environmental problems and reduces the pollution of air, water, soil and food."

We are safe in concluding that there can be considerable differences in tomatoes and other vegetables depending on the soils in which they are grown. Unfortunately, there is no "quality control" or label attesting to their nutrients. Our trip through the produce section of a supermarket is thus a gamble and looks may be deceptive. As I am sure many readers will attest, there are other, non-nutrient values in plants, including the tomato. There is much current interest in phytochemicals such as lycopene, contained in the tomato and apparently valuable as an anti-cancer agent.

Organic produce is expensive. While some (Clancy, 1968; Gussow, 1996; Hornick, 1992) may feel that the jury is still out on the nutritional benefits, the freedom from toxins (herbicide and pesticides, some of which are cumulative in the body), make organically grown products well worth the extra cost. Some producers even go further. I spoke to the chemist at Walnut Acres who described their testing procedure for the deadly aflatoxin that oc curs in peanuts. They wanted to be well below the FDA limit in their peanut butter.

With agribusiness "factory farms" we can't know how much nitrogen has been over applied to the crops. Then there is the annoying lack of knowledge about how long and at what temperature those supermarket vegetables have been kept. Frozen products may well be superior in this regard. In any event, your purchase of organic products is a vote toward returning the soil to sustainability, for the organic farmer must revert to the "older" techniques of maintaining fertility, practiced for centuries by other cultures throughout the world, such as recycling wastes and using cover crops, fallow composting, rotation and green manure crops.

It all comes back to our relationship with the soil, as the four volumes of William Albrecht's work (1975, 1975, 1989, and 1992) abundantly testify. It would seem that some commercial agriculture more and more resembles hydroponics in that the "soil," whatever its structure, simply supports the plant while the artificially derived nutrients and much of the water are simply pumped through it. What organic matter remains is rapidly used up by soil organisms starved for cellulose. The farmer becomes industry dependent. An exception are the mid-western chernozem soils with deep organic layers built by centuries of prairie grass with insufficient rainfall to leach out the nutrients, unlike soils in the east, with more than thirty inches of rainfall. The "ideal" soils with a balance between rainfall and evaporation occur along the 98th meridian, west (Figure 29). Organic farming seeks to preserve or even enhance organic matter (dead plant and animal tissues). It is dependent on being recycled by soil organisms, large in both numbers and diversity. There are more species below ground than above and " . . . decomposition is on a par with productivity in terms of global importance. . . ." (Wardle *et al.*, 2000.)

A good critique of organic versus conventional or "mineral" fertilization is given by Knorr and Vogtmann (1983) who prefer the term "eco-foods" or "ecologically grown foods" to "organic" and define them "as those foods which result from environmentally sound, resource efficient and sustainable (over the long term) agricultural systems." They also reviewed studies starting with McCarrison's (1926) data on pigeons and rats, which found that millet fertilized by cattle manure, was markedly superior to that fed by "chemical manure." Knorr and Vogtmann discuss research that showed that organic diets significantly affected rabbit reproduction as well as sterility rates in cattle. They cited evidence from MacLeod (1965) and Schuphan (1974, 1976) that while crude protein may increase with increasing inorganic fertilizers, the concentration of essential amino acids actually decreases. Pettersson (1978) found that organically grown potatoes had both higher true protein content and higher essential amino acid index. One is reminded that the Irish with their potato patch may not have been able to survive without the cow that supplied their organic fertilizer.

Crude protein rose but biological protein values fell in spinach and lettuce with increasing inorganic fertilizer. Both

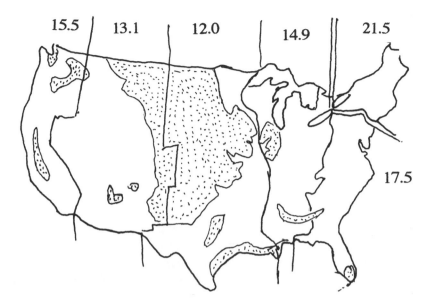

Figure 29. Number of dental caries (cavities plus fillings) in 70,000 Navy inductees in World War I, by sections of the United States, superimposed on the former location of short and long grass plant communities (stippled). Maximum nutrition is afforded by the grasslands soil along the 98th Meridian of longitude West. The acid podzol soils of New England afford the poorest nutrient base. Inductees there had 75% more cavities than those from Texas. Interestingly, the mineral-rich, chernozem prairie soils along the 98th Meridian are the finest areas for livestock growth, as they were for the bison before them. (After Albrecht, 1975.

McCarrison and Pettersson showed that true protein was lower after the application of inorganic NPK fertilizer. Long term experiments by Schuphan (1976) found higher vitamin C concentrates in eco-foods. Knorr and Vogtmann caution that high amounts of either organic or inorganic fertilizer may deteriorate plant quality. These authors also give actual storage losses from decay and shrinkage (54 percent) and 10.5 percent higher weight losses averaged for potatoes, carrots, turnips and beets grown on inorganic-fertilized soil.

If the quality of a food is low, (i.e., less nutrients in a given portion) then comes the question of how much food you have to eat to get what you need. I have not seen the data from which Senate Document #264 was prepared but can only quote what

Wallach (1993) wrote that it said in 1936: "The alarming fact is that foods—fruits and vegetables and grains—now being raised on millions of acres of land that no longer contain enough of certain needed minerals, are starving us, no matter how much of them we eat!"

It is true that the early settlers in the eastern United States exhausted the land's fertility rather rapidly, then moved west. (Compared to western soils our eastern soils have a thin topsoil layer with limited organic matter.) Areas of Georgia Piedmont soils were exhausted by 1850 and wagonloads of settlers set out for the "new" soils of Alabama and Mississippi. When they reached the prairie soils of the Midwest, they could tarry longer for the fertile organic horizon was deep and thick. The richest soils remaining in the east were in the wetland floodplains, certain relict Pleistocene soils high in mountain valleys and on broad ridge tops, certain bluffs of loess, and acres underlain by carbonate rocks.

One approach to a more natural fertilization of soil is that prescribed by Hamaker and Weaver (1982), whose thesis was that soil is best restored by adding finely ground rock, presumably obtained from a local quarry. They published lab reports indicating that soils given rock powder produced plants richer in protein, with gains of phosphorus (57 percent), calcium (47 percent), and magnesium (60 percent), over soils given "chemical" fertilizers. An interesting variant of this was an effort by a Lithonia, Georgia, firm to market granite "flour," plain ("Hybrotite") or with soil bacteria added ("Activated Hybrotite") derived from species gleaned from the granite outcrop soils where they naturally broke down the Lithonia granite-gneiss into its twenty-two component minerals. It was claimed that the bacteria enriched rock flour, when mixed with the manure layer in a chicken house, would, if turned and watered, quickly compost the smelly mess into a non odorous and rich organic product within a few days.

Before we scoff at such ideas, we must acknowledge that nature herself contributes much water and airborne fertilizing substances. Airborne deposits are less well known. Volcanic eruptions can send mineral-rich ash to distant continents and have contributed to soil fertility, especially in Central America and the East Indies. Pfeiffer (1947) documented the contribution of airborne (aolian) deposits: the Sahara contributes to Europe a layer five millimeters thick in 100 years; in our mid-west, one inch of topsoil has been blown from western prairies to the Mississippi Basin; China has wind-blown loess deposits several hundred feet thick; the productive black earth of Morocco and southern Russia are wind-blown loess; and the soil of Alpine meadows is said to be derived from dust deposits, of 1.8 to 3.7 pounds per square yard per year. Modern ecology recognizes that many substances, including iodine, chlorine, sulfur and nitrogen, are brought in by rainwater to augment the release of other essential nutrients from the rocks.

CHAPTER TEN

Genetics

"As humans specialized in different environments, the digestive, absorptive, metabolic and excretory functions of different groups underwent differential selection, leading to enormous variability in nutritional processes and needs at the population and individual level. . . ."

—Leslie Sue Lieberman

As man indulged his zest for exploration, he eventually settled down in various environments of Eurasia where local resources could support him, providing he could adapt. Having recently abandoned his hunting and gathering heritage, his generalized foraging behavior with its wide nutritional scope was replaced by a specialized use of local plants and animals in agriculture and pastoralism. Efforts to adapt are still going on and have apparently spawned a surfeit of problems, many of genetic origin.

It seems a wasted effort to try to determine your biochemical type if you suffer from a legacy of inherited conditions, such as might be due to the consumption of grains and dairy products from the relatively new pursuits of agriculture and pastoralism. Perhaps we have expected too much of our body's ability to adapt. Evidence of non-adaptation is common. To take an example, our ears and nervous system have not adapted to loud, continuous noises, which still destroy our hearing, because apparently even the deaf can survive in modern society, whereas primitive man depended on his ears for survival. Ask a war veteran with post-traumatic stress syndrome how well he has "adapted" to those terrible audio-visual impacts many years ago. Food-wise, we live on in spite of all manners of allergies to all manners of proteins and chemicals, thanks to modern medicine. What particularly concerns us here are our adaptations to foods to which some of us have partially adapted and others not at all.

Randolph Nesse and George Williams (1998) have summarized some interesting facts about non-adaptation. Most hunter-gatherers found salt and fat to be scarce. Seasonal things like honey and ripe fruit might also be in short supply. Individuals who could gorge on fat (and sugar) when it was available could survive famines better than those individuals who could not readily store much excess energy. Unfortunately, we have not had enough time to adapt to a *continuous* high intake of fat, like every day. Neither have we adapted to a high intake of concentrated carbohydrates (flours, fruit juices, extra sugar, etc.) which are converted to fat, but we still have the urge (partly inherited and partly taste-conditioned) to eat these foods. Nesse and Williams state: "The proportion of overweight Americans is one third and rising." Corporate America, of course, favors increased consumption, not restraint.

High-calorie modern foods, by fostering premature fat stores, are apparently shifting the menarche of United States females closer to age twelve. In eighteenth and nineteenth century Europe, girls reached menarche at about seventeen, and in foraging societies, girls were in their mid twenties before they had accumulated enough fat reserves to accommodate pregnancy. (Hardy, 1999.)

Nesse and Williams discuss the conclusion of Boyd Eaton and his colleagues at Emory University, who deemed the prevalence of breast cancer in our society may be due to this early onset of reproductive ability in females, coupled with the long delay until and between pregnancies. This allows longer periods of high levels of menstruation related hormones, sometimes leading to breast cancer. It seems that in modern societies, females will average 400 or more "periods" in their lifetime, in contrast with the 150 endured by female hunter-gatherers.

There are strong suggestions that the nausea of morning sickness confers survival advantage in that it makes the pregnant female less likely to eat substances potentially damaging to the fetus. Another interesting observation on adaptation concerns gout, caused by an excess of uric acid. Because uric acid is a potent anti-oxidant, evolution may have favored high levels, which would slow tissue aging in most individuals but in some, producing gout, Nesse and Williams (1998)

Another difference between individuals and perhaps populations is due to the amount and activity of thermogenic brown fat we inherited. This means that individuals can have different metabolic rates, making it easier for some to lose weight. (Lieberman, 1987.)

Before we can intelligently assess our own metabolic status we need to look at what is known about the genetics of our reactions to foods and the nutrients and minerals they contain. We need look no further than the common mineral *iron,* to realize our body's genetic wisdom. Bacterial growth, it seems, is severely iron dependent. Eggs have iron so tightly bound in the albumin (white) that bacteria invading the porous shell cannot use it to multiply. It has been demonstrated that infections in people are also iron dependent. It is awesome to consider that the human liver has evolved to sequester iron during an infection so as to deprive the invading bacteria of this needed nutrient. Thus, Zulu tribesmen get amoebic infections after drinking beer brewed in iron containers and so do Masai warriors when given iron supplements. Milk affords the Masai some protection, since the lactoferrin in human milk (20 percent) and cow milk (2 percent) binds the iron in the body (transferrin also binds it). Many physicians do not realize that iron may harm patients with infections, especially if they are on low-protein diets. (Neese and Williams, 1994.) These authors state that the influenza-sick person may reject iron-rich ham and eggs (iron is available in the yolk) in favor of tea and toast. Genetic traits for extra iron early in life may benefit anemic individuals and menstruating women but harm middle aged men.

We and other animals have had to develop defenses against disease-producing organisms as well as counter the wide variety of toxins that plants produce to keep from being eaten. Neese and Williams review some facts and theories that indicate this constant genetic interplay between plants and animals. Mentioned elsewhere are protease inhibitors that prevent protein digestion and the phytates and oxalates that tie up minerals like calcium. Plant defenses get even more sophisticated and threats to them are communicated to the entire plant and even between plants. These authors mention that damage to tomato and potato leaves increases protease inhibitors throughout the plant, which would render the plant proteins less digestible. I am reminded of the discovery by Dr. Joe Lewis of the USDA Agricultural Research Laboratory in Tifton, Georgia (Martens, 1999), who found that the saliva of an attacking insect causes some plants to secrete specific volatile substances to attract the predators of that particular pest. The plant world has formidable defenses against predation by animals, incidentally including man (some to prevent premature self-digestion).

Some 15 percent of potato proteins block digestive enzymes, and these defensive proteins had to be "bred out" by Andean natives (white potatoes originated in the Andes). Humans have also had to develop genetic means to detect the presence of health-threatening substances in plants. Plants of the guns *Brassica* (cabbage genus) grow wild in the Andes and may produce goiter in such iodine-deficient areas. Ninety-three percent of Andean natives can detect the bitter taste of PTC (phenylthiocarbamate) which simulates that of the cabbage genera plants; only 70 percent of Americans can detect it (this test is given to biology students to illustrate the genetics involved).

In addition to genetic response, humans in the Northern Hemisphere have had to develop cultural means to cope with plant toxins, protein inhibitors and mineral blockers. It is supposed that tannins and alkaloids of acorns would have killed or discouraged Stone Age Europeans until they learned how to get rid of the toxins—the same with cassava (manioc) south of the equator. The Pomo Indians mix acorns with red clay to bind the tannin, other groups pound the nuts up, leach them with water or boil them to extract the toxin. (We still like a little of the bitter tannin taste in our teas and red wines.) Nesse and Williams also cite a theory that Stone Age people supposedly ate twice the calcium we do, and thus had enough in their systems to bind up the oxalates which would have made minerals in their vegetable foods unavailable.

Apparently we are even attempting to adapt to environmental toxins such as the common organophosphate pesticides. This was brought out in the Gulf War when some soldiers proved to be nine times more likely than others to incur the "Gulf War Syndrome" which is theorized to be a genetic inability to produce high blood levels of an enzyme which destroys organophosphate poisons. (Nesmith, 1999.)

Since we are still trying to adapt to both plant and animal foods some of us, depending on our genetic origin, inherit medical problems when trying to eat certain foods. It involves our enzymes.

Enzymes are proteins made by specialized body cells. They control vital bodily functions, such as energy release from the foods we eat. Happily, for the human story, there is some diversity of enzymes in humans, and sometimes even among individuals. These variants, or slight differences in enzyme chemistry, constitute a molecular basis for biochemical individuality. (Aebi, 1981.) Dietary conditions, quantity and quality of food, frequency and size of meals and length of fasting periods apparently cause codes written in the cell's DNA to instruct enzymes to establish metabolic blocks or intolerance reactions to certain foods, resulting in sickness or weakened immunity. Intolerance to milk and dairy products containing milk sugar (lactose) is a case in point.

The newborn of almost all mammals (seals are an exception) use milk sugar as an energy source, along with varying amounts of fat. The ability to digest lactose sugar is lost at weaning, leaving many of us unable to enjoy dairy products. The digestion of milk sugar or lactose is made possible by the enzyme lactase (enzymes generally have an "a" in their last syllable). Although lactase is normally lost at weaning, in areas of the world where cattle and milk drinking have been a part of local nutrition, adults by natural selection are genetically adapted to retain the lactase enzymes. It is not only the ability to digest milk sugar. Lactose-tolerant individuals may have a 78 percent advantage over those who are non-lactose-tolerant in their ability to absorb calcium. (Harris, 1985.) If you can't use dairy products that means eating a lot more green leafy vegetables as a calcium source.

Most Caucasians can handle dairy products but most Africans and Orientals cannot. Africans who herd cattle (Ibo, Masai, Dinka, Tussi, Fulani, Nuer, and Hima) are genetically milk-tolerant as adults. And so are Bedouins, Saudi Arabians and the peoples of northwest India and Pakistan. In Europe the highest levels of lactase occur in the north, 95 percent in the Dutch, Danes and Swedes. South of the Alps, they range from high to intermediate, with low levels in Spain, Italy, Greece, Israel and in city-dwelling Arabs.

Favism is an even more serious genetic enzyme difference found in humans. It comes from eating the fava or broad bean (*Vicia fava*)[9] and is the most common known genetic disorder in the world. (Katz, 1987.) It is a sex-linked genetic deficiency of a red blood cell enzyme and causes a severe hemolytic anemia, resulting in death in one out of twelve cases. It occurs throughout

---

[9] The Greek philosopher Pythagorus is credited with saying, "Do not eat broad beans." About one-third of the population of southern Italy and Greece has the favism gene. "Malaria was probably endemic in southern Italy from ancient times until the 1940s. . . ." (Cochran and Ewald, 1999.)

Europe, northern and equatorial Africa, the southern Caspian region, the entire Middle East, India, Southeast Asia, southern China, Indonesia and New Guinea. Although many populations consume the beans raw, most ethnic groups are said to soak them, which removes the water-soluble toxin. You wonder why anyone eats them at all. One reason may be that one copy of the gene prevents the malarial parasite from efficiently invading red blood cells. Two copies of the gene, however, cause abnormal sensitivity to the toxic components of fava beans. Katz thought that it works somewhat like a serious depletion of vitamin E, a deficiency of which causes damage to the red blood cells that are infected with the malarial parasite.

Another genetic "affliction" is the presence or absence of an enzyme that breaks down alcohol (alcohol dehydrogenase), a deficiency high in Orientals and Native Americans and low in Caucasians. It causes flushing, nausea, rapid heart beat and muscle weakness due to an accumulation of acetaldehyde.

A fourth genetic change emphasizes the danger of introducing non-traditional foods. It is a congenital inability to digest certain sugars (sucrase-isomaltase enzyme deficiency). It is found in people who do not traditionally eat sucrose. It occurs in American whites (2 percent), Greenland Eskimos (10 percent), Canadian Eskimos (7 percent) and Canadian Indians (4 percent).

It is revealing to look at another major medical condition resulting from a reaction to a common food, celiac disease, an adverse reaction to gluten (the major protein of grains like wheat). It causes damage to the cells lining the intestines (mucosa) and is a response of the immune system. It also increases the chance of a malignancy in the gut. Its distribution follows wheat-eating people much as lactose tolerance follows people who keep cattle. It occurs on an interesting gradient from Israel to Ireland, the incidence being lowest in Israel where it has existed for a longer time. Apparently the longer people dwell in a wheat-eating zone, the more opportunity for those susceptible to die off, so you wind up with a population that is more tolerant. Celiac disease strikes young people before they have had a chance to reproduce. This speeds up natural selection. Recent research also links gluten intolerance with multiple sclerosis. (Fallon, 1995.)

Incidentally, the more cereals in the diet, the more schizophrenia. "Overt schizophrenia is uncommon in societies whose diets include little or no cereal." (Simmons, 1981.)

Celiac disease is important because it documents the rapidity by which nature can accommodate to the relatively sudden changes we have asked our bodies to undergo in the past 10,000 years since the agricultural revolution. This may be significant in searching for our own personal nutrition, for it is an example of an adjustment to a novel food not available during our very long tenure as hunter-gatherers. It appears that we can impose changes on our Paleolithic bodies in as short a time frame as 6,000 to 8,000 years. People carrying the celiac disease gene that reacts to gluten left Turkey and the eastern Mediterranean 6000 B.C. (antigen levels 7 percent) and spread to England, western France and the Basque region by 3000 B.C. (antigen levels 31 percent).

The distribution of celiac disease or "sprue" in the British Isles is illuminating. It is high in Ireland because wheat was not a staple food there until after the potato blight in the mid-nineteenth century. It is lower in southern England, whose inhabitants have been eating wheat since the Roman period. More gluten intolerance would be expected from peoples coming from Wales and southwest England where barley was the preferred food or from northern England and Scotland where oats predominated.

We begin to see that identifying your exact place of origin can be important in understanding what you should eat, since how and what we eat alters our hormones, hormones regulate enzymes, and enzymes control homeostasis.

We need to understand that reactions to certain foods can be inherited. In prior times, the "family physician" knew at least your immediate genetic background. Today, unfortunately, physicians do not have the time or opportunity to learn your family history and most people no longer live in close proximity to their parents and grandparents.

Krause (1995) states that the role of genetics is not emphasized in medical schools and Reading (1998) makes the point that the medical profession treats the isolated individual and does not consider his or her genetic background.

The next question that we need to answer is exactly how certain foods damage the body and set the stage for degenerative disease.

In a nutshell, here is how it works: classic food allergies such as to dairy products and grains are inherited. By damaging the

walls of the small intestine, they prevent the absorption of critical vitamins and minerals. This in turn weakens or damages the
immune system, which in turn predisposes the body to degenerative disease such as cancer and autoimmune diseases (Figure 30).

Also, if the damaged and inflamed gut "leaks" large undigested protein particles into the blood stream, as Sherry Rogers
points out, the immune system makes antibodies against them.
Since some healthy body tissues have antigen recognition sites
that resemble these unwanted "rogue" protein particles, these
"new" antibodies attack them. If this is in a joint, inflammation,
swelling and pain result.

Likewise, eating improperly creates a "biological night-
mare": The excess production of arachidonic acid in the metabo-

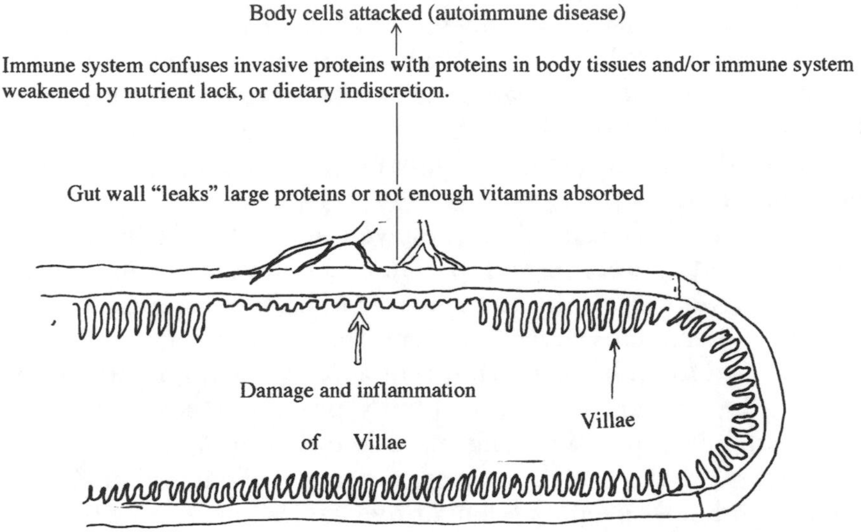

Body cells attacked (autoimmune disease)

Immune system confuses invasive proteins with proteins in body tissues and/or immune system
weakened by nutrient lack, or dietary indiscretion.

Gut wall "leaks" large proteins or not enough vitamins absorbed

Damage and inflammation

of   Villae

Villae

Figure 30   Autoimmune disease seems to arise from damage to the
intestinal wall (fingerlike villae in this case) by its sensitivity to certain
foods, such as wheat gluten or *Candida* overgrowth. The damage may
either allow the gut wall to "leak" large protein molecules into the blood
and confuse the immune cells or inhibit the absorption of nutrients
(such as vitamins C and B and minerals like zinc) essential for proper
immune function. Dietary indiscretion (too much sugar, not enough fish
oils) may also cripple immune function, when "good" eicosanoids (PGE
1) are depressed by sugar and lose the ability to either stimulate (by release of lymphokines) or control the proliferation of immune system
cells in the blood, as Sears (1995) has indicated.

lism of fatty acids (Sears 1995) leads to the underproduction of "good" eicosanoids (PGE 1) and the over production of "bad" eicosanoids (PGE 2), thus leading to autoimmune disease, especially with reduced levels of vitamins C, B1, B3, B6, zinc, magnesium and manganese.

Thus our ancestral inheritance, coupled with gustatory sins of eating forbidden foods, can set the stage for autoimmune disease in which the guardian white blood cells turn on our own tissues instead of protecting them. If they attack a joint, it is called rheumatoid arthritis.

According to Reading (1988), autoimmune diseases in your family tree are manifest if one or more of the following afflictions are present: pernicious anemia, celiac disease or systemic lupus erythematosis (SLE). Pernicious anemia is due to a massive vitamin B12 deficiency. Celiac disease, with damage to the intestinal walls, is the allergic response to either whole grains or their fractions (gluten and alpha gliadin). It is treated with a grain-free diet and heavy doses of vitamins and minerals that test low in the patient. SLE is a degeneration of the connective tissue under attack by the autoimmune system and is treated by discovering the allergy to certain foods such as milk, eggs, beef or grains and then eliminating them. During SLE, the body is apparently unable to absorb vitamin B and C supplements needed by the normal immune system.

Celiac disease leads to a host of maladies including pernicious anemia, gastrointestinal and breast cancer, colitis, diverticulitis and psychiatric symptoms of CNS degeneration with depression. Seventeen of eighteen victims of Down's Syndrome had celiac disease. (Reading, 1988.) In fact, Reading theorizes that Alzheimer's disease may be due to celiac disease which, although it causes malabsorption of vitamins and minerals, also allows toxic metals such as aluminum to be absorbed and concentrated in the brain.

Reading also believes that Multiple Sclerosis (MS), grain allergies, celiac disease, low B12 and low folate can cause atrophy of the brain's cerebellum as well as degeneration of the spinal cord. He implicates malabsorption of B1, B3, B6, B12, folate and trace elements essential for the health of nerve sheathes, as well as the absorption of toxic metals so railed about by Sherry Rogers.

Reading states that if cancer is frequent in families, its most likely cause is hereditary autoimmune disease, especially celiac disease and SLE. He urges that every cancer patient be tested for the presence of autoimmune bodies in the blood and for reactions to fractions of grains, eggs, beef and yeast. Symptoms of autoimmune disease, other than cancer and leukemia, are severe depression, thyroid problems, frequent infections, tuberculosis and vitiligo (piebald skin).

To summarize: According to Reading, you need tests for food allergies and autoimmune disease if you have any of the following classic symptoms; pernicious anemia, celiac disease, SLE, bowel cancer, rheumatoid arthritis, thyroid problems, chronic indigestion, diabetes, frequent diarrhea (or, yes) premature gray hair or premature balding.

Thus we see that a number of human problems, such as allergies to milk and grains, are of recent genetic origin, being failed attempts to adapt to the rapid and drastic changes imposed by the agricultural revolution some 10,000 years ago. This is not to discount the fact that some of us have successfully adapted. The Industrial Revolution that followed has only seemed to compound and confuse the dilemma. Perhaps one solution lies in disbursing and sharing our knowledge via the electronics of the Information Age.

Of course, there are other less obvious allergies to substances in the food we eat, the air we breathe and the fluids we drink. Or, as we are increasingly aware, we react to the *lack* of certain nutrients in food and fluid.

Other genes, not necessarily related to foods, also have apparently helped people adapt to deadly diseases. One of the best known is a mutant involving genes for sickle cell anemia in Africa, which in a single form (in a heterozygous individual—paired with a normal gene) confers protection from malaria. Katz (1980) proposed that the rapid spread of manioc in sub-Saharan Africa over the past 400 years has been due to its ability to reduce the frequency and severity of sickle cell anemia.

Diseases, which we do not normally think of any value at all often can, or have in the past, conferred protection against disease. While two copies of another gene causes cystic fibrosis, only one copy in an individual apparently protects against typhoid fever, a disease that regularly killed between 5 percent and 15 percent of northern Europeans. Other mutations of hemoglobin C (in Northwest Africa) and hemoglobin E (Southeast Asia) also defend against malaria. Such anti-malarial traits have survival advantage until the gene becomes so common that children begin inheriting it from both parents, thus pairing the two abnormal genes. (Cochran and Ewald, 1999.)

We hear a lot these days about "strengthening the immune system" and eating anti-oxidants. Tons of these highly touted supplements won't do you much good if they can't be absorbed due to a food allergy you have inherited or otherwise have acquired. Before we can fine-tune our diet, such basic issues must be addressed. Our genes determine our ability to extract nutrients from foods and at the same time not absorb toxic non-nutrients so prevalent in today's environment. At the same time, genetics can control our behavior by altering levels of neurochemical transmitters in the brain. Clinical depression, for example, can be the result of either inherited food malabsorption or inherited alterations in brain chemistry.

Our genes control and organize all organs and tissues towards the efficient use of energy. Unhealthy aging is said to be the loss of this efficiency, accelerated by poor quality diets. An inadequate intake of specific nutrients, especially after age forty, can cause the inherited genes to faultily express themselves. (Bland, 1998.) Diets and specific nutrients can therefore modify gene expression as well as promote and improve our bodies so that we age healthily.

According to Bland, genetic research indicates that while we all possess the same number of physical attributes such as legs, eyes, ears, fingers and toes, internally our genes are coded for vast functional differences at the biochemical level. Enzyme production (related to detoxification), for example, is said to vary from four to seven fold among individuals. Such enzymes are strongly influenced by nutrients. Cruciferous vegetables such as cabbage, broccoli and cauliflower can increase enzymes that detoxify cells.

As we have seen in a previous chapter, tiny organelles in every cell called mitochondria, are the energy factories of the cell. They also contain a genetic code, mitochondrial DNA (mDNA) which, unlike that of the cell's nucleus, is derived solely from the mother. mDNA is twenty times more likely, however, to be damaged by free radical oxidation than the chromosomal DNA in the nucleus. Such injuries cause it to mutate, produce energy less efficiently, and thus deteriorate the entire body. It has been discovered that individuals differ markedly in their susceptibility to such damage.

Evidence has been presented that how genes express themselves (by enzyme or otherwise) can be strongly altered by stress. (Pert *et al.*, 1998.) In fact, these authors indicate that we must now broaden our definition of our healing system to include emotions, neuropeptides, endocrine glands and secretions and immune system components-all can influence gene expression and the regulation of gene products within the cell.

Genetics and the Brain

I can think of no better way to begin this section than to look at the broad picture of genetic change in the human brain. Jared Diamond brought out some humbling conclusions in his book on the fates of human societies. (*Guns, Germs and Steel,* 1997.) Basically, he attests to the concept that ecology is indeed the most fundamental science in understanding our relationship with the world, and that human history is determined by environment, not biological differences in people themselves.

He has expressed something that many of us who have worked among "uncivilized" people have suspected but never verbalized. From his thirty-three years of experience, Diamond concluded that the native New Guinea people were on the average more intelligent, alert, expressive and "more interested in things and people around them than the average European or American." To explain why the New Guinea natives are probably genetically superior to Westerners and better at escaping disadvantages that accrue to children of industrialized societies, he suggests that natural selection for intelligence has been "far more ruthless in New Guinea than in more densely populated politically complex societies where natural selection for body chemistry was instead more potent." Diamond gives an example of the latter: genetic resistance to disease where people with Type O or Type B blood are more resistant to smallpox than those with blood Type A.

Apparently, brains of New Guinea natives have responded to natural selection, by enabling the individual to avoid death from the most dangerous threats in his environment such as murder, tribal warfare, accidents and problems over food. Early man in the savannas of Africa and during his peregrinations in Eurasia surely was subject to the same traumatic events that troubled the New Guineans. Therefore, it stands to reason that the more intelligent early men survived, leading us to surmise that, genetically speaking, this process, over millennia, might lead to better, if not larger brains.

Anyone who watches the daily news is doubtless aware that we still have the traumas of murder, war, accident and food problems, some of which are now part of the phenomena of a nation, rather than of a tribe or extended family (band).

If Diamond is correct, today we reproduce regardless of intelligence or the gene pool within our cells. Perhaps our survival in a literate and button-pushing society is now dependent on how we use the capacity for intelligent behavior we have inherited, and how we employ it to exploit the enormous store of knowledge we have accumulated since the written record began.

Reflecting on the lack of any organic change in the human brain in the past 30,000 years, LaChapelle (1988) published a presumed quote from Konrad Lorenz: *The difference between modern and Paleolithic Man is "one of cerebral training and not of biological or anatomical advance. In later Paleolithic Man there was already all the room for memories, all the associative capacity, the reasoning power, the ability to learn, and the perceptive acuity of modern man."* LaChapelle concludes: "The main difference is that primitive man used all his capacities in relationship with all of nature while modern humans concentrate on the artificial world which we have created for ourselves."

Trying to live in an artificial world, possibly by interfering with natural selection that would have removed them, we have wound up with genetic or environmental changes in brain hormone levels that mess up our lives and lead to aggression, migraine headaches and depression. (Thomas Murray, pers. comm.)

Depression seems to run in families (Krause 1995) and evidence is mounting that it has a genetic basis. Several brain transmitters are involved. Although an over-simplification, gene-induced, low levels of serotonin contribute to a host of problems in addition to clinical depression: aggression, bulimia, migraine headaches, PMS, and violent behavior. Excessively high levels contribute to autism, manic depressive disorder and schizophrenia. Receptors hypersensitive to serotonin cause obsessive-compulsive disorder and panic attacks. (Krause, 1995.) How our genetic heritage influences appetite through serotonin and how fat gain is programmed in our genes is discussed in the chapter "Introduction to Metabolic Typing."

Interestingly, the Scottish scientist Margaret Patterson stated (LaChapelle, 1988, p. 49) that low frequency electric currents can "cause as much as a three-fold elevation in endorphin levels" and that a 10-Hertz signal speeds up the production and turnover rate of serotonin.

It would be interesting to know whether our endorphin levels relate to the resonant standing radio waves (Schumann waves) of low frequency (8-30 Hz) that resonate between the earth and the ionosphere, and that are said (Callahan, 1995) to correspond with human brain wave patterns (8, 14, 21, 27, 33 Hz).

Patterson also commented that heroin drastically elevates brain opiate endorphins "subjectively interpreted as ecstasy" and may also interact directly through opioid receptors. Incidentally, pepper-hot foods that cause irritation in the mouth and gut may increase endorphin secretion. (Rozin, 1987.)

Another brain chemical important in behavior is dopamine. It regulates motor activity and apparently stimulates the brain's pleasure areas too much causing impulsive behavior and possibly schizophrenia, and too little linked to dopamine abnormalities such as attention deficit disorder (ADD) and Parkinson's disease.

If you stimulate dopamine or inhibit serotonin artificially, you get increased aggression and sexual activity. Addictive drugs, such as nicotine, cause a sudden release of dopamine and addicts may be trying to correct low levels.

A brief summary of the relationships of our senses and brain to some chemistry may be in order, since panic and other anxiety disorders and abnormal reactivity to the environment appear to run in families. (Charney, 1999.)

Commonly, drugs such as Prozac are used as antidepressants. They boost serotonin levels by preventing its normal degradation by transporter substances at the nerve synapse. Neurotransmitters must be turned off as readily as they are turned on. Drugs like Valium, Xanax, Librium, and Miltown are also used in panic disorders. These drugs enhance another neurotransmitter, GABA, which dampens anxiety and fear.

There are other genetically acquired levels of hormones that strongly influence behavior and directly relate to survival. Fortunately, we don't need them often any more. Unfortunately, they still function just as powerfully as they did in our primate ancestors, especially in fear and anger. In the brain, noradrenaline transmits messages from the limbic center to enhance our thought processes. Secreted from the Locus Ceruleus, it inhibits or quiets cortical activity so that the animal becomes more sensitive to incoming sensory stimuli like sights and sounds made by potential enemies or prey. (Glantz and Pearce, 1989.)

Noradrenalin (norepinephrine) and adrenalin (epinephrine) provide a "high" that was essential for survival. Elsewhere, we discuss their importance in speeding up the heart and stopping digestion in situations of fear and anger. (Recall that anxiety is low- grade fear and that resentment and frustration represent low-grade anger). Some people may actually give themselves an adrenalin "high" by invoking situations which incite them to anger and sometimes rage. Adrenalin addiction may be a component to life-threatening recreations such as rock-climbing, white water kayaking and parachute jumping, assisting in inducing superhuman strength and endurance.[10]

A corresponding mental reward is the exhilarating euphoria or "high" produced by the brain's analgesic substances, beta-endorphins and enkephalins, the effect of which may last for hours. Aerobic exercise, such as running for twenty minutes, produces an endorphin release ("runner's high"). More anaerobic, weight-training routines used by bodybuilders may result in a 60 to 70 percent increase in beta-endorphins. (Stout, 2000.) Together, these hormones make the dangers of life including war, tolerable, if not rewarding. Both adrenalin and/or dopamine seem to be involved in some people's attraction to urgencies and crises and they may have inherited an increased susceptibility to stimulation. It is said that sensation seeking is up to 60 percent genotic, confirmed by experiments in England (Zuckerman, 1998) and involves dopamine receptors. Thrill-seekers may have low levels of a brain substance (MAO, monoamineoxidase) that destroys adrenalin and dopamine. If true, it follows that young people would have low levels of MAO and higher levels in older folks would explain their diminished desire to seek stimulating experiences and account for their increased levels of fear and anxiety.

---

[10] Cocaine apparently orks by potentiating the effects of neurotransmitters by inhibiting the re-uptake of dopamine at the synapse between brain cells. It has been said that the motivation for both cocaine and parachuting have a common shared pathway in the brain. (Zuckerman, 1998.)

It seems that dopamine, serotonin and the activation of the brain's pleasures center are an everyday concern. In the "wild state" it is argued that the human body was adapted to moderately high levels of "sensation seeking" but not too much and not too little. This has been translated to support our once necessary need to roam, and to "expand our horizons" by "exploratory aggression" which is another way of saying "zest for adventure." Both the adrenalin rush from the anticipated danger of the unknown and the deeply rewarding pleasures of the discovery of new sights and smells, along with pride in one's ability to find food, water and security, are factors in the exploratory urge that motivates most primates. Since man is a highly social primate, you could also expect some pleasure seeking in being recognized as a dependable, loyal and courageous member of a family, tribe, neighborhood, industry, government or military unit.

Let us see what early research had to say about pleasure seeking and, incidentally, reflecting on how, why and what we eat. H. J. Campbell (1973) experimented with different types of animals from fish to humans and formulated a theory of how the brain controls our behavior. (Prior paragraphs have examined behavior controlled by organic chemicals).

One author concluded that we possess what he calls a "triune" or three-part brain. (MacLean, 1973.) The oldest of the three parts, which surrounds the ancient mid brain, he calls a "Reptilian Complex,"[11] The Reptilian Complex directs reptiles in aggressive behavior, territoriality, ritual and the establishment of social hierarchies. The implications that some human activities are of reptilian origin may be unsettling to some.

The next area to evolve, the "limbic system" surrounds the reptilian complex. Campbell considered the limbic system to be the highest brain center in fishes. Certainly parts of it, such as the olfactory lobes, were vital to the survival of fishes. Ornstein and Sobel (1987) thought that the limbic system evolved into a unified control center around 300 million years ago, about the time amphibians crawled out of Carboniferous swamps and evolved into the first reptiles. Another spurt of change in the limbic system may have occurred in the first mammal-like reptiles of the Mesozoic Era. (Sagan, 1977.) In any event, Campbell developed a theory that the limbic system of all vertebrates, how-

---

[11] Consisting of an olfacto striatum, corpus striatum, and globus pallidus.

ever primitive, contained what he called "pleasure centers" which supposedly "reward" animals for agreeable (and survival enhancing) things they do. They lie adjacent to limbic areas that cause displeasure and thusly inhibit disagreeable behavior.

In rats, the pleasure areas compose 35 percent of their brains. Humans still possess these centers[12] and they still control our behavior. The difference is that humans have a third part of the brain, the neocortex, which now has a two-way communication with the pleasure areas of the limbic system.[13] Campbell's theory is that the only clear, undeniable difference between man and the lower animals is his ability to stimulate the limbic pleasure areas by mere thought, whereas in lower animals, the limbic centers were activated only by stimulation via the external receptors: eyes, ears, nose and skin.

His evidence for the antiquity of the limbic system stemmed from a fascinating series of experiments with vertebrates. Fish, he discovered, will continuously dart back and forth between electrodes placed in their tank. Inactive crocodiles, instead of lying motionless all day, would lumber back and forth between similar electrodes because the weak electric currents stimulated their skin receptors and "felt good" (i.e., had activated pleasure areas in the limbic system). His squirrel monkeys would manually switch a 500-watt light bulb on and off, hour after hour, by reaching outside the cage to press a switch up to 500 times in fifteen minutes. The intermittent light flashes in their eyes apparently stimulated their pleasure centers, incredible as it may seem. This could also attest to the boring life of caged animals. Incidentally, the male hormone testosterone caused a remarkable increase in response to stimuli in both sexes (females secrete testosterone from the adrenal gland) from fish to primates. Campbell called such response to peripheral receptor stimuli "sub human." And it isn't a large jump to conclude that our often hypnotic staring at the flashing lights and colors of the TV set is not markedly advanced over the behavior of squirrel monkeys (Figure 32).

---

[12] Amygdala, septum pellucidum and parts of the hypothalamus.

[13] While, with the rat, 90% of its cerebral cortex is involved in sensory processing and voluntary movement, in humans only 15% is utilized for these purposes. The bulk of the remaining 85% of the human cortex is devoted to learning, memory, speech and language, conceptualization, abstraction and association of input from several senses simultaneously.

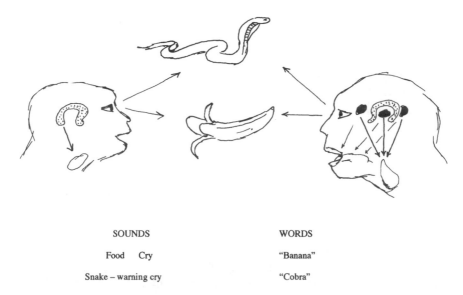

SOUNDS	WORDS
Food Cry	"Banana"
Snake – warning cry	"Cobra"

Figure 31. Illustrating the enormous advantage of human speech in identifying and conveying information about objects important to survival. Sounds and cries of monkeys and apes arise from the primitive limbic area (stippled), whereas in humans the huge cerebral cortex has three areas adapted to associate words with objects seen, felt or heard. Sensory information (sight, sound, touch, smell) goes to three specialized areas in the human brain (solid) where it is integrated by the angular gyrus, matched with a word retrieved from the brain's filing cabinet by Wernicke's area, then to Broca's area which activates the nerves controlling face, lips, tongue and larynx. The three areas are connected by a pathway of nerve fibers (not shown). The limbic system of the human brain still participates in our daily lives. With deep emotion, one may be "speechless" or utter only non-verbal cries, moans or grunts.

It is interesting that people's activities use varying degrees of stimulation from both sense organs and higher brain centers. Mountain climbers and white water kayakers get rewards from challenge and danger. Part of this may be due to the adrenalin "high" and, if sustained or strenuous enough, from an endorphin-enkephalin rush (runners' high). The higher brain centers contribute by evaluating the strategies of staying alive. An added benefit to a rock climber would be a cerebral appreciation of rock, its origin in the furnaces of space and why we must eat its minerals to stay alive. It must be neocortex involvement to activate the pleasure areas of a kayaker who uses his sensory receptors,

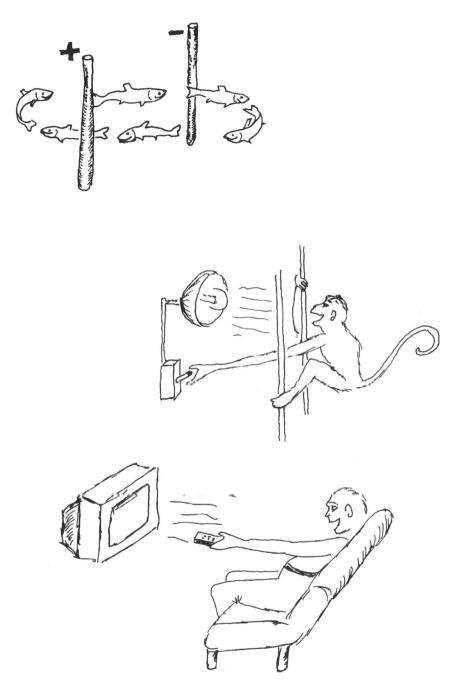

Figure 32.

brain and body movements to maximum and exquisite efficiency. This "conquering" of powerful natural forces brings a glowing pride, entirely apart from the various chemical "highs" brought about by the sights and sounds and demands of roaring water. By the same token, an Olympic gymnast, with absolute control of beautiful movement, evokes in us admiration and pleasure to the intensity of tears.

Campbell quotes the great animal behaviorist Konrad Lorenz: "Most people, however, are in such an early stage of evolution (stimulating their pleasure centers by external sense organs rather than using the neocortex to think) that they should be called *Homo sensorians* (sensory man) rather than *Homo sapiens* (thinking man)." Campbell's plea is that good changes will accelerate if people recognize the neural basis of behavior and "choose to behave as human beings rather than as clever apes."

A rewarding life may be the balance of "simple" sensory joys with the intellectual input of the cerebral cortex. According to Campbell, painters, musicians, architects and film producers may use both. They make their considerable contributions with their thinking brain but may use the public's sense organs to help get their message across. "Pure" thinkers would probably be philosophers, lawyers, theoretical physicists, theologians and sociologists.

The pathways from the neocortex to the more ancient brain regions, such as the limbic system, apparently need repetitive experiences of the non-sensory type. To establish full control by the higher brain centers and to build a full repertoire of appropriate responses to varied environments and social situations takes a long childhood. (Campbell, 1973.) There is also a need for parents who teach beyond the sensory level, presenting intellectual (thinking) challenges to enable the child to develop the full potential of the human brain. In early man, children and adults must have regularly faced intellectual challenges with survival benefits.

While we have gotten a little afield from nutrition, the knowledge of how the brain is stimulated and programmed is relevant to our understanding of both our prehistory and our food preferences. Campbell would say that, in our search for new food tastes, odors and appearances, we are obeying an ancestral command to stimulate the pleasure center of the brain, all a part of our incessant search for stimulation. Campbell's theory then, is that nerve impulses from the peripheral receptors, eyes, ears, nose, sense of touch on skin and taste in mouth, activate the limbic pleasure areas, causing animals to constantly try to find situations where these organs are stimulated. Food, according to this theory, is sought primarily because it activates limbic pleasure areas. Its appearance, odor or taste-nourishment is incidental to the limbic reward.

Man's large brain has made it easier to rapidly adapt to a wide variety of foods and to preserve this information by learning and teaching. Presumably, pleasure center rewards were still valid but overlaid with the fact that while something didn't taste as good as something else, it was necessary to eat it to survive. Fermented and soured foods may not titillate the taste buds so pleasurably but the pleasure of survival and having sufficient energy must have overridden the desire for a more pleasant taste.

While Campbell says that pleasure in eating has had enormous survival value in the life of higher vertebrates, it is difficult to see how some animals can get much gustatory stimulation from some foods eaten repetitively, such as birds eating the same seeds, or a dog wolfing his dry ration in five minutes, or people eating rice three times a day. This would work if we relate the hunger center to the pleasure centers of the limbic brain. We have to recognize that the limbic centers in the hypothalamus are essential to maintaining sufficient energy to keep us alive and kicking. This is done by an "appestat" that monitors blood sugar levels and sends a "hunger" message if they start dropping, as for example, if we do not eat a balanced meal with some protein.

You might ask why our ancestors acquired such a large brain with the subsequent ability to direct our choice of foods, not just by sight, odor and taste but by thinking about the consequences. Obviously, thinking brain centers do not always override the sensory appeal of modern foods, fast or otherwise.

Recall that Milton theorized that the complexity of food gathering gave the more active and individualistic spider monkeys large brains and more intelligence than the slow, stodgy howler monkeys. It is tempting to believe that larger brains had survival advantage when, sometime prior to the Australopithecines, primates left stable forest habitats and invaded the various types of savannas.[14] In these new habitats, they had to deal with a greater variety of large and dangerous predators and prey by means of an intensely cooperative social structure. At the same time, they had to adapt rapidly to a less dependable and year-round environment relative to shelter, food and water. Baboons are about the only primates with small brains that have been able to survive successfully in this type of environment, and only by virtue of a strong social organization.

We can further theorize that the large brains, whose development was hastened by the demands of adapting rapidly to the exploration and expansion of early man in the Rift Valley and throughout Africa, prepared *Homo erectus* to leave Africa altogether for the new and even more stimulating and demanding environments and climates of Europe and Asia. Modern man, *Homo sapiens,* had more variation in brain size than his predecessor, *Homo erectus.* This might be expected if one considers the enormous regional differences and environmental challenges imposed by the intense cold and the great beasts of the Pleistocene Ice Ages.

The Brain—Mental and Physical Health

The human brain originally evolved to maintain the stability of the body, functioning both as a pharmacy and computer. The most recent genetic brain addition, the neocortex, can, however, strongly modify brain chemistry by mere thought. It has been said that we can think ourselves sick or well. This is probably the

---

[14] Brain weight in primates is only roughly proportional to body weight. Gorillas, however, with brain volumes of 500 cc are quite a bit heavier than chimpanzees with 400 cc. While the robust Australopithecines were roughly the weight of chimps, their brains were gorilla-sized. The gracile Australopithecines of six million years ago were smaller (45 to 65 pounds) but had larger brains (430 to 600 cc). (Sagan, 1977.) The earest *Homo (habilis)* had a brain not dramatically larger (500 to 800 cc) at a heavier body weight (65 to 100 pounds) and was allegedly the first completely bipedal savanna dweller. Next in line, *Homo erectus* and *H. sapiens* had similar body weights. *H. erectus* (750 to 1250 cc) had, according to Sagan, *varied* stone tools and lived in *varied* habitats, while its successor, *H. sapiens,* had a larger brain (1100 to 2200 cc) lived in a *global* habitat and whose tools included metal and now, of course, chemical, electronic, and nuclear "tools."

downside of the many advantages of a larger brain in higher mammals. It is difficult to imagine that rabbits worry day and night whether a fox will ambush them on the next hop or two. But humans do worry that things will get worse or believe that they will get better. Being told that a placebo pill decreased pain, the brains of a group of patients secreted endorphins equivalent to 8 mg of morphine. (Ornstein and Sobel, 1987.) Even the recitation of a prayer can apparently trigger profound physiological effects. Tribal shamans, as well as modern physicians, transform frightening unknowns into things knowable, named and explained, thus quieting the brain's alarm reactions. A study of Japanese migrants in California revealed that, in spite of Western food, high cholesterol, cigarettes and high blood pressure, those who had maintained their traditional social relations had one-fifth the heart disease suffered by Japanese who had adopted a pattern of Western social life.

The hypothalamus and other parts of the limbic system are strongly involved in emotional reactions and appear to regulate the immune system as well. Appropriate stimulation of the hypothalamus leads to enhanced immune function. In turn, stress-produced endorphins decrease the tumor fighting ability of natural killer cells. The stress of social instability proves to be life threatening, internally or externally.

Recent research has expanded this theme and defined a precise relationship between the brain, nervous system and immune systems. (Pert *et al.*, 1998.) The surprising part of this is the participation of the immune system which can now be thought of as sort of a "liquid brain." Immune system cells occur in blood and lymph passages and on organs and tissue cells throughout the body. There are now two recognizable means of communication throughout the body. One is the hard-wired brain-nerve system, the other being the substances in blood and body fluids called neuropeptides, some seventy or eighty of which are identified. Together they form a network that controls both the operation and health of our body, physically and mentally. Neuropeptides can be thought of as "messengers" that transmit information to organs and cells just as surely as do the nerves themselves. Relative to nutrition and energy production, the entire gastrointestinal tract is lined with cells that contain neuropeptides and their receptors. (Receptors are areas on the surface membranes of cells that are "unlocked" by the neuropetide "keys.") By means of the messenger neuropeptides gut cells can "speak" and "listen" to the brain. So, according to Candace Pert, and others, "gut feelings" are truly emotional phenomena, just like brain feelings.

In fact, immune cell products, such as Interleukin-1 can instruct the brain to direct a "cautious avoidance" behavior that causes us to "stay out of harm's way" until healing occurs. (Humans may not be the sole beneficiaries. "Something" tells deer when sick to quit eating and rest in a safe place). Conversely, what is running through the brain can have profound effects on the immune system such as altering cell function by messages straight to the cell nucleus. Accordingly, chronic states of distress, such as helplessness, unresolved "loss," hopelessness and depression deter healing and promote disease. Pert and others also state that habitual repression of strong emotions (by increasing opioid peptides) causes deficits in the immune system leading to "reduced resistance to infection and neoplastic disease."

So all pervasive and controlling is this biochemical network that we may need to add it to the conventional neural-endocrine-oxidative control systems that most researchers use in metabolic typing. Illness then becomes an imbalance, not just of nutritional and physiological factors, but of psychosocial and emotional factors as well.

Pert *et al.* review concepts that the entity we blithely call the "mind" could be defined as the flowing and changing network of messenger substances and the cells of both brain and body that together orchestrate all the processes of life. Similarly, they suggest that "spirit" or "soul" could be defined as the non-material life force that energizes and animates this ceaseless flowing network of information. To this latter definition I might add the effect of a presence or power that pervades the universe and all the life forms within it, and which has delineated the rules by which our earthly life-support systems function; rules that each of us must play by in our respective biomes and ecosystems.

The tremendous power of the mind authenticated by Candace Pert and others, lends solid credence to the philosophy that underlies many Eastern religions. It behooves us all to reconsider the enormous impact on our health and longevity of the stresses we subject ourselves to in the race for the "good" life that "developed" societies extol.

Since it evolved to control stability (homeostasis), the brain has a sophisticated system for monitoring food intake and body weight. Calories in and calories out is too simplistic. Fat calories differ from carbohydrate calories in how they are handled. The brain has an all-important "set point" that determines body weight. People with excess fat cells acquired during their first two years of life have a high set point and are constantly hungry, trying to conform to "normal" weights. As one reduces, weight loss becomes more difficult as one approaches the set point.

Two things can lower the set point. One is starvation, when life-saving metabolic set point changes occur. This saved the lives of hunter-gatherers and prisoners in concentration camps. Exercise, which approaches the workload of the hunter-gatherer, such as walking twenty-five miles a week, burns more calories and is said to lower the set point. A day-long hunting or fishing trip or playing a hard game of football will increase metabolism for several days, but is compensated for by increased appetite so that body weight remains relatively stable.

Our genetic endowment of brain and biology evolved for a different and stable world where change was gradual. Today, we are forced to try to adapt to unprecedented changes, not the least of which are in the foods we eat, the fluids we drink and the air we breathe. Medical institutions are full of non-adapters. There is a paradox here, however. The brain has evolved also to constantly explore (and later to analyze) the environment. It is thus easily bored. There is even a theory that some cancers are promoted by insufficient information input (boredom). (de la Peña, 1983.) Foods, of course, affect the brain. Carbohydrates will increase the secretion of relaxing serotonin; eggs will increase the neurotransmitter acetylcholine.

Ornstein and Sobel concluded that, to promote health, we must believe that life is meaningful, that we have adequate resources to cope and that it is orderly and predictable. This would include understanding our own metabolism. The trick is to balance stimulation with the body's need for stability. What is common to most major religions seems to be to introduce a stable, complete view of life on Earth, which, in spite of change, loss and death, promises (as Ornstein and Sobel say) that "life itself and our contribution to it will continue."

The Gene Wars

The battlefield is DNA within the chromosomes. One battle is between "good" and "bad" genes within us. The other battle pits the slowly changing genes of one organism, us, against the fast changing genes of other organisms such as viruses and bacteria. The outcome is death and degenerative disease if we lose and life, health and longevity if we win. We are finding out that our genes now influence many diseases. They may turn on disease or turn on inhibitors. Generally, defective genes seem to work against us probably through weakened enzyme or immune systems.

The Human Genome project is currently mapping our 23 chromosomes. In 1995, only two had been mapped (the "Y" and number 21).[15] Recently, Shreeve (1999) presented the latest finding of the various teams of the Genome Project. At that time some 1,200 disorders had been identified. All twenty-three human chromosomes have acquired the ability to influence the probability or course of either metabolic/endocrine problems (such as congenital hypothyroidism, diabetes and fructose intolerance) or neurological/psychiatric disorders (such as Alzheimer's, Huntington's Disease and schizophrenia). At least elven chromosomes carry genes for different types of cancers. Chromosome 17 alone carries genes for leukemia, breast, ovarian and small-cell lung cancer.

The Human Tumor Gene Index of the National Cancer Institute has identified more than 50,000 genes active in one or more cancers. Some 5,692 are active in breast cancer cells. (Ezzsell, 2000.) A genetic predisposition for cancer does not mean that we will necessarily get it. The immune system has evolved to eliminate any cell that "gets out of hand," so we must enhance, not inhibit, our immune system function. This is done by close attention to diet, not just to the right food for our metabolisms but also for the phytochemicals that they contain. In addition, we need to carefully watch our stress levels from physical and chemical agents in the food we eat, the water we drink and the air we breathe. Furthermore, even given with the best intentions, our drugs are suspect. Scientists now believe that tiny, genetic variations in only 0.1 percent of our genes influence whether, in 30 to 50 percent of the human population, a given drug will be effective or, conversely, act as a poison. (Brown, 2000.)

---

[15] Chromosome 21 seems to be the site for Down's Syndrome (Mongolism) and Alzheimer's Disease, according to Krause (1995). Krause also discussed both the frequency of known inheritance (5% to 10% for breast cancer) and the frequency of its running in families (25% in both breast cancer and diabetes), which to him, suggested an inherited weakness or susceptibility.

If we had only inbred ourselves on an island somewhere, we would have by now seen a more rapid degeneration of general health. This "experiment" has already been conducted. In Iceland, osteoarthritis is five times more common than elsewhere. Owing to 1,100 years of isolation and a fourteenth century plague, Icelanders are more genetically homogeneous than any other industrial society. (Gibbs, 1998.) It is thought that the defective gene for osteoarthritis was imported by one of the original immigrants in the middle of the ninth century.

Unlike Iceland, in the United States, at least, we have diluted and modified our gene pool by out-breeding with wave after wave of immigrants from all over the world. Since some of these immigrants brought defective genes, we have now incorporated them into our gene pool and have mixed them around.

In a society living close to nature, as in hunters-gatherers or localized horticulturists (as in the Amazon), death, inability to breed or produce viable offspring, or infanticide would soon eliminate defective genes.

It must be clear by now that medical and surgical intervention has allowed many humans to survive so that, unlike the rest of the animal kingdom, they are free to spread their defective genes throughout the population. The compassionate humanitarianism of medical science is heart-warming, and to deny anyone the alleviation of suffering is unacceptable. But we will make no real progress in understanding the deterioration of our national health ($100 billion yearly for diabetes alone) until we view our dilemma objectively.

As individuals, we cannot change our genes (yet). But we can use our knowledge of nutrition and life style to counteract our unwelcome susceptibilities to disease produced by the "bad" genes we may have gotten in the lottery of life. And technology may yet find a way to alter, control or eliminate defective genes.

Another epic battle of the gene wars is people versus other forms of life, notably viruses and bacteria. We know we are in for a fight when Western Nile Fever invades New York City. Hemorrhagic viruses, such as Ebola and Hanta, suddenly appear and spread wildly. Hospitals are in a life and death struggle with "bugs" which are now drug-resistant. Formerly benign microorganisms, such as *E. coli* now turn vicious killers. This is due to the incredible short life cycles of these organisms which can spread an advantageous mutation like wildfire, sometimes within a single individual (such as AIDS is thought to do). We, on the other hand, breed so slowly and our mutation rate is so low that our defensive gene change is inconsequential. Given time, of course, human genes can change, such as the one for sickle cell anemia, which occurred in Africa and is protective against malaria.

The bottom line in these battles appears to be that it often boils down to the lifestyle of each of us as a "soldier" and what we as individuals, eat, drink and breathe. Since most of society seems to be ignoring our biological roots we, as individuals, must find them again. Millions of little independent victories may not win the war, but it will allow enough of us to survive to support the general offensive.

CHAPTER ELEVEN

Supermarket

"The organism (animal or human) is the 'biochemical photograph' of the environment in which it lives, particularly of the soil which manufactures the nutrients for it."

—Andre Voisin

Credit for coining the phrase "hunting and gathering in the supermarket" goes to Eaton *et al.* (1988). Recently, I spent an entire afternoon not doing much gathering but a lot of hunting through a local store, reading mostly labels. I don't believe I saw another person read a label all afternoon. I thought of natives in the tropical rainforests and their intimate knowledge of hundreds of plants and animals gained through millennia of experience and perpetuated throughout verbal history. I thought of my neighbors, former settlers with their gardens, livestock and knowledge of edible and medicinal wild plants. Then I looked at my fellow citizens in the store, hunting and gathering the only way that most of them knew, in the produce bins, the meat counters and along the aisles of the supermarket. How much did they really know about the soils where these products were grown, the vitamin content and toxins used on the produce, the hormones fed the cattle, and, above all, the processes, preservatives and additives that created those colorful rows of packages, canned goods and frozen meals? One can only hope that the FDA and the USDA have done a good enough job, for they are apparently the only replacement most of us have for the collective wisdom of tribal cultures, where man knew what to eat and what not to eat and everything was natural and organic.

Perhaps the largest overall problem facing the supermarket customer is that for convenience, carbohydrate sources such as starch and sugar have been processed, refined and concentrated until they are crammed with calories. They lack the natural coatings, husks, skins and pulp that once provided essential fiber, but more importantly, limited the amount an individual could eat at one time. They also quite often lost their vitamins and minerals during processing or storage. Some domesticated grains have been bred for more calories and less fiber. Oils with over twice the calories of carbohydrate or proteins are added to many products to give them a "rich" taste. Soybean oils seem to predominate, supplanting the olive, pig and cow (and the coconut) which yielded fats which did not readily oxidize, unlike the polyunsaturated fats of soy, corn and other seeds. Thus we wind up with foods we were not designed to handle, substances more in the nature of high-energy emergency rations that may or may not keep well on the grocery shelves.

We won't have much trouble identifying the major food categories, carbohydrates, proteins and fats, as we wheel down the aisle with our grocery carts. But even these gross categories have been tampered with and some modified to our detriment. Carbohydrates are now more and more sweetened with "high fructose corn syrup." It's natural in corn, but added to other products, it apparently triggers a deleterious response. Worse is the presence of "partially hydrogenated vegetable oils" in almost everything, from breakfast cereals, crackers and cookies and frozen dinners, to margarine and microwave popcorn. When vegetable oils are "hardened" with hydrogen, they change chemically from a good "cis" form to a bad "trans" fatty acid. From 1890 to 1990 there was a major shift from naturally saturated fats (animal fats, coconut and palm oils) to partially hydrogenated vegetable oils. (Enig, 1993, 1995.) Trans-fats not only act, (as do saturated fats) in excess to produce cardiovascular problems, but cannot be used by the body to produce essential prostaglandins. They also impair the use of normal fatty acids and "deprive the body of its weight loss capability." (Gittleman, 1988.) Trans-fats also create weakened cell walls. Unfortunately, vegetable oils reused by fast food restaurants increase in both trans-fats and rancidity. French-fries and doughnuts are about 40 percent trans-fat, cookies and crackers up to 50 percent. (Gittleman, 1988.)

Even more subversive for the modern civilized hunter-gatherer among the grocery shelves are the additives that titillate our taste buds. Blaylock (1994) has thoroughly documented the danger of taste-enhancing substances. The leading culprit is MSG

(Monosodium glutamate). It is among a group of substances that cause damage to the retina and hypothalamus of the brain, especially in young animals. Called an "excitotoxin," it excites brain cells to die by blocking open their calcium channels. Excitotoxins are strongly suspected of playing a major role in degenerative brain diseases in adults, such as Parkinson's and Alzheimer's.

Major excitotoxins are MSG and aspartame, the sugar substitute. Unfortunately, because of competition, the processed food industry has disguised these substances, especially MSG, which is found in harmless sounding "hydrolyzed vegetable protein," "vegetable protein," "natural flavorings" and even "spices." The first three in particular may contain 12 to 40 percent MSG. (Schwartz, 1988.) Hydrolyzed vegetable protein is especially dangerous since it contains "three known excitotoxins and has added MSG." (Blaylock, 1994.) It was added to baby foods for years. Although no longer added to most, Blaylock indicates that excitotoxins are still added to some baby foods today. Babies are especially vulnerable.

As my bleary eyes kept focussing on label after label, I kept asking myself, *With all those flavorful ingredients in those jars and cans, why in the world would anyone need to add "natural flavorings?"* I suppose it is for the same reason that restaurants add sugar to sweet potatoes. It appears that "natural flavorings" may contain from 20 to 40 percent MSG. (Blaylock, 1994.)

In all fairness, we have to be careful in reading labels. Not all labels are deceptive. For example: In the use of words like "natural flavoring" (singular) and just plain "flavoring." Since I eat a lot of canned beans, I critiqued the labels of two leading companies. The same company that puts out a bean with bacon soup, clearly labeled to contain MSG, has a pork and beans product that contains no MSG—the word "flavoring" on the label means the addition of beef or pork only. The words "natural flavoring" (singular), on the label of another leading company's Original Baked Beans, means only a single harmless spice has been added, *not* MSG.

Artificial sweeteners, according to Blaylock, contain 40 percent of the powerful brain toxin aspartate (aspartame). While, he says, there is little evidence that such excitotoxins actually cause things like Parkinson's and Alzheimer's, Huntington's and Amyotrophic Lateral Sclerosis "there is growing evidence that they can aggravate these conditions and that they may even precipitate them in sensitive individuals." It is my understanding that it takes quite a few years to destroy enough brain cells to notice the difference, but by then, it is too late. Blaylock's final advice is to use skill in reading labels and willpower to resist your favorite chips, sauces, soups, pizzas and frozen dinners. Fortunately, antioxidant vitamins and minerals, adequate magnesium, branched chain amino acids and zinc "have all been shown to offer varying degrees of protection," according to Blaylock.

Overreaction to foods and additives is even involved in weight loss. One theory is that blood levels of the neurotransmitter, serotonin, drop after eating certain foods, initiating a craving for serotonin-restoring sugars and starches. Our allergic reactions to foods can directly trigger cellular responses or cause the intestinal lining to "leak" incompletely digested food proteins into the blood stream, where they generate cell toxins and inflammation. Thus: "Due to dietary insufficiency or another defect in one of the body's detoxification systems, any one or more of the artificial additives, or naturally occurring pharmacoactive agent in a food may cause a . . . disruption to the immune system and metabolic function." (AMTL Corp., 1999.)

Our cravings for sugars and starches or proteins may not be totally due to childhood conditioning or the seductive products on grocery shelves. There are little recognized hormonal adjustments that help us balance our diet between carbohydrate and protein sources. It is known that a high protein meal reduces the amino acid tryptophan and thus levels of the brain neurotransmitter serotonin, which causes us to desire more carbohydrates. Conversely, an increase in serotonin reduces our desire for them. Two important amino acids (tryptophan, tyrosine) and lecithin have all been shown to affect levels of the brain's principal neurotransmitters (serotonin, norepinephrine, epinephrine, acetylcholine). (Wurtman, 1982.)

Tryptophan, tyrosine and lecithin are food substances (precursors) from which these vital brain transmitters are formed. These same precursors are also implicated in the aging process and can be used in preventing senile afflictions. Brain neurons are lost with aging. In Parkinson's disease, up to half of the nerve cells involved can be lost before symptoms appear. This same phenomenon may be present in other conditions, perhaps in Alzheimer's. How the elderly person eats then becomes increasingly important. Wurtman, speaking of diets to which the precursor food substances (tryptophan, tyrosine, lecithin) can be added, said that the continued reliance of the elderly "on normal but unenriched diets" might be construed as poor nutrition.

So, a successful hunting and gathering trip in the supermarket would avoid any food carrying on its label: partially hydrogenated vegetable oils, Aspartame, MSG, hydrolyzed vegetable protein, vegetable protein or natural flavorings. It is understandable that food processors do not wish to reveal a proprietary recipe that may involve seasonings. If they list such simple things as salt as an ingredient, surely the other things could be named.

Most of our shopping fervor ought to be confined to the produce bins (and their frozen counterparts), the meat counters and the dairy and eggs section. And speaking of dairy, it has been claimed that homogenization is the leading culprit, rendering fat droplets small enough to pass through the gut wall. (Douglass, 1985.) It is indeed unfortunate that certified raw milk is no longer available. It keeps much longer. Eventually, unlike pasteurized milk, it only sours, while pasteurized milk turns putrid.

The FDA would surely bring to our attention foods that are toxic or contain dangerous chemicals, but I'm not so sure that these regulatory agencies warn us about substances added to foods that cause slow and subtle degeneration of the body tissues, weaken the immune system or subvert normal metabolism.

It would be blatant to endorse the words of another health-conscious consumer: "The world is going to hell in a grocery basket." But, as you become more conscious of food values, simply stand by the check-out counter of a local supermarket and note how few of the products in the grocery carts provide good solid nutrition, such as unprocessed fresh meats and sea food, butter, buttermilk and yogurt, whole grain products like oatmeal and raw vegetables and fruits.

Our ancient limbic desires to appease our appetites for food, made tasty by fats, salt and natural sugars, is now being exploited by manufacturers and retailers. In this commercial world, food is viewed as a commodity rather than a nutrient source. This commercialization has led to transnational food firms which have replaced the old means of exploitation by colonialism. (Franke, 1987.) It is said that only 25 percent of us have adapted to the high-density carbohydrates so highly touted by the food industry, while 25 percent of us have not adapted to them at all. (Sears, 1995.) If true, advertising refined flour and sugar products is detrimental to the national health, to which legions of diabetics and other unhealthy individuals can attest.

As we enter the new millenium we realize that the earth's ecosystems are host to six billion uninvited guests in human form. An idea of how they must live sustainably and might live healthily has hopefully been conveyed.

How we eat is an important part of a larger picture. Recently, faced with the new millenium, some visionary environmental advocates (including the head of AFL-CIO) expressed how we might "get it right" for the coming centuries ahead (Sierra, 2000) (our environmental record for the last 1,000 years has been dismal indeed). A lot of what they say is addressed in Part I. Paul Hawken comments on the astonishing concentration of corporate power: "Three companies—Monsanto, DuPont and Novartis . . . strive to control 90 percent of the germ plasm that provides the world with 90 percent of its caloric intake." John Sweeney (AFL-CIO) states "It is going to take hard and sophisticated work to overcome the increasing power of fewer and fewer giant corporations that control the work and the resources that sustain both the planet and the people on it."

As the Ehrlichs say (Sierra, 2000) you cannot use the GNP to assess society's prosperity because most economists fail to recognize the value of natural capital inherent in "biodiversity, productive land and fresh water." With all living systems declining we are using more of what we have less of—natural capital— in order to use less of what we have more of—people. Industry makes people more productive but at the expense of resources and services of living natural systems.

This section closes with the unsettling words of Claire Cummings (1999): "A revolution has taken place in our eating habits, and its implications for agriculture, health and the environment are enormous. The interests of agribusiness and fast food corporations are now merging with those of the media and entertainment industries, and the result is an unprecedented corporate takeover of our food supply which is transforming not only how we eat, but also how we think. Food has lost its significance, has been wholly de-ritualized, and has become little more than pre-packaged family entertainment." Strong words but perhaps helpful in enabling us to glimpse the big picture of nutrition in America.

PART II

THE SEARCH FOR A PERSONAL NUTRITION

CHAPTER TWELVE

Introduction

"Every person has a nutritional-metabolic pattern that is characteristic, indeed as unique as a fingerprint."

—René Dubos

From Part I we have seen that we evolved from omnivorous primates with group behavior and large brains. Adapting to new African environments we perfected cooperative hunting and gathering and acquired even larger brains. This allowed us to spread and adapt to cold climates as carnivore dominants and to warm climates as herbivore dominants. In a strong seasonal climate Europeans fortuitously managed to domesticate both plants and animals. In Southeast Asia, in parts of Africa and in Central America other grain-bearing plants were developed. The agriculture that resulted led to man-managed instead of nature-managed ecosystems. High energy, storable, new plant foods allowed sedentary cultures and unlimited population growth, while domesticated animals in the Old World permitted more restricted populations to exploit the native vegetation of vast steppes and grasslands. Certain cultures in Southeast Asia and the Pacific Rim region, by simulating nature's plant communities and her method of maintaining soil fertility, were able to develop a sustainable production of quality foods. The clever control of water allowed even larger concentrations of humans. In many areas of the world the traditional agriculture and diets that evolved enabled many indigenous groups to adapt to local soils and climates in harmony and health with the almost complete absence of degenerative disease.

This working bond between people and their sustainably fertile soils was broken by cash-crop agriculture, migration into towns, the abandonment of traditional diets and the purchase of food from distribution centers out of their control. With dietary needs now modified by taste and convenience, refined and processed foods provided by profit-motivated industry replaced the nutrient-rich productivity of subsistence farms and gardens. Some human cultures were able to adapt their Paleolithic bodies to endemic disease and novel high-energy plant foods. But substituting our own quality control over that of nature's set the stage in some affluent nations for a litany of health problems. Faced with an almost daily indulgence in an unlimited supply of tasty and concentrated calories, we prepared our Paleolithic bodies for starvation that never came. The end result has been a national epidemic of chronic obesity, a growing rise in degenerative disease, and rapid aging.

As Part II emphasized, through Paleolithic man at least, our bodies were adapted to a dietary regime of protein and fat, largely from animal sources and, from the plant world, complex (roots, seeds, nuts) and simple (fruits, honey) carbohydrates. These bodies we inherited essentially unchanged were the end result of several million years of adaptation to the forests and savannas of Africa, as well as from a brief but substantial sojourn in ice-age Eurasia.

What has drastically changed are the dietary regimes. Since the advent of agriculture 10,000 years ago, the physiology of the body for some cultures has been forced to try to adapt to novel "new" foods in a tiny fraction of the time spent as humans of the genus *Homo.* This forced natural selection resulted in a rapid adaptation to the special environments of particular regions of the earth. Today, we find adaptation to the various foods available in each region: milk (central Asian nomads, north Africa), wheat, barley, pulse (mid-east, northern India), rice-fish (southeast Asia), millet, rice, soybean (China), yams-taro (Pacific area), beans-corn-pepper (southern North America), white potato-quinoa-bean (Andes area). Those who could not survive on the foods in their environment did not pass their genes along.[16] The Arctic Eskimos,

---

[16] This is similar to the regional adaptation to germs during the past 10,000 years. For example, Europeans have acquired some genetic resistance to smallpox but, in another region, North America, the natives had never adapted to this disease and had no resistance to it.

as an example of hunter-gatherers, were probably adapted to their extreme high fat/protein diet long before Neolithic times.

Thus we face the final phase of the story. In nations such as the United States, the genotypes from regions adapted to specific foods were brought together by emigration and immigration, and subsequently bred with one another indiscriminately. In the nutritional pot pourri that resulted, the best solution for each of us seems to be to find out the foods to which we are individually adapted.

The Roman philosopher Lucretius is credited with the saying that "one man's meat is another man's poison." If so, he was perhaps the first person to state the central tenet for a personal nutrition, often called, for convenience, "metabolic typing." Science and medicine have for so many years been wrestling with the mechanics of multiple diseases and their myriad causes that we may have lost sight of the wisdom behind that ancient idea that individuals are different. We look different externally, so why shouldn't we be different internally?

The theme of having a personalized nutrition is that you treat the person who has the disease, not the disease who has the person. This is a conceptual revolution in human health, a revelation that needs to supplant years of indoctrination by conventional medicine.

As René Dubos says: "The public health services themselves, despite their misleading name, are concerned less with health than with the control of specific diseases. . . . " (Dubos, 1965.)

The rising tide of *degenerative* disease, which now comprises about 80 percent of our medical problems, emphasizes the need for a new paradigm. Our latest afflictions are insidious and have hardly given us time enough to die off in adaptation to them. In 1900 the two great killers were pneumonia (11.7 percent) and tuberculosis (11.3 percent). In 1994 it was heart disease (32.1 percent) and cancer (23.5 percent) (CDC, National Center for Health Statistics). In 1959 48.8 percent of men were rejected as unfit for military service and of 300 soldiers autopsied in the Korean War, 77.3 percent had heart disease. They averaged twenty-two years of age. (Page, 1972.) Young people may just appear healthy, apparently degenerative disease begins in the teens or earlier. Recent (Strong *et al.*, 1999) figures from 2,876 people indicate that atherosclerosis begins in youth, 23 percent of males had coronary arterial plaque by age fifteen to nineteen.

There is one thing that impresses above all the rest: the fact that degenerative disease is so *slow*. It is the insidious accumulation of many small incidents of abuse, the gradual and imperceptible weakening of glands, enzyme systems and immune functions. It is like aging before your time.

In spite of our current mismanagement of what we eat, drink, breathe and think, our ancient body machinery should be able to reverse much abuse and still heal itself. Theoretically, all it asks are the nutrient substances its progenitors had for millions of years and freedom from any new substances, such as toxins, to which neither it or its fore-bears have had time to adapt. A stark example of the effects of the lack of adaptation is courtesy of the reptile world. When the Atlanta Zoo built an expensive new reptile house, hundreds of valuable reptiles from all over the world began dying off. Distraught officials finally discovered the cause. Formaldehyde fumes (undetectable by the human nose) were offgassing from the plywood used in constructing the cages. Eventually, the cages had to be torn out and completely rebuilt. The reptilian body had never had to cope with even minute traces of this toxic substance. This leads to a logical theory that noxious gases, either by being inhaled or by changing the climate, led to the extinction of the dinosaurs, especially if we assume that neither the warm or cold-blooded species were able to hibernate. The ancestors of living reptiles (all cold-blooded) could have survived by breathing under water (as do some modern turtles) or by hibernating in underground chambers, as many reptiles do today.

Now, here is a perplexing thing: some people can abuse their bodies horribly and survive what most of us cannot. This tells us that something drastic has happened to the human genotype in the short span of 10,000 years, perhaps accelerated in the last 1,000 or even 300 years. For most of us, our magnificent inheritance from the prehistoric past simply has not had time to change our genes to adapt to modern life. In addition, modern medicine, as wonderful as it is, has used its expertise to save each and every defective genotype from dying according to nature's plan, which is the cornerstone of Darwinian evolution. Women with pelvises too genetically narrow for the baby to pass frequently died in childbirth but are now saved along with the child by caesarean section. This defective gene would have been stopped cold in the world of our past. Saving lives this way seems morally commendable. The brutal truth is that the children thus saved can spread the defective gene at will. Degeneration of the entire population has to be the result with more and more dependence on medicine and surgery. Such factors must account for much of the individuality of our body chemistry, in particular the spread of aberrations of our internal biochemistry, leading us to become more and more divergent from our "primitive" past. On top of this, we add the complex genetics from the Caucasian melting pot. Finding our nutritional or metabolic type may be the only way to determine our true identity at the cellular, endocrine and enzymatic levels where it counts.

Beginning with Bieler and Watson, comparatively few have extolled the merits of biochemical individuality. A later surveyor of nutrition, Eleanor Eckstein (1980) said that what we "can't do yet, is to identify the most appropriate modality of management for individual patients, based on the specific abnormalities each person has," a formal way of stating it. The Bible is not much help. Before the flood man was instructed to eat along vegetarian lines (Genesis 1:29). In postdeluvian days Noah was instructed to be more carnivorous: "Every moving thing that liveth shall be meat for you. . . . " (Genesis 9:3)

Metabolic typing addresses the variability of human metabolisms. It is probably considered "alternative medicine," a field that is expanding so rapidly that even your friendly neighborhood physician may be beginning to use some of it. As you know, alternative or integrative medicine seeks to use "natural" and supposedly more wholesome nutrients and to use drugs from herbs rather than from pharmacies. It also embraces the latest findings in mind-body relationships, including Far Eastern practices, spirituality and modern psychoneuroimmunology.

If modern medicine seeks to treat the symptom and not the underlying cause, this is a somewhat disrespectful view of the healing power of natural forces. Many physicians do understand the healing powers of the body. Unfortunately, the patient wants a quick fix. "Take two aspirin and call me in the morning" is probably an acknowledgement that nature needs a little more time before human intervention.

No one has more ably established the human bodies' remarkable ability to heal itself than Andrew Weil, M.D. (1995). According to Weil, in ancient Greece doctors worked under their patron Asklepios, the god of medicine, while healers served his daughter Hygeia, goddess of health. Asklepians are said to emphasize treatment while Hygeians favor healing. Treatment originating outside the body, healing coming from within. The Hygeian philosophy, strengthening the body to heal itself, underlies most Eastern medicine. In the West, the incredibly expensive "interventions of technological medicine" are escalating the cost of being ill. (Weil, 1995.)

Weil reiterates that the followers of Hygeia "maintain that health results from living in harmony with natural law." His book, Spontaneous Healing, is a testament to the fact that spontaneous healing is a common occurrence. As I see it, to heal ones self from within is a residual ability inherited from the pre-agricultural eons of our existence in nature, where our survival demanded total compliance with natural laws. Today, we must re-learn the rules of correct living that our ancestors had no choice but to obey.

While there is a current fad to beat up on the medical profession, the "new" metabolic-typing paradigm also exposes to attack devotees of alternative medicine. Kristal and Wolcott subscribe to the idea that, in treating degenerative disease, modern alternative medicine is not to be congratulated any more than current allopathic medicine. The flaw in both, they say, is the failure to recognize the biochemical individuality championed by Roger Williams. According to Kristal (1998) alternative practitioners are, like orthodox medical doctors, "still treating the disease, the system, the deficiency or condition, the organ, the dysfunction, albeit using natural methods." We try to interpret lab results from analyses of blood, urine or hair in terms of what we think are excesses or deficiencies. (Kristal, 1998.) And, according to Kristal, "almost as many people are not being helped in the alternative field as are not being helped in the orthodox field." This is unsettling news.

As you read the contributions of the researchers and clinicians in the sections that follow, perhaps you can see how the principle of biochemical individuality begins to create order out of chaos. An ultimate goal is to enable you to realize your unique potential as a one-of-a-kind person. This is not to lose sight of the fact that (deep down) there is a fundamental biological organization that we all share, such as an autonomic (automatic) nervous system and an endocrine, or hormone delivery system. These ancient systems are absolutely essential to maintain a balance. Stick your hand in a glass of ice water. In a little while the hand muscles become almost useless as the chemical reactions and enzymes in a mammal can function only within a narrow range of temperature, not too hot and not too cold.

The animal body seeks homeostasis or balance in all things, including the blood. The blood must be neither too acid nor too alkaline and blood sugar must be held close to a certain level. This balance is apparently achieved by a few fundamental control "mechanisms." In metabolic theory disease exists because of a loss of balance (imbalance) by one or more of these controls, most of which, like yin and yang, have opposing effects. Those in metabolic typing believe that every food or nutrient can either stimulate or inhibit one (or more) of these systems. Implications are that what you're eating could be deleterious to your health. Can you really separate cravings from the subtle signals that your body needs a certain food? If you eat red meat and fats you may want sweets. Restrain yourself for twenty minutes and this craving goes away. Meanwhile, you have paid your bill and have left the restaurant so temptation is behind you. Do our bodies say that we need more carbohydrate or is it that we have developed, over a lifetime, a "sweet tooth?" The last chapter addresses such questions.

Besides the enticing menus with endless taste sensations, there is another important factor that influences our decisions as to what to eat. Agronomy, coupled with modern agricultural science, is a huge and powerful force in what DeChapelle (1988) calls the "IGS" or Industrial Growth Society. We endure a veritable media blitz of advertisements extolling what to eat or drink and our incomparable food industry leads the world in processing and presenting foods for human (and animal) consumption.

Since we were anthropoids, we have obtained our foods like all other animals: gleaning wild biomes for the fruits of the earth. For a tiny portion of that immense experience, we have become not-for-profit subsistence cultivators and herders. Now, the major problem seems to be the complete for-profit commercialization of our diet. Large corporate organizations have "taken over" our foods. We are, by and large, supermarket dependent.

Surely there is no effort, conscious or otherwise, to devitalize our foods by anyone in the food industry. After all, Kellogg and Post started their companies by recognizing the health value of grains, as did Graham with his whole grain crackers.

Can we have some plain talk here? Since we all have taste buds, who is to blame for their perversion by making foods sweeter, spicier or deliciously fatter and exploiting an ancient primate food bias. If we agree that there is no industrial conspiracy to undermine our health, then we have to believe that it is the profit motive because everybody has to eat and the market is enormous. For the vast bulk of foods offered for sale the quality of the "merchandise" has suffered. Diligent hunting and gathering in the supermarket can still bag you some highly nutritious foods. Fierce competition for the food dollar has surely been the reason for more and more sugar added to breakfast cereals. Cost cutting is another aspect. Why did a large food company remove the delectable tamarind fruit from its steak sauce (they kept the color)? Perhaps for the same reason the highly effective herb *hydrastine* (from the golden seal plant) was removed from a leading eye solution. Native Americans were using this (now rare) herb for their eyes long before we burst on the scene.

We seem to be slowly acknowledging that vital substances essential for our health can be economically derived from actual living plants and animals, albeit from often exotic environments. Why does it seem odd to us that "primitive" cultures found all their daily needs supplied by the plants and animals they lived with? Maybe we are the ones who are "out of step" with reality. We need a map through a trackless forest of information and misinformation.

It would seem like nirvana if we could take a pill so that we could continue eating and drinking as we always have done. It is what you eat regularly that determines health and longevity, not the occasional banana split or chocolate "pig-out." Finally, we must search for that special metabolism we possess as individuals. We are not created equal for all foodstuffs. This part of the book goes into the details of finding your way through the modern dietary morass.

In the sections which follow, you will note certain specialties (degrees) following the names of researchers. Since this is a new field and orthodox medicine often has a lag time in adopting new things, the leaders in biochemical individuality are mostly either chiropractors (D.C.), naturopathic physicians (N.D.), dentists (D.D.S.) or specialists or generalists in one field or another (Ph.D.). Since I am one of the latter and a southerner, I am authorized to tell you what the elderly southern lady said when I told her I had a Ph.D. She said, "Is you one of them kind of doctors who don't do nobody no good?" Many fine physicians (M.D.s) now practice in fields variously called "alternative," "integrative," "holistic" or "preventive" medicine. The reader is urged to seek their help and guidance.

CHAPTER THIRTEEN

Feeling Good

A Brief Look at the Biochemical Basis behind Your Individuality

"What will it be, 'Good morning Lord or, good Lord it's morning?'"

—Morgan Raiford

Ann Louise Gittleman says that assessing your biochemical individuality is the next paradigm in the search for human health. This chapter addresses some of the basic biology behind this concept.

You don't have to look much further than the work of scientists like George Watson to discover that "feeling good" is simply a reflection of the inner energy flows that affect your organ systems and particularly your brain. The flow of energy, from foodstuffs to feelings, is what this is really all about. The need to define a metabolic type is simply a way to limit the confusion when confronted with the zillions of individual responses to environment, especially foods. It is a way of putting up a few signs to guide you along the pathway through a formidable jungle, a mix of inherited and acquired adaptations you have extracted from your long historical and pre-historical journey.

Unfortunately, dealing with the complex result of such a long struggle trying to live with the soils, waters, air, plants and other animals that make up our planet is not an exact science. Unless cloning is seriously conducted, each person is going to be slightly different, from everyone else. One way out of this evolutionary saga is to look at the flow of energy through our bodies, something we all share. In fact, everything is organized around energy flow, from the smoker vents in the deep sea to rockets reaching for the depths of space.

Feeling good boils down to whether or not the energy-generating process within our body's cells is supplied with the appropriate nutrients that we evolved to use. Minerals, such as the element calcium and the combination of the elements, carbon, hydrogen and oxygen into a compound such as sugar, all fall under the title of "nutrients." Our cells need a balance of the right kind of nutrients, balanced amounts of each, and foods that supply the right mineral and vitamin content, before we can confidently wheel that grocery cart down the aisles of the local supermarket.

Except for the final chapter, Part II of the book deals with individual researchers and practitioners of metabolic typing, starting with Williams (1956) through Baum (2000). In order to understand their studies and theories, what follows is a short review of cell biology. Since it is somewhat technical, you may wish to use it more as a reference. As you read about the various authors in the rest of Part II, the diagrams that show the cell's energy pathways and the difference between fast and slow oxidizers will be especially useful.

Body Balance–Within the Cells

Figure 33 seeks to present the main routes by which the nutrients in our foods result in chemical compounds that, either with or without oxygen, yield the energy that holds their molecules together. Here are some unfamiliar words but we need them to understand the sophisticated chemistry that enables us to live. Energy-yielding reactions take place in two different places in the cell (be it muscle, liver or kidney). The release of energy without oxygen (anaerobic) takes place in the gelatinous matrix (cytosol) filling most of a cell. This reaction nets only two energy-rich molecules of ATP, an ancient phosphorus-rich compound that energizes all life on earth. An important intermediary, pyruvic acid, created by this oxygenless procedure is conveyed into little bodies or organelles within the cell called mitochondria, the cell's major energy factory. Here, in two turns of a chemical "wheel" or cycle involving oxaloacetic acid and acetyl co-enzyme A, two more ATP molecules are generated. Though not shown in the diagram, this Krebs Cycle, as it is called, does require oxygen (aerobic) as does the breakdown of fatty acids.

During both the aerobic and anaerobic phases, hydrogen atoms are given off and conveyed into the final, and major, energy-yielding step in the mitochondria (called the electron transfer phase). Here the hydrogen atoms are essentially ionized and their

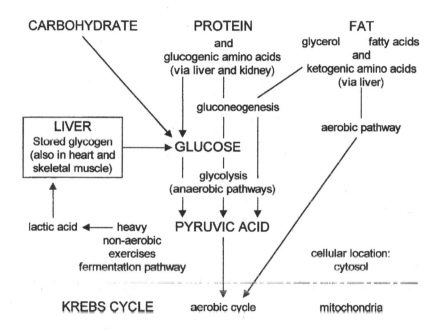

Figure 33. The fate of foodstuffs in the body; energy producing pathways, not requiring oxygen (anaerobic), except for fats and the Krebs Cycle. In aerobic exercise both fat and sugar-burning enzymes are working; in anaerobic exercise (when muscles hurt or "burn") only sugar-burning pathways are operative. Glucose stores are limited to fifteen to twenty grams (three to eight hours supply), principally in the liver but in other cells also. Stored liver glycogen (normal adult) is seventy grams (average). Fasting or exercise without adequate rest initiates conversion of muscle protein to amino acids (gluconeogenesis) which become the sole source of glucose production within twenty-four to forty-eight hours. (Watson, 1972; Bailey, 1994; Pryor and Polonsky, 1998.)

free electrons are used to produce thirty-four ATP molecules, yielding a total cellular energy output of thirty-eight ATP molecules. These drive all life processes and apparently have done so for at least a billion years since this invention in some of the first independent cells floating in the ocean. To shy away from accepting adenosine triphosphate (ATP) into our vocabulary would ignore one of the most significant molecules ever to evolve on earth, for it originated in ancestral primitive, single-celled organisms (prokaryotes) from which all later life evolved. This stunning fact led Lynn Margulis of the University of Massachusetts to propose a now widely-accepted theory that small free-living cells that had become able to use oxygen to produce ATP were devoured by larger free-living cells but, instead of being digested, were held inside and nurtured as a beneficial part of the host that had eaten them. This symbiotic arrangement was so mutually beneficial that life forms used it—the smaller, ingested former free-ranging cells are now called mitochondria. As advanced and complex animals as we are, our billions of diverse cells still use this very ancient method of supplying and storing energy inherent in the chemical bonds holding three phosphate molecules together.

With Figure 33 as a basic theme, Figures 34 and 35 contrast the energy flow in two major metabolic types that almost everyone agrees on: slow oxidizers burning carbohydrates (sugars and starches) too slowly and fast oxidizers burning them too quickly. These two figures show that these two metabolic types have, in the Krebs cycle within the mitochondria, either too much of one and not enough of the other of the two principal compounds from our foods. As Watson indicates, it is a matter of balancing the energy input from these two major sources, carbohydrates and fats.

These figures are intended also to show exactly where some of the vitamins "plug in" to either speed up or slow down the supply of energy from food molecules to either oxaloacetic acid or acetyl coenzyme A ("O-acetate" or "acetate" as Watson calls them). You will see why you shouldn't give (except in minimal quantities perhaps) the same large doses of the same vitamins to both slow and fast oxidizers. Each metabolic type needs to take a special formula tailored for that specific metabolism. This was determined by Watson through many years of empirical observation and diet manipulation on real live patients, most of whom had mild to severe mental and emotional problems. Most multivitamin preparations on today's market, as you may now realize, are designed really for the shotgun effect and most of the time they work to some degree because most of us fall somewhere between the two extremes of being either slow or fast sugar burners.

And, in many cases, we are deficient in maybe just one essential vitamin or mineral in which case the multi-vitamin-mineral pill rectifies the deficiency. Sometimes even a single vitamin can do remarkable things to alter energy flow, especially to the brain which, after all, is where "feelings" come from. For example, a B-vitamin, niacin, participates in the enzymes that break down glucose (sugar). Acetate contains pantothenic acid. The absence of these vitamins can have profound effects on the cell's effort to

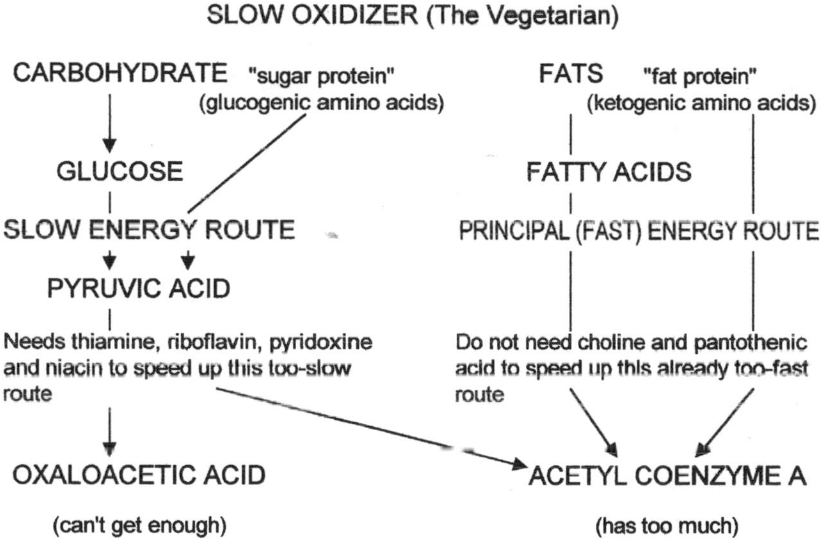

Figure 34. The slow oxidizer needs certain vitamins to "speed up" energy flow from glucose and must avoid certain vitamins that "speed up" energy flow from fats (and ketogenic amino acids). The slow oxidizer has insufficient oxaloacetic acid to combine with acetyl coenzyme A to efficiently operate the remainder, of, and principal phases of energy production (Krebs Cycle, electron transfer). Clearly, the slow oxidizer needs foods that generate glucose and needs to "go light" on fats and proteins. Lower carbon dioxide and carbonic acid levels alkalize (raise pH) the blood. (Based primarily on Watson, 1965, 1972.)

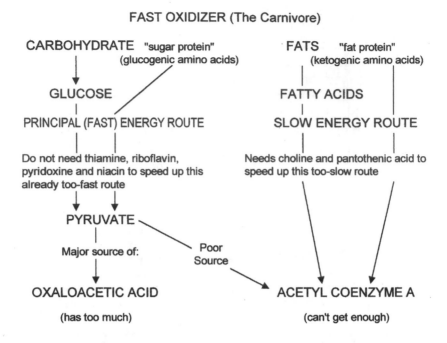

FAST OXIDIZER (The Carnivore)

CARBOHYDRATE "sugar protein"   · FATS   "fat protein"
                (glucogenic amino acids)   (ketogenic amino acids)

GLUCOSE   FATTY ACIDS

PRINCIPAL (FAST) ENERGY ROUTE   SLOW ENERGY ROUTE

Do not need thiamine, riboflavin,   Needs choline and pantothenic acid to
pyridoxine and niacin to speed up this speed up this too-slow route
already too-fast route

PYRUVATE

Major source of: Poor
                        Source

OXALOACETIC ACID   ACETYL COENZYME A

(has too much)   (can't get enough)

Figure 35.   The fast oxidizer needs certain vitamins to "speed up" energy flow from fats (and ketogenic amino acids) and avoid those which "speed up" an already too-fast glucose oxidation. The fast oxidizer has insufficient acetyl coenzyme A to combine with the large amount of oxaloacetic acid in order to efficiently operate the remainder of, and principal, phases of energy production (Krebs Cycle, electron transfer). Clearly, the fast oxidizer needs fats and protein-rich foods and must "go light" on those that generate glucose (sugars, starches). The increase in carbon dioxide and carbonic acid acidifies (lowers pH) the blood. (Based largely on Watson, 1965, 1972.)

extract energy (ATP) from what you eat. Even balanced metabolisms can be boosted and personalities changed by "adjusting" the intake of single nutrients. Watson cites (1972) the remarkable story of his patient Bob Walsh, considered to be a balanced metabolic type, which he calls "sub oxidizer." This twenty-five-year old man was formerly highly active, read books avidly, attended plays and concerts and loved mathematics and was going for an advanced degree. He suddenly dropped out of college, became bereft of goals and ambitions, read no more, and went into intellectual hibernation. Following a daily dose of 100 mg (later 300) of pantothenic acid, Walsh's life completely turned around. He quit his current paper-shuffling job, re-enrolled in graduate school, and earned his Ph.D. in math in two years, writing his dissertation in three months. One lesson in this is that you don't have to be necessarily sick or have any obvious symptoms of ill health to be a victim of poor eating habits. You just operate far below your potential just because of your dietary choices. By poor eating habits you have essentially choked off the energy flow to body and brain, thus becoming sort of a mental and emotional cripple.

Most of us are not fortunate enough to have a Dr. Watson at beck and call. We just keep plugging along day after day and not accomplishing very much. Certainly not making our dreams and fantasies come true, in the name of action, as Hamlet put it. To claim some portion of a sense of self-worth we drive ourselves into a state of over-commitment, trying to meet everybody's demands to earn the accolades of our fellow man. Trouble is, we push ourselves beyond our mental, emotional and physical reserves. Watson blames it on "the sick life patterns of large cities" citing prolonged driving to work and back, the job and all the things at home that push us to exceed our ability to "absorb stress and recover fully within a twenty-four hour period." Add unnaturally long evenings under artificial illumination staring at TV and few people can restore body and brain with only five or six hours of sleep. We are a little more tired each morning, thanking God for Friday. According to Watson, a few years of this gradual biochemical erosion and we begin the inevitable physical and psychological troubles.

The more extreme slow or fast oxidizers truly need to know their type because they can not eat a "normal" diet and avoid ill health or a suboptimal life. Not only are the abnormal reactors affected by diet but their problems are compounded by environmental factors which adversely affect the production of energy in the brain and other components of the central nervous system. The arrival of a cold front, napthalene (moth balls) in your closet, new carpeting on the floor or the arrival of a flu or cold virus on your respiratory membranes, all exacerbate the basic metabolic problem. For example, if as a fast oxidizer you don't cut your carbohydrate down and eat more fat and protein following a sharp shift in the weather your already marginal stores of acetate will be reduced making you an even faster oxidizer and worsening all symptoms. It is a well-known phenomenon that during periods of sharp weather changes people start hacking and coughing and hospital deaths increase.

If we can become sad, apprehensive and fearful and have weakened immune systems when climatic or other stressful events in our daily lives have unduly lowered our blood sugar, then what about those people with chronic mental and emotional problems? Since their physicians can find nothing physically wrong with them they are trundled off to see a psychologist or psychiatrist.

Watson's conclusions are enlightening. He found that, following dietary change, the "rate of improvement we have found among those suffering from virtually every kind of mental illness is very high—about 80 percent." He did find a small but resistant core group of people with minimal or no improvement who had formerly been treated unsuccessfully with electroshock, drugs and "analysis" and suggested a genetic origin for their difficulties. After surveying the various psychoanalists with different theories as to the causes of mental illness, including Freud, Jung, Adler, Rank and Fromm, Watson was forced to conclude that their basic belief and practice could only be explained by facing the reality that there "is simply no foundation of scientific fact to support *all* of these contradictory schools of psychotherapeutic thought." His summation was "we have found functional mental illness to be a reflection of disordered metabolism, principally involving the malfunction of enzyme systems."

Body Balance–The Autonomic Nervous System

One major structure that enforces balance in body processes is the autonomic nervous system with its two sets of nerves (sympathetic and parasympathetic) whose secretions have opposite effects on target glands and organs. If you are frightened, one branch (sympathetic) prepares you to instantly respond to attack by bear or mugger with particular attention to heart rate, brain and muscles, things you need immediately. At the same time organs that you don't need to be sending blood to, like the digestive tract, are rudely shut down and the sugar-rich, oxygenated blood is sent to where it is needed.

Unfortunately, anxiety can be low grade fear, and frustration can be low-grade anger so that either of these, if chronic, can continually signal the adrenal glands to secrete the mobilizing hormones and can exhaust them, wreaking havoc with your body. Persistent stress mobilizes another hormone, cortisol, a characteristic of only certain mammals, including man.

Incidentally, actions like eating, sleeping and sex are done under dominance of the para-sympathetic system. The heartbeat is slowed by a parasympathetic nerve (vagus). Here blood flow is not needed to the skeletal muscles for external movement but to the smooth muscles which surround the internal organs, which can sustain slow and powerful contractions. Interestingly, while penile erection is produced by the contraction of smooth muscle from the continued input of parasympathetic secretion (acetylcholine), ejaculation is a sudden reversal, caused by a quick release of antagonistic sympathetic system hormones.

Basically then, what you see, hear, smell, taste, touch and even remember does its number via the autonomic system.

Body Balance–The Endocrine System

We have seen that the autonomic nerves dictate to the endocrine glands, which then secrete the appropriate hormone. It so happens that some of these hormones affect our health by controlling mineral metabolism. For example, the adrenal cortex, in addition to the glucocorticoids previously mentioned (like cortisol) that affect energy production also secretes another type of hormone called "mineralocorticoids" whose job it is to regulate the balance of two metals that control fluid levels in the blood and cells, sodium and potassium, the so-called "electrolytes." One such hormone, aldosterone, is usually higher in the fast metabolizer than in the slow.

Some authors consider the hormones (often called "steroids") "anabolic" in that they "build up" cells and tissues, rather than "tearing down" or "using up" (called catabolic) cells and tissues. Calcium and magnesium are considered anabolic and "calming" minerals. It so happens that when these are augmented or retained in the body, sodium, potassium and phosphorus levels are lowered or "lost" according to Watts. Conversely, under catabolic conditions there is a retention of sodium, potassium and phosphorus and a "loss" of calcium and magnesium. You would feel stimulated rather than calmed with the latter situation.

Apart from building and maintaining the nerves and glands, the purpose of food is to provide energy so that everything "works." As we have seen, energy is the use of a common element of the atmosphere, oxygen, and its effects on other common elements in a process called oxidation.

Oxidation consists of the low-heat "burning" of sugars, the object of which is to keep our organs and muscles fueled with energy. The blood sugar is held at a level close to 100 (mg per l00 cc). Consistently high blood sugar spells diabetes. Since the brain uses a relatively huge amount of energy and influences how we "feel," the all important balance is obtained by adjusting the rate of creation of blood sugar or its removal by the liver instructed by various hormones. This is the famous glycolytic cycle. Various cells such as those in muscle tissue can also store and release sugar.

The body has evolved to sacrifice parts of itself to maintain the all important blood sugar, of which the brain is a major consumer (25 percent). The adrenal cortex is prepared, under the duress of prolonged stress or starvation, to do the following: cause your lymphatic system to atrophy, convert your muscle tissue to glucose, remove the protein matrix of the bones (followed by calcium loss and osteoporosis), and thin the skin. This unwelcome but necessary process is called gluconeogenesis, and the hormones that convert your body tissues to glucose are called glucocorticoids. They have one other depressing function: they can decrease the absorption of calcium. You may recall that low levels of the sedative mineral calcium is characteristic of fast oxidizers.

An important gland which characterizes fast oxidizers is the thyroid, which unquestionably increases the basal metabolic rate of the speed at which you "burn" sugar (glucose). It does this in response to environmental factors such as cold temperatures (you'll eat more in cold weather) or when it is "overactive" (hyperthyroidism). The thyroid and the adrenal medulla in particular thus produce "catabolic" hormones, "using up" body resources to enable you to do something, keep warm or run from a bear. It is a good time to note that Bieler, Abravanel and Cooper are about the only researchers who use the endocrine glands in their classification of metabolic types.

Some foods have gross effects on the glands and metabolism: Protein can stimulate your metabolic rate between 30 percent and 70 percent. Others (cabbage, cassava, apricots, soy) can inhibit glands such as the thyroid.

Among glands presumed dominant in slow oxidizers, the gastrointestinal tract consists of everything from salivary glands to cells lining the stomach and intestines and the bulk of the pancreas, to the bile delivery system. There will be little argument if we state that the action of the parasympathetic nerves is to stimulate the gut and associated glands and organs, just as surely as epinephrine from the adrenal medulla will inhibit these same organs and glands. You can't concentrate your blood and energy in the abdomen digesting a meal when you need that blood and energy in the heart and muscles to resist a mugger.

While the main bulk of the pancreas can be thought of as a component of the digestive system, it is confusing to list it as characteristic of either slow or fast oxidizers because it has two sets of glandular tissues whose actions oppose one another to achieve the sought after "balance" of blood sugar. One of these patches of endocrine tissue, located in the Islets of Langerhans, secretes insulin. When the pituitary gland detects an increase in blood sugar from something you've eaten it instructs the release of insulin to bring it down to normal. Insulin causes glucose to be gotten out of the blood stream and to be stored in the liver as glycogen. It can also instruct storage of glucose in fat cells as triglycerides and amino acids in muscle as protein. (Gilman *et al.*, 1990.) Just as importantly, insulin blocks the breakdown of glycogen as well as inhibiting its antagonist glucagon. Glucagon is secreted by another group of Islet cells in the pancreas, either signaled by a drop in blood sugar or by the sympathetic nerves. Amino acids in the blood can also stimulate the release of glucagon. Apparently too much protein will also increase insulin levels, which is one reason it is recommended to eat some protein at each meal, not all at one meal. High intensity exercise can also increase glucagon, as well as reduce insulin, thus exhausting all the stored glucose and, again, glucose levels must be maintained at all costs.

As you will read in the chapter of William Wolcott, the interplay and balance of the autonomic nervous system and the relevant endocrine glands is important in metabolic typing. The following two paragraphs, partly fact and partly presumption, suggests how the autonomic system can influence the endocrine system.

If overly active, your sympathetic nerves can suppress digestion and assimilation and can accelerate cellular metabolism by stimulating the thyroid and adrenal glands. This double whammy may cause you to run out of gas. You may need, or crave, carbohydrates, foods that are easily converted to energy, not the slowly-digesting proteins and fats. Theoretically, ancestors in the warm tropics may have adapted to more carbohydrates and less protein.

If, on the other hand, your parasympathetic nerves are over active, digestion and assimilation are augmented. Proteins and fats are adequately processed to provide sufficient energy. Presumably, less stimulation by the thyroid and adrenals is necessary. As one theory goes, your ancestors may have come from colder climates. Certainly, cold weather stimulates the endocrine glands to speed up metabolism. Fast-digesting carbohydrates are hard-pressed to supply the long-term energy flow demanded by cold weather, nor can they compete with fats that yield twice as many calories per gram. In fact, adult Eskimos do very well without any appreciable source of carbohydrates.

While on the subject of energy, glucagon and insulin, you might be interested to know that an understanding of their action is absolutely essential to appreciating the popular Zonal Diet of Barry Sears (1995). According to Sears, glucagon (and EPA) are vital to the proper release of energy from the cellular machinery. In the all-important Krebs or citric acid cycle, glucagon inhibits a vital enzyme (Delta 5 Desaturase), which converts a fatty acid (a form of gamma linolenic acid or GLA) into the infamous and, in quantity, undesirable arachidonic acid (which leads to the "bad" eicosanoid hormones). Glucagon's antagonist insulin, on the other hand, appears to encourage or activate this potentially dangerous biochemical pathway, and this is where blood sugar needs to be balanced by the interplay of these two hormones, glucagon and insulin. This is another reason for learning your metabolic type, so that you can consume the appropriate amount of carbohydrates, thus avoiding a big dose of insulin, which drops your blood sugar so that you grab something sweet to feel good again. Thus, if you feast on carbohydrate-rich foods, snacks and soft drinks all day after you have stored all the sugar you can in the liver and muscle cells, the rest will go to adipose (fat) tissue. At the same time, since insulin inhibits glucagon, the body can't draw on that glucose from the liver and muscle cells already filled to the brim from your previous meals. This can be a vicious and deadly cycle. If you have a strong constitution you just get fatter and fatter. If you have a genetic weakness or for some reason have damaged your organs or glands, the stage is set for a host of degenerative diseases.

Sears (1995) has contributed to the concept of individualized biochemistry. He found that the fatty acid ratios (GLA/EPA) had to be constantly adjusted for each individual. This led him to emphasize the concept that food is the best thing to normalize and balance the metabolism because it can precisely control the production of both insulin and glucagon. Thus it is the best and most economical route to health. Sears was also impressed with the fact that, in his experience, women on their low-fat-high-carbohydrate diets with their perpetual quest for weight control, needed more and more Omega-3 oils and less and less GLA (Gamma linolenic acid). He found that the indiscriminate self-dosing of nutrients including fatty acids, vitamins and minerals, was often counter-productive; food was the way to go. In other words, "Never let the tail wag the dog," as he puts it.

While he doesn't discuss distinct metabolic types Sears does concede that individuals differ greatly in their metabolism. He indicated (1995) that only 25 percent of people were adapted to high density carbohydrates while another 25 percent get a "very elevated insulin response" to such foods, the balance of us lying in between. In a later work (1999), he reiterated this difference; some people might tolerate 60 percent carbohydrates without consequence.

We can be grateful to Sears for elucidating the metabolism of essential fatty acids, especially omega-6, beginning with linoleic acid (found in almost all foods), carried around the body by LDL (Low density lipoprotein) and converted by a key enzyme to the important activated fatty acid GLA (gamma linolenic acid), rarely found in foods (except oatmeal, cooked, not instant, three to five times per week). The impact of the human environment on this critical fatty acid can be summarized: It's production (from linoleic acid) is reduced by too much sugar, too much Omega-3 oils, and trans-fatty acids (as in products containing partially hydrogenated vegetable oils). It is also suppressed by viral diseases and stress. Stress does its damage by elevating adrenalin and/or by raising cortisol (which raises insulin and depresses glucagon). Last but not least, GLA production is depressed by aging, especially past the age of thirty. The ability to make "good" eicosanoids (and PGE 1 prostaglandins) at age sixty-five is one-third that at age twenty-five.

Since insulin inhibits the burning of fats, many overweight people with consistently high levels of circulating insulin keep storing carbohydrates as fat and, unless they drastically reduce their intake of sugars and starches, the insulin levels will always stay high. Atkins (1998) calls these people "keto-resistant" because they don't have ketone bodies in their blood, which are released when the body uses stored fat. Atkins cites research that indicates that some tissues, such as the brain, actually prefer ketone bodies over glucose as a fuel source. Apparently, you need about two days without any carbohydrate intake to start burning your fat stores in abdomen, thighs, buttocks or wherever.

Increased insulin and cortisol are responsible for most of the ill effects of eating excessive amounts of grain-derived processed carbohydrates (cereals, breads, pasta), fruits, fruit juices and other sources of sugar. Sears (1999) is credited with saying that insulin is our "passport to accelerated aging." Elsewhere, cortisol has been called the "death hormone."

It appears that the hormone serotonin may control and balance the type of foods we eat. According to Ross (1987) a high protein-low carbohydrate diet lowers serotonin and produces a desire for carbohydrates while a low protein-high carbohydrate diet increases serotonin and elicits a "craving" for protein.

Regarding appetite in general, it is unfortunate that the "on" switch is far more sensitive than the "off" switch. (Harris, 1987.) Three million years of natural selection has resulted in humans who could store fat to survive periods of starvation. Now, with periodic starvation no longer a threat, this attribute becomes a contemporary defect in the human genome. In the meantime our weak shut-off system is a standing invitation to the food industry to manipulate aversions and preferences regardless of their damage to our health. (Harris, 1987.)

Quantity of Food: What's All This About "Calorie Restriction?"

How much you eat of certain foods is as important as what types of food you eat. When I studied nutrition at Cornell University in the 1950s, I was impressed by the research of Clive McCay published with the title "the thin rats bury the fat rats." This was apparently the first research that showed that calorie-restricted animals outlived their cagemates that ate all they wanted. Most of the experiments on calorie restriction has been done with mice in the laboratory. One dramatic human experiment has been conducted. In the famed Biosphere II experiment (September 1991 to September 1993), Roy Walford, gerontologist and expert authority on calorie restriction, was one of eight individuals who locked themselves in this giant terrarium. On a very nutrient-rich and fiber-rich diet of 1,800 calories per day (western diet has 2,360) the eight people lost from fourteen to fifty pounds in six months, with body fat declining to 6 to 10 percent in males and 10 to 15 percent in females. The average 148-pound man dropped to an average 126 pounds. The Walfords made two statements regarding individual variation: one 120-pound woman may need 1,800 calories per day to maintain "normal" weight, another 2,400; and "naturally thin people tend to be 'burners', i.e., they burn off excess calorie intake as waste heat." Individual variation in the eight Biospherians was not discussed *per se,* but the changes in certain physiological parameters were detailed. The Walfords made significant statements about dietary variability: "There is no exactitude in the realm of human nutrition" and "Diet programs that pretend to allow you to estimate your basal calorie needs . . . , then to add the amount of calories expended in different types of exercise," are misguided. (Walford and Walford, 1994.)

The Sear's Zonal Diet, also known as a 40-30-30 (40 percent carbohydrate, 30 percent each of fats and proteins) has a number of devotees. Personally I have followed it rigorously for two years since I appear to be somewhere in the mid-range metabolically speaking. The Zonal Diet has a lot going for it and is based on sound physiological principles, but it is apparently not for everyone, especially those true slow and fast oxidizers. Even thin people may lose weight. Sears himself (1995, p. 201) admits that the caloric intake of the zone-favorable diet (800 to 1,200 calories for the average person) is close to that of "classic dietary-restriction experiments."

Low-calorie diets may do more than cause weight loss. Watson cites (1972, p.15) a six-month study of thirty volunteers, psychologically normal males at the University of Minnesota. Their semi-starvation diet permitted 1,600 calories daily, mainly carbohydrates but including fifty grams protein and thirty grams fat daily. The group as a whole showed marked neurotic and psychotic personality changes, some so disturbed that they "inflicted physical damage on themselves."

As said elsewhere, the most sensitive and personal arenas of human behavior seem to deal with sex or food preferences. We have to be highly motivated to change either. It would seem that those who make any drastic change in their diet are either health nuts, elite athletes who would do anything to win, or terminally ill patients. Fear of AIDS certainly drastically modified the sexual behavior of many individuals, perhaps fear of disease and premature aging will enable others of us to adopt a deprivation diet—eliminating some delicious and easily obtainable foods to which we have unfortunately grown addicted. It isn't easy, but the alternative is worse.

Supplements and Body Balance

Let's delve briefly into how supplements are involved in balancing body chemistry, choosing minerals as an example, largely from Watts (1990, 1993, 1994, 1995). Figure 62 summarizes the unhealthy effects of ingesting too much of various vitamins and minerals. How do we handle this in everyday life? Well, just to pick a few examples, how do you get too high levels of iron? You could get it from your drinking water, that favorite iron pot you cook in or from too much red wine (white wine is low in iron). Or you can kill two birds with one stone and drink beer, white wine and eat shellfish, all low in iron and high in copper. Getting more copper lowers your iron levels. You could supplement with copper but risk lowering your zinc to reduce copper. You could cut your intake of vitamin C, or you could increase zinc intake. But, watch out, you don't want to tamper with the zinc-copper ratio (ideally 8:1) because too much copper cuts your zinc. Remember some ninety-plus enzymes are zinc-dependent.

You've got common minerals in fairly large quantities (calcium, magnesium, sodium, potassium, phosphorus) and minerals in tiny amounts (trace minerals) such as zinc, molybdenum, copper and chromium. It is common knowledge that the vast majority of the elements in our bodies are metals, probably having originated in the explosions of super-novae and, furthermore, hold key positions in enzymes without which life would not be possible.

It is impressive that a single metallic mineral, magnesium, recommended by Sherry Rogers, M.D., has been known to relieve muscle spasms of the lower back so severe that patients are often unable to proceed to the bathroom under their own power.[17] (We get only 40 percent of enough magnesium in the average American diet. In addition, anti-hypertensive drugs accelerate its loss).

Metals like calcium are used to build bones: trace minerals don't build anything you can see but build molecules, usually enzymes. Enzymes cause every body function to happen. Without them, cells and tissue would be lifeless blobs. Molecules containing trace elements (and to some extent vitamins) are actually in control of our life functions. The metals are in charge. Zinc is necessary in over 100 enzymes. You can't smell without zinc nor conduct credible sex. It is to researchers such as Watts that we owe so much for trying to make sense out of the absolutely bewildering interactions between minerals, vitamins and glandular secretions.

So it's risky business rushing out to buy more of this or that vitamin or mineral in hopes that where a little is good, more will be better. How in the world do the multivitamin-mineral companies figure out just the right proportions? The truth is they can't, especially for you. They can put out a *general* dose of each for the "average" person. Problem is, you may not be average. Happily, we may be able to get you into some metabolic type where the basic foods and supplements your own body needs can be supplied.

We all make changes in our life styles, in eating and in taking supplements. It is for this reason that organizations who determine your metabolism suggest periodic re-testing.

Even with outside tests and assistance, we are the only ones who can fine-tune our own body chemistry. Unlike animals, we cannot analyze our food and drink with our noses and mouths. In an experiment, dogs chose water to drink from a water dish containing a piece of copper tubing, over a dish with just plain water. (Coleby, 1997.)

---

[17] Magnesium chloride solution (18%), 1 tsp. 4 times a day with 8 oz. water plus one capsule (20 mg) of manganese picolinate each day. The only place I've found the magnesium solution is N.E.E.D.S. (1-800-634-1380). Rogers suggests also a trial avoidance of nightshade family plants (potato, tomato, pepper, eggplant, tobacco).

Not long ago, I began having severe night cramps in my calf muscles. I adjusted calcium and magnesium levels back and forth without results. Then, on a long trip, having forgotten to bring enough extra calcium, I tried to buy some in a local drugstore to augment my supplement routine. I could not find any that did not contain vitamin D, so I bought some and took it, along with the 400 units of vitamin D that it contained. Like magic, my leg cramps disappeared. The 100 units of vitamin D in my excellent supplement formula was simply not enough. While this is anecdotal, it is an example of fine-tuning one's metabolism.

Most of the writers in the field agree that there can be no one protocol of vitamins and minerals that will keep everyone healthy. Do not, however, toss your pet formula in the wastebasket yet. You might be just one of those lucky middle-of-the-roaders with a beautifully balanced metabolism, a stunning genetic gift of nature, because it will permit you to eat almost anything you want and be healthy, and almost any concoction of supplements will work for you. Unfortunately, the gene-mixings from our ancestral heritage in Eurasia coupled with the results of our proud and fabled ethnic melting pot here in the United States have blurred nice, distinctive metabolisms we may have evolved when we dwelt apart for so long in remote portions of the northern hemisphere. You can join me in wishing that there was some pill or magic bullet that we could swallow and go on eating just like we love to do.

These complex interrelationships of autonomic nerves, endocrine glands and foods and the substances therein (like vitamins and minerals) makes a clear picture of your individual metabolism difficult or impossible for the layman and most orthodox physicians to determine. There are, happily, certain tests that can help us establish our biochemical individuality. You can do this, of course, by using trial and error eating and supplementing, along with perceptive judging of how you "feel." But most of us do not live in a controlled environment, and are constantly exposed to different foods, fluids and stresses and often forget to take our supplement pills. So yes, to put your mind at rest, there is a way out of all of this. Otherwise, you must constantly guard against the many pitfalls and traps laid for you in almost everything you read and hear. "Just take this or that and you will feel like a new person." So off you go down the same old road with the same old lifestyle eating the same foods and goodies, traipsing the same supermarket aisle and making the same visits to your doctor and dentist.

It will be helpful to review the research and writings of those who have contributed to trying to make sense out of the complexity of our individual biochemistries. The brief discussions that follow are roughly in chronological order.

CHAPTER FOURTEEN

The Father of Biological Individuality

Roger Williams, Ph.D.

Regarded as the father of biochemical individuality, Roger Williams, a noted biochemist at the University of Texas (1940-1963), did research that discovered pantothenic acid. He also gave folic acid its name. In 1956 he established the "Genetotrophic Principle," which stated that: "Every individual organism that has a distinctive genetic background has distinctive nutritional needs which must be met for optimal well-being."

A personal nutrition is founded on biochemical individuality. It can hardly be divorced from inherited variations in body parts, organs, and glands. It is instructive to briefly review the tremen dous variability of the human organism. This is partly because we are indiscriminate breeders, mating across all ethnic, cultural and racial boundaries and organizing into highly mobile groups that can sweep across continents and oceans. Other mammals are much less variable, partly because they are rigid conformists when it comes to what they eat, selecting only what nature offers in their particular niche within the natural world. Yet, surprisingly, as Williams points out, at least in rabbits, rats and cows, there is remarkable biochemical individuality concealed under their look-alike furry coats and facial features.

Hippocrates spoke of man as infinitely variable. (Grey, 1941.) Differences in appearance of the various divisions of the human race, based on skin color, body form and proportions, height, weight and the distribution of fat storage depots such as the protruding buttocks of the African Bushman (steatopygia), have long been recognized. Differences in internal organ composition, size and function have been less obvious, especially when dealing with the ethnic and cultural mix of Europe and the Americas.

Just to take one organ group as an example, as early as 1885, an English surgeon, Frederich Traves (F.R.C.S.), measured human intestinal lengths from fresh cadavers and found that the longest small intestine in males (31.10 feet) was more than double that of the shortest (15.5 feet). (Females varied by only a third). The shortest and longest colons in both sexes were 3.3 and 6.5 feet, again the longest being twice the length of the shortest. These measurements were independent of age, height or weight. It is tempting to speculate on how this affected the ability of these individuals to digest salad or meats, since it is obvious that vegetarian rabbits have enormously long guts, while carnivorous cats have extremely short ones.

It remained for Roger Williams to document the relatively huge anatomical variations in other human organ sizes and shapes. He determined (1956) that some human stomachs could hold six to eight times the volume of others and that stomachs varied more in size and shape than mouths or noses. He noted that "normal" features of human anatomy were copied from one textbook to another, but probably applied to only 15 percent of the population. Such differences extend to glandular tissue. For example, the insulin-secreting tissues of the cells of the pancreas (Islets of Langerhans) he found to vary from 200,000 to 2,500,000 per individual. Relating this anatomical variation to function (physiology), he stated that those individuals with islet tissue less than 0.9 percent of pancreatic tissue were liable to be diabetics; those with 3.5 percent of their pancreas devoted to the secretive islets were likely to have too much insulin (hyperinsulinism). He said (1956, p. 95) that: "Each individual, normal or not, it appears, must have a distinctive endocrine pattern which is based upon the anatomical and physiological potentialities of each gland and the intricate balances which exist between the different endocrine agents."

Williams went on to say that the acceptance and understanding of individual variation was the only way to avoid prejudice, racial or otherwise. The tremendous factual variability within individuals precludes lumping people into categories. Equally as disturbing to him was the acceptance of a "Pollyanna doctrine of human uniformity." He considered that the pressure to "conform," as relates to students in the academic world or workers in the business world, was a deadly aspect of the fallacious idea that everybody is so similar that you can demand uniform behavior. Williams expressed this when he said that: "The vague idea that almost anyone can do almost anything" has brought devastation to millions of lives. The only failures, Williams noted, were those who did not take advantage of their inborn capabilities. Williams moved from discussing the fact that one person's frontal sinus may have twenty times the volume of another's, to detailing the very large variation in biochemical physiology, such as dealing with the endocrine gland secretions.

Williams considered that peoples of extreme eastern Asia and Japan may have been genetically selected to be healthy with a low calcium intake. One bottom line of his work was the recognition that all of us can't eat the same things and be healthy, either racially or locally. He alluded to the 2,000-year old wisdom of the Roman Lucretius who wrote "What is food for one man may be fierce poison to others." Because of man's innate variability, Williams brought to our attention an idea apparently originating with an English physician, Perry of Bath (quoted by Sir William Osler) that one must treat the patient that has the disease rather than the disease that has the patient. William Kelley, Harold Kristal, William Wolcott, and others have carried this battle cry forward.

CHAPTER FIFTEEN

Are You Lashing Your Tired Adrenals?

Henry Bieler, M.D.

"Modern man ends up a vitamin-taking, anti-acid consuming, barbiturate-sedated, aspirin-alleviated, Benzedrine-stimulated, psychosomatically-diseased, surgically despoiled animal: nature's highest product turns out to be a fatigued, peptic-ulcerated, tense, headachy, over-stimulated, neurotic, tonsil-less creature."

—Herbert Ratner

The work of Henry Bieler (1965) has impressed many in the field of individualized nutrition. Abravanel and King (1985) acknowledged his influence on their approach to the subject. Bieler was a modern day disciple who followed Hippocrates' admonition: "Thy food shall be thy remedy." He was convinced that, given adequate raw, natural materials, the primitive instinct of animals allows their bodies to repair themselves. This *vis medicatrix naturae* is at the root of all healing arts, ancient as life itself. "Why," Bieler asks, "have we forgotten it?"

Reviewing the statistics, like the fact that 40 percent of young men were unfit for military service in World War II, Bieler eventually concluded that "A truly healthy person is as rare as a pearl in a barrel of oysters." Americans, he said, have no concept of normal good health since they have never known it. He concluded that food eaten today (in the 1950s and 1960s) "is about as far removed from the natural diet of man as man is from his primitive jungle." But, he emphasized, man still has the same digestive apparatus and liver as his remote ancestors. He often made reference to our "cave man liver."

Bieler concentrated on the endocrine glands and the chemistry of food and metabolism. After fifty years of experience in this arena he still considered himself a student and never lost an insatiable curiosity about the role nutrition played in the health of the human organism. However, before he began his studies in nutrition and the chemistry of the endocrine system, he ate atrociously and heavily used salt as a stimulus to "lash his tired adrenals" and eventually had a health crisis himself. He said that: "Lunch and dinner were incomplete without a heavy dessert and a quart of milk. . . ." Bieler was thus aware of our obsession with food from the cradle to the grave and the "tenacity" of food habits. When he changed his own diet, his medical colleagues whispered that "Bieler is starving himself to death, he is going crazy." A year or so later he stopped using medicines entirely in his practice and began to get better results through altering the chemistry of foods and glands.

He was so successful that he was appointed to the Tilden-Weger-Bieler Chair of Dietetic Medicine at Columbia University's Goldwater Memorial Hospital. He remarks that many of his medical colleagues lost interest in the growing science of endocrinology when adrenal and thyroid extracts failed to compensate for weakened glands. Humorously he recounted Osler's statement that we live on a quarter of what we swallow and doctors live off the other three-quarters.

While changes in growth and temperament resulted from the over stimulation of endocrine glands, to Bieler the most important finding was that one could predict and understand the cause and progress of many diseases with symptoms arising from glandular-controlled avenues dealing with the elimination of toxins. Bieler believed that most illness is an attempt to rid the body of toxic matter, whether from improper or incompletely digested proteins or other more obvious sources, i.e., disease is evidence of an unnatural elimination process. Bieler soon discovered that the treatment of many afflictions could be accomplished by simply giving the body R & R either by abstaining from food or abstaining from foods creating patterns of toxicity. The science of endocrinology paved the way for Bieler to classify individuals into three classic gland types: Adrenal, thyroid and pituitary (Figures 36 and 37). Most of us, Bieler noted, are a combination of all three, but, he states, one type is always dominant.

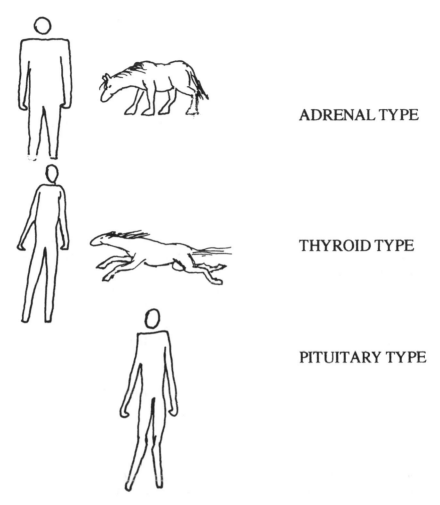

ADRENAL TYPE

THYROID TYPE

PITUITARY TYPE

Figure 36. Bieler's metabolic types. Bieler's adrenal "draft horse" types often have a "hairy ape" appearance. With boundless physical energy, they are the "bubbas" of the world and the "working men" of our society. The "race horse" thyroid types have high sensory development; often dissatisfied with everything and everybody, they may be society's movers and shakers. The often flat-footed and knock-kneed pituitary types contribute creative and artistic efforts to society, but can wind up thin, brooding and dour.

ADRENAL TYPE: Adrenal glands determine whether oxidative "fires" will burn or not. Draft horse type. Perfect oxidation of phosphorus in nervous system and carbon in muscles. Often a "hairy ape" appearance. Palate low, arched and wide. Body parts large, wide, stubby or thick (bones, shoulders, waist, ear lobes, skin, genitals). Peristalsis rapid, body temperature above 98.8, physical energy seemingly inexhaustible, with great endurance. I.Q. usually in lower range (the "bubbas" of the world), predominantly peasant-worker and unskilled labor types. Typical gland function ratio: P50, T25, A100.

THYROID TYPE: Thyroid glands determine how fast the oxidative "fires" burn. Race horse type. Burns food too fast, increased secretion by salivary and other glands, including liver, kidney and sweat glands. Palate V-shaped, steeply arched. Heart rate above seventy-two. High strung, senses highly developed, always listening, watching, smelling. Frequently fatigued, often dissatisfied with surroundings, home, friends, etc. Several streams of thought swirl through brain; dreams a lot. Seldom hungry for breakfast (toxic bile hangover). May eat lightly, usually stays thin. Afflicted with gas, constipation and champion night sweats. Sexual sensations exquisitely developed. Typical gland function ratio: P75, T100, A50.

PITUITARY TYPE: Research on this type limited in Bieler's day. Bieler's most conjectural type. Central incisors large, head large, upper lip longer, joints lax, knock knees and flat feet common; legs and arms may be long. Over-secretion creates giants; under-secretion, dwarfs. Rich in "soul" qualities, very creative and artistic. Has strong sex drive. Can wind up thin, brooding and dour. Typical gland function ratio: P100, T75, A25.

Figure 37.   Bieler's types.

Well-rounded individuals cannot be easily classified under a specific glandular type, according to Bieler. While his techniques for determining metabolic type in such cases are not entirely clear, Bieler states that "there is a method for deciding which gland is truly dominant." If 100 is the normal value of any gland, then the "normal" individual would have the equation: pituitary

100, thyroid 100, adrenals 100. A pituitary type deficient in either thyroid or adrenals might be: P150, T50, A100 and be a "lazy, impractical dreamer." But, Bieler says, if we find this formula: P150, T100, A50, we have an individual known as a genius. Because of his subnormal adrenals, he must constantly stimulate them by the use of meat, coffee, tea, salt, alcohol, or even narcotic drugs. After thus lashing his adrenals he would read P200, T150, A100. The result would be some masterpiece of creativity—a symphony, poem, painting, sculpture or heroic literature, but almost invariably followed by depression up to and including a truly suicidal state. Without these non-creative periods of depression, Bieler states that the adrenals of this genius would become exhausted, resulting in a "tragic, too early death. . . ."

The thyroid type (P75, T100, A50) with impaired pituitary and adrenals would have exaggerated thyroid characteristics, so that the person is high strung, "wired," nervous, and changes his mind (and doctor) frequently. This type can be alarmingly gaunt and may be accused of anorexic behavior.

The pituitary type (P100, T75, A25) is apparently a trial for the physician. Depleted adrenals "give him his characteristic weakness, cold hands and feet, poor digestion and constipation." His over stimulated pituitary makes him brood a lot about his occupation, wondering and speculating endlessly. His inordinate craving for coffee, alcohol or narcotics is serious and his inexhaustible sexual energy constitutes an added drain on his weak adrenals as well as a problem for the "target of his lascivious barrage."

Bieler's studies in both the United States and Europe pointed to the importance of the liver, an organ that excretes wastes through the bile (via the gall bladder and bile duct into the duodenum or small intestine). It is thus a major player in the body's defense against disease. That idea was later echoed by Max Gerson and William Kelley when they emphasized that the first step in curing cancer was to restore normal liver function. At this point, it may be profitable to review some of the interactions of the liver, kidneys and endocrine glands, any of which may be impacted by the products from overcooked, improper proteins, toxic metals, excess salt and drugs. (The latter ought to be called "drug-drugs" in contrast to "food-drugs.") When the liver fails as a blood filter, toxic material, detected by the pituitary gland, stimulates the endocrine glands, the "third line of defense against disease," to over activity. This leads to all manner of problems. If the thyroid gland goes into overdrive, for example, it may force toxins out through the serous membranes of the lungs or abdominal cavity in what Bieler calls "vicarious elimination of toxins." If the adrenals were strong, the kidneys and bowel would handle the elimination of toxins, but if they are weak, or the thyroid is over-secreting, the body may try to eliminate elsewhere such as the lungs, and as Bieler says, the lungs make poor kidneys. Then there is the question of too much pressure on the kidneys. The chemical process of filtration of toxins through the kidneys depends on the degree of oxidation and, under duress, according to Bieler, the kidneys can be forced into the function of vicarious elimination to the point of destroying themselves and/or elevating the blood pressure dangerously. The adrenal cortex, Bieler notes, controls oxidation of phosphorus in nervous tissue and carbon in the muscles, as well as in the liver, kidney and body cells. Our civilized diet, he states, has put extra work on the adrenals to facilitate waste elimination from the kidney, both of which can themselves be exhausted and shorten life.

For those who would try to "flush out" toxins via the kidney by drinking a lot of water, Bieler has a cautionary caveat. He states that in 30 minutes following excessive water intake, toxins no longer appear in the sweat or the urine. This, he explains, is because toxins in the blood are always at a fairly low level, and it just takes time to rid the body of them. He advises that a "small daily increase" places less load on the heart and does the job better than the copious swilling of glass after glass of water. The colon, incidentally, appears to absorb water only in the amount needed. This suggests that enemas would be the ideal way to augment body fluids. I suspect, however, that there will be no rush to the drug store to purchase enema bags for this purpose.

Since the liver appears to be so vitally important and must be "got right" before the endocrine glands will coordinate their effects: the primary step towards health, according to Bieler, is to take the dietary burden off the liver, which then restores the balance between the pituitary, thyroid, and adrenal glands. The first practical step would be to stop ingesting "ordinary" foods heavy with proteins, sugars, starches, and fats. Bieler's "therapeutic antidotes" are water, diluted fruit juices, dilute vegetable soups and dilute raw vegetable juices. He advises short fasts while supplying dilute vegetable broths and soups of non-starchy vegetables. Incidentally, Bieler says that if no food at all is eaten it will take the following times to clean out the body's toxins: bowel (with physic or enema) fourteen hours; blood, three days; liver, five days. As the patient improves one may include lightly cooked meats (rare lamb, rare lean beef) balanced with generous amounts of raw and cooked non-starchy vegetables *at the same meal.* Bieler repeatedly admonished against overcooking meats, stating that raw meat (unlike cooked meat) forms no putrefactive acids in the urine and (unlike cooked meat) is a hydrophilic (water-soluble) protein similar to raw egg whites. Both cooked egg white and meat become hydrophobic (water insoluble) colloidal proteins. Bieler emphasizes that cooked protein impairs the liver. He cites Stefannson's experiments with young Caucasians taken to the Arctic and fed only on raw meat, even stating that, remarkably, they had no problems with elimination on what is presumed to be a fiberless diet. One is reminded here of the efficacy of the macrobiotic diet for some individuals. Bieler was big on potassium-rich vegetables such as celery, parsley, zucchini, leafy greens and string beans, liquefied in a blender and used as a soup. He was emphatic in insisting that only one type of protein be given at a single meal (i.e., don't mix dairy with meat or fish). He was equally adamant about the dangers of our treated (pasteurized and homogenized) dairy products. He also had a thing against ice cream and salt.

In his emphasis on eating healthy, natural foods like unadulterated meats, marrow, brains, fats, raw eggs and raw milk from animal sources and beans, nuts, seeds, avocado and coconut from the plant kingdom, Bieler was ahead of his time. As we can see from the writings of Gittleman, Fallon and Enig, we are just now getting around to his recommendations.

CHAPTER SIXTEEN

33,000 Cancer Patients Can't be Wrong

William Donald Kelley, D.D.S.

In 1967, William Donald Kelley published an approach to curing cancer. During the course of the work he developed what became known as the "Kelley metabolic paradigm" which related individual metabolisms to the autonomic nervous system. (Kelley, 1977, 1999.) Kelley was one of the earliest practitioners to treat people based on their individual metabolic needs, treating the patient who has the disease rather than the disease that has the patient. When an interviewer (Healthview,1977) asked Kelley why so many of their readers asked, "I'm eating the best foods, taking the right supplements, and watching my health in general, yet I still feel miserable. Why is this?" Kelley replied: "A person may be following a program of the best foods, the best supplements and plenty of exercise—but how does he or she know that these are the *best* foods for them? How does he or she know those foods are good for them at all?"

Assuming he began about 1955, by 1977 he had treated over 10,000 patients from all over the world. The last figure I read was nearer 33,000. Steve McQueen is perhaps his best-known cancer patient. (McQueen apparently died of surgical complications). Nick Gonzalez, reporting to Robert Good, M.D. of the Medical Research Foundation, who investigated Kelley's claims, found a survival rate of 93 percent among 139 terminal patients he was checking on. Kelley was prosecuted for practicing medicine without a license and is still not recognized in medical circles, though widely respected by many health care practitioners. His work (reprinted in 1977, 1999) is revered by Kristal and Wolcott, and John Lawder wrote to me that he considered Kelley a genius.

While he ran the Nutritional Counseling Service in Dallas, Texas, Kelley apparently required clients to fill out a 3,200-question form. It is claimed that he was one of the first to use a computer to analyze such data. When I took his program in 1986, there were 1,444 questions, 114 of which required laboratory test results. The others addressed individual history, health problems, medications, dietary intake and so on.

Kelley recognized a total of 10 nutritional or metabolic types, which he organized into three groups: vegetarian, meat-eating and balanced metabolizers. (Figures 38 and 39.) Like Rogers did later, Kelley also produced a type of "metabolic cross." (Appendix A.) His horizontal line went from Type I, a strict vegetarian (extreme sympathetic dominant, acid, slow oxidizer) to a Type II carnivore (extreme parasympathetic dominant, alkaline, fast oxidizer). All types on Kelley's vertical axis had balanced autonomic systems but varied in their metabolic efficiency, ranging from Type III (extremely inefficient) to Type X (extremely efficient). Accordingly, types above the horizontal line are efficient, those below, inefficient.

Kelley's theories on the historical development of metabolic types are worth a brief review. He felt man originated as a Type I vegetarian who, on moving to the Mediterranean area, ate more

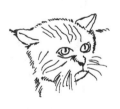   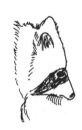   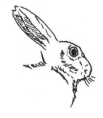

CARNIVORE TYPE
Types II, V, VII

BALANCED TYPE
Types III, VIII, IX, X

VEGETARIAN TYPE
Types I, IV, VI

Figure 38.   Kelley's metabolic types. Type II needs up to fourteen ounces of meat daily (said to be of northern European origin); Type V needs meat only two to three times weekly. Of the vegetarians (herbivores), Type I are strict, Type IV are 60% (Mediterranean types). Of the balanced (omnivore) types, Type VIII has more people than any other category among the three types.

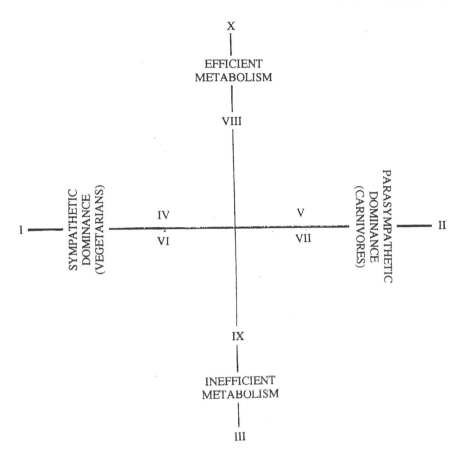

Figure 39. Kelley's "metabolic cross." (Compare with that of Sherry Rogers, Fig. 57). Unlike Rogers, Kelley's vegetarians are acid, his carnivores alkaline. Roger's cross did not deal with the autonomic system. While Kelley's categories I and II are strict as to food, IV and V are nonstrict, and are able to eat a wider variety of foods. Categories VI and VII, however, are poor at metabolizing and assimilating and likely to be sickly. Categories on the vertical axis have perfect autonomic balance but range widely in metabolic efficiency. Category VIII has the most people and these can do well on supermarket and even fast foods. (Modified from Kelley, 1999.)

grains and gradually became Type IV. Climates there were colder and grains were more available, as well as small animals. Type V emerged as civilization moved further north and larger mammals became more important food items. He claims that people who populated India, China and the Pacific had to become Type

IV or stay as Type I because of the available food resources. Types II, V and VII could not survive, because religious sects forbade animal products. He brings out an important point that: "East Indian teachers come to America and think that all Americans should be on vegetarian diets because everyone in their homeland is. " Kelley felt that it would take 8 generations to make any effective genetic changes. His bottom line was that only harm can come from ignoring metabolic type and "basing one's diet on a particular philosophy or religion."

Because of intermarriage between different nationalities, cultures and religions, Kelley realized that in America's melting pot there could be few 100 percent pure metabolic types. He stated that, until the early 1900s our ethnic and cultural groups remained relatively stable and pure but, by the 1940s, the mix of genetic backgrounds had given rise to percentage mixes of metabolic types. By the 1950s, he said, so many infants had been saved by medical science that the incidence of defective types III, VI and VII had become common and their defective genes widespread. By the 1960s, Kelley claims that modern stressful lifestyles and poor nutrition were exhausting even genetically dominant types.

Reviewing thousands of case histories, Kelley was able to say that an individual could change their metabolic type under certain conditions. For example, with sequential exhaustion of sympathetic and parasympathetically enervated glands, a person could change from a Type VI through a Type VII to a Type III, essentially a basket case. If a strong parasympathetic dominant would exhaust his parasympathetic glands, and eventually his sympathetic ones, he could flip through Types VII, VI and into III. Kelley also claims that his system became sophisticated enough so that he could tell what percentage of a person's function was in each of the 10 categories (i.e., Type II-1 percent, Type IV-33 percent, Type VI-11 percent, etc.).

Happily, for those who could not take his detailed program, he offered, as did Wiley (1986), two simple do-it-yourself tests, not infallible but reasonably accurate indicators of your major metabolic group. The first involved swallowing fifty milligrams of niacin on an empty stomach. If your skin turns red in one-half hour and you feel very hot and itchy, you probably have a meat-eating metabolism. If you only feel warmer and have a little facial color, you are probably a balanced individual. If you don't feel anything you are probably a vegetarian. The second test involves taking eight grams of Ascorbic Acid (Vitamin C) for three days in a row. If this makes you feel depressed, lethargic, exhausted and irritable then you are a carnivore. No change and you have a balanced metabolism. If you feel better—more energy, better sleep— then you are likely a vegetarian.

As early as 1986, Tom and Carole Valentine published the first book for the general public specifically devoted to metabolic typing in both text and title. Basically, their well-written book describes Kelley's theories, studies and programs. As a news journalist, Tom Valentine first wrote about Kelley's approach to cancer in 1941 and in 1977 his family enrolled in the Kelley Metabolic Ecology Program. These authors are astute observers and present the details of Kelley's program in understandable language. They describe Kelley's ten metabolic types, as well as his recommendations on eating and cleansing the system of toxins with often controversial methods, such as involve purging and coffee enemas.

Because William Wolcott was Kelley's chief assistant, the Valentines also discuss Wolcott's contributions in a chapter titled "Fast, Slow and Mixed Oxidizers." They describe the consternation among nutritional therapists when Wolcott announced that a small segment of the population can be sympathetic, fast oxidizers or slow-oxidizing parasympathetics, just the opposite of Kelley's findings. The Valentines elucidate the all-important question of acid-base balance: that the oxidation rate (the faster the rate, the more acidic you become) tends to balance a strong autonomic influence (parasympathetic) that tends to make you alkaline. When the oxidation rate is slowed, however, the individual becomes more alkaline with adverse effects. They quote Wolcott: "Whereas the autonomic balance may play a primary role in the existence of the myriad characteristics of the metabolic type, the oxidation rate can enhance, support, overshadow or even negate the autonomic based symptom."

Further, the Valentines related how Kelley used calcium to determine autonomic dominance (calcium is high in slow oxidizing sympathetics, low in fast oxidizing parasympathetics). They cite Wolcott as reporting that calcium works synergistically with magnesium and in opposition to potassium and sodium. Thus calcium levels tend to rise in slow oxidizers while potassium is lowered. Conversely, calcium levels fall with fast oxidation while potassium is elevated. Foods that speed the oxidation rate increase parasympathetic control, thus fruits and vegetables (high in potassium) worsen mineral imbalance of fast oxidizers by lowering calcium and raising potassium. The Valentines recount an interesting anecdote of Wolcott's therapy. A sixty-one-year-old man had called, crying uncontrollably and in a suicidal mood. His dietary program was pushing him towards sympathetic, slow oxidation with a calcium-rich diet that only exacerbated his problems. The quickly assimilated calcium in one-half teaspoon of cream of tarter brought him back to normal within twenty minutes. This incident points out how rapidly the proper nutrients can sometimes work.

Kelley and Wolcott, along with a psychiatrist, John Rhinehart, M.D., studied the social behavior of metabolic types. They contrasted the hard driving, logical and action-oriented sympathetic dominant with the more intuitive "people person" personality of the parasympathetic dominant executive. They went so far as to state that when two parasympathetics meet, as sales manager and purchaser for example, "the sale is virtually assured." At the same time, the logical, left brain dominant sympathetic may find the intuitive, feeling-oriented, right brain dominated parasympathetic intolerable, and the deal is off. These authors also indicated potential conflicts when a school teacher of one dominance deals with a child of another autonomic dominance.

CHAPTER SEVENTEEN

How to Become Mentally Ill on 1,600 Calories

George Watson, Ph.D.

Of the pioneers in the field of individualized nutrition, few can equal the contributions of George Watson who studied, for thirty years, the way body tissue converts food into energy. Since the brain required 25 percent of the body's main energy source, glucose, problems in energy supply rapidly and strongly affect the brain. Watson concentrated on the psychochemical aspects of biochemistry—how feelings and emotions are dramatically influenced by what we eat. He subsequently published (1965) the scientific basis for his psychochemical (metabolic) types.

His first book, *Nutrition and Your Mind* (1972),[18] directed towards the understanding of abnormal behavior, was required reading for pre-medical students and over 500 psychiatric clinics and psychiatrists as a textbook on the biochemical treatment of behavioral disorders. His second book (1979), was based upon research done more with "normal" individuals who, while not particularly ill, just felt "there was something wrong." They didn't feel "up to snuff," as we say, even though their doctors told them that they were in good health. Watson titled his approach "orthonutrition," defined as the optimum amount of the right nutrients at the right time.

---

[18] 1972 book not in print; 1979 available, order #E901, Edom Laboratories, Deer Park, NY 11729. The odor test is also available from Edom.

How Watson first discovered that people could be grouped into metabolically different categories is interesting. On day, on a whim, he tried ingesting a 100 mg tablet of thiamine hydrochloride (vitamin B-1) and found to his surprise that, thirty minutes later, the odor of a crushed thiamine tablet had changed, and at the end of the long work day, he no longer felt as tired. This led him to test a panel of twenty subjects with the same odor. He found to his surprise that they fell into two groups. The Type Is, subsequently known as slow oxidizers, found the odor of thiamine to be featureless at 10 mg but sweet and pleasant at 100 mg, and further, their mood went from low to high. Type IIs (fast oxidizers) found the thiamine odor to be strong, sharp and unpleasant at 10 mg and hardly detectable at 100 mg (except for gassy or prickly sensations), and *their* mood went from feeling good to depression. Two decades of research followed to confirm with high validity (over 90 percent), correlation between blood tests, psychological test scores and patients' improvement. Eventually, about 1961, he devised a kit of six substances, which he called the Psychochemical Odor Test. A look at Figures 34 and 35 will show you where thiamine is "good" for the slow oxidizer and "bad" for the fast. This led Watson to recommend different supplements for each type.

Watson called his metabolic types "psychochemical types" determined by the manner by which the body transforms foods into energy. He eventually recognized four such types: slow, fast, sub and variable oxidizers, each type requiring a different suite of supplements (Figure 40 and Appendix B).

Unlike routine blood tests the odor tests proved to be a reliable means for diagnosis and recommended therapy for psychiatrists and psychologists. These tests, however, reached a limited market. I bought my first in the early 1980s. Other than a short questionnaire, Watson relied principally on the odor test, but supported by blood parameters, especially dissolved carbon dioxide and carbonic acid levels of the blood.

Watson's two major metabolic types, slow (Type I) and fast (Type II) oxidizers describe the rate of oxidation (burning) of sugar in the body. Slow oxidizers don't burn it fast enough or in quantity enough (in either the glycolitic or citric acid (Krebs) cycle), while fast oxidizers burn sugar too fast and in too large amounts. His many years of research documented the effects of

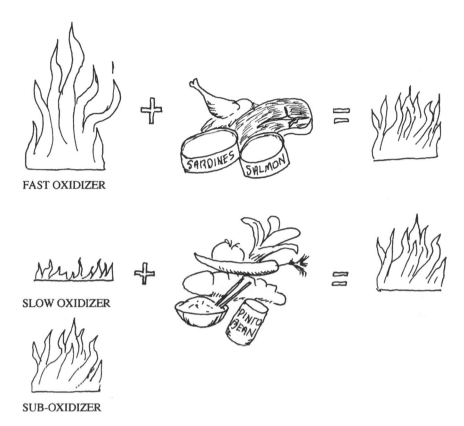

Figure 40. Watson's psychochemical types illustrating the high protein/fat diet needed to normalize the fast oxidizer and the high carbohydrate diet to "speed up" the slow oxidizer. The balanced sub-oxidizer needs, obviously, a "balanced" diet consisting of optimum protein (some high purine forms), whole grain cereals, sufficient fruits and vegetables, and proper supplements.

different foods and supplements on real-life people passing through his office and lab.

Among my friends, several of them, in fact most, seldom eat protein with each meal, especially breakfast. After a skimpy breakfast of a bran muffin and tea, or cereal and coffee, or (horrors) a doughnut and coffee, they invariably run out of steam before lunchtime and keep asking me "when do we eat?" Since they apparently lean towards fast oxidation, I tell them, "well, what do you expect, you didn't have much if any protein for breakfast."

They look at me as if to say: *"this is the way I eat and this is the way I'm going to keep on eating."* One soon discovers that eating is almost as personal as sex and dissecting a friend's diet apparently constitutes invasion of privacy.

It so happens, as Watson explains, that while the body can use only one-half the protein eaten to make glucose (blood sugar), it is the gradual digestion of protein over several hours that keeps a constant supply stored in the liver (as glycogen) to be slowly released all morning long as necessary to keep blood sugar levels stable. Starch, sugar and caffeine, on the other hand, are assimilated, stored and burned too fast to last very long. At the same time, you must, however, eat enough carbohydrate to enable the liver to convert protein into stored sugar (glycogen). Neither fat nor alcohol can substitute for either sugar or protein. As a corollary to this, fat can't burn and yield energy without the burning of *both* carbohydrate (starch or sugar) and protein. Watson grapples briefly with the question of how weight is successfully lost: weight is healthily lost (not to exceed one pound per week) when you maintain a blood sugar level high enough so that you are not always hungry and constantly reaching for some sort of snack or sweet drink. How do you do this? By eating the correct amounts of carbohydrates, proteins and fats so that their total caloric yield is less than you burn. This deficit in calories forces your body to burn fat from your abdominal stores (if you are apple shaped) or from your thighs and hips (if you are pear shaped). What is the correct amount of protein? According to Watson it is approximately one gram for each 2.2 pounds of body weight. Take your ideal weight (NOT what you weigh now) and divide by fifteen. This gives you the ounces of cooked, lean meat you need daily, translating to about three and one-half ounces for each of three meals. Don't eat it all in one meal or you'll be reaching for a cookie or soft drink and defeat yourself. Only slow oxidizers can "get by" with skipping breakfast or with juice and coffee or if they do eat a low-fat, high-starch meal (dry cereal, milk). Obviously, you need to know your metabolic type.

Watson warns against starvation-type diets, especially if unsupervised by a physician. He recounts the story of one middle-aged woman who was so emotionally upset she would get up and iron her bed sheets as many as twenty-five times in one night because she felt a wrinkle. She had put herself on an almost fat-free diet with only one-half the amount of protein she needed.

The consequences of not knowing your nutritional type and thus eating improperly or taking the wrong supplements can apparently cause an astounding array of behavioral symptoms. Most are due to an improper ratio of carbohydrates, proteins and fats that interfere with the cellular machinery of the glycolytic and citric acid cycles. The outcome is a change in the blood sugar level. This one simple event can send you to a psychiatrist or worse. The brain needs that 25 percent of blood sugar produced and provided at a steady level of around 90 to 100 (mg per 100 mL). While physicians are prone to say that your blood sugar is in the "normal" range (65 to 105), Watson found that a low reading of 65 could produce severe anxiety and depression in some individuals and a reading of 105 could cause a slow oxidizer to be depressed to a point of suicide.

Watson concluded that four categories of things adversely affected the body's ability to create energy normally (mediated by the nervous system): 1) inadequate nutrition; 2) chemical interference (drugs, biocides, toxins, infections, allergics; 3) stress; and 4) failure of tissue repair due to lack of sleep. Inadequate nutrition includes suppressing the healthy bacterial "flora" of the bowel, which normally synthesizes such essentials as riboflavin, biotin and vitamin K. Watson stated that mental depression was the first abnormal reaction and that *it was impossible to substitute vitamins by mouth to restore the damaged bacterial community.* He advanced the interesting news that *any* abrupt changes in the environment, such as a climatic cold front, disturbs metabolism adversely, apart from increasing or reducing the pressure of oxygen entering your lungs.

Watson even went so far as to say that your energy levels determine whether you're an introvert or an extrovert. He says that systematically manipulating your food and supplements is the only direct way to determine the best nutrition for you. Missed periods and loss of libido, according to him, involve failure of the body to produce "new" cells due to suboptimal diet.

Regarding mental health, Watson devotes quite a bit of space to the inadequacies of psychotherapy that will not endear him to psychologists. He has watched groups of healthy young volunteers on a diet of 1,600 calories with controlled ratios of carbohydrates, proteins and fats, undergo in six months marked personality changes, both neurotic and psychotic. One of his cases (with a plasma pH of 7.35) was read by her physician as normal. She was a schizophrenic, however, and when her diet was adjusted to yield a pH of 7.45, she no longer had the affliction. Watson followed 300 subjects for five years and by manipulating their diet and supplements obtained an 80 percent improvement rate. He attributed the other 20 percent to possible genetic influences. He stated that schizophrenia, manic depression and anxiety neuroses tell us nothing about the physical state of the patient and lead us to believe that all anxiety problems are biochemically similar. In the absence of a "sniff test" or in conjunction with it, Watson advises a biochemical backup test. He considered the best to be tests for pH, plasma bicarbonate and dissolved oxygen, the best other test being a glucose tolerance test.[19]

He noted that the following variables were affected by his Group 1 or Group 2 supplements: blood glucose, total plasma lipids, cholesterol, plasma pH and related bicarbonate/carbonic acid ratios, urinary and salivary pH, blood pressure and pulse. He found that these two groups of vitamin-mineral combinations could have opposite effects and, surprisingly, he discovered that a large enough dose could "produce symptoms clinically resembling mental illness."

Furthermore, Watson found that energy systems were not always under the control of endocrine glands such as the thyroid, where the net effect is to raise blood sugar. He found few abnormal conditions due to thyroid problems. One severely disturbed patient at the furniture-smashing stage had a pH of 7.55 and very low carbonic acid levels. By giving thiamine and other vitamins, he was able to drop her pH to 7.42 and nearly double the other parameters, immediately normalizing her behavior.

Watson emphasizes the importance of protein quality. Proteins are probably the least known of our nutrients. Most of us know that there are "complete" proteins contained largely in meat, fish, fowl, eggs and dairy products. Vegetarians and slow oxidizers in general need to be especially aware of the amino acid

---

[19] In case you wish to take a lab test: A *slow oxidizer* has a venous plasma pH higher than 7.47 (average about 7.54) and a level of dissolved carbon dioxide and carbonic acid averaging about 0.73 mM/liter, while a *fast oxidizer* has a pH lower than 7.45 (average about 7.36) and a CO/carbonic acid level averaging about 1.27 mM/L. A healthy "normal" adult should have a pH of 7.43, with acid levels of 1.35 mM/L.

content of vegetables so that they can be "combined" so as to provide "complete" protein with all eight essential ones (that cannot be synthesized in the body). This presumes you don't cheat with animal sources like eggs (ovo-vegetarian), eggs and milk (ovo-lacto-vegetarian) or eggs, milk and fish (ovo-lacto-pisco-vegetarian).

Watson makes particular reference to another class of proteins he calls "nucleoproteins." These are the valuable nucleotide bases, adenine, guanine, cytosine, thymine and uracil. The first four comprise the genetic code in DNA. Their availability is critical to one's total personality strength. Watson considers the most important of these bases to be adenine and guanine (called by the chemist "purines"). Elsewhere we discuss "purine-rich" proteins such as herring, mussels and sardines.

The information storage and message conveyance system of cells is made up of various kinds of nucleic acids. As you may be aware, one of these, the famed DNA (deoxyribonucleic acid) in the cell nucleus issues precise instructions as to what kind of cells to make and where to make them. Another nucleic acid such as mRNA (ribonucleic acid, where uracil substitutes for thymine) carries messages from the blueprint DNA throughout the cell.

Unfortunately, the quality of these nucleic acids seems to deteriorate as we age. Along comes Benjamin Frank (M.D., 1975, 1976) credited with bringing to our attention the novel discovery that high quality DNA and RNA can be supplied our cells from outside the body to enable us to stay healthier far longer than expected from the general experience of the human race.

It so happens that the nucleotide bases form the rungs in the spiral staircase of the DNA molecule as well as the links by which RNA copies their sequence (message) by which tasks within the cell are carried out. All this is powered within the citric acid cycle in which a special compound, ATP, loses a phosphate and becomes ADP, which becomes ATP again, over and over. Nucleic acids in the diet apparently increase ATP productivity, which is, of course, the ultimate energy source for running our bodies.[20]

---

[20] According to a table published by Frank, foods with the highest content of nucleic acid (analyzed from RNA) are canned sardines 590, pinto beans 485, lentils 484, chicken liver 402, garbanzo beans 356, fresh sardines 343, black-eyed peas 306, fresh salmon 289. (Frank, 1976.)

Since the nucleic acid content of foods is of great value in the critical citric (Krebs) cycle where the bulk of cellular energy is produced, only with this cycle operating at peak efficiency can you slow down the aging process and combat degenerative diseases. This is the legacy handed down by men like George Watson and his contemporary, Benjamin Frank.

CHAPTER EIGHTEEN

How to Relieve Nervous Tension with Alcohol and Sugar—and Lose Your Teeth

Melvin Page, D.D.S.

"It is store food which has given us store teeth."

—E. A. Hooton

Like his contemporary, Weston Price, Melvin Page (1949, 1954, 1974) was a dentist. Teeth seem to be one of the first things to degenerate from faulty nutrition and remarkable men like Page have been led to try to understand body chemistry because they deal day to day with these visible manifestations of poor nutrition. Page went on to implicate and test the relationship of two minerals important in tooth formation and maintenance, calcium and phosphorus which, he found out, are both influenced by our day to day intake of minerals in our foods. He, like Price, came to reflect on what we must have eaten in our collective past. He titled the many centuries old diet of our fathers "the biologic diet." Later researchers in the field of individual biochemistry owe Page recognition for working out the relationships not only of calcium-phosphorus to our health but in relating these minerals to the two major branches of the autonomic nervous system, which, in turn, signal the endocrine glands.

Over a period of twenty years and 20,000 blood tests later, Page had enough data to make it possible to graph and understand

a patient's calcium-phosphorus balance. From a dentist's stand-
point he could confidently state that the critical point is reached
when the calcium-phosphorus ratio is 8.75:3.5 mg per 100 cc of
blood. Below these amounts for either mineral, calcium or phos-
phorous is withdrawn from the internal substance of teeth and
bones.

Relating a person's ratio with the prevalence of cavities, later
(1974) called the Page Method, represented the degree of efficiency of body function expressed by the calcium-phosphorus ratio
and the amount of sugar in the blood, the ideal ratio being calcium 10 and phosphorus 4 (or 2.5 parts calcium to one part phosphorus) per 100 cc of blood.

Page found that tooth decay varied when normal body metabolism varied, and that this metabolism was controlled by the endocrine glands and the autonomic nervous system. Since the
endocrine secretions control growth he was eventually able to determine that body proportions could be used as a visual cue to an
individual's body chemistry.

To make a long story shorter, he found that he could group
people into two main metabolic types, each dominated by one or
the other of the opposing branches of the autonomic nervous system. He found that sympathetic dominants as he called them,
had greater weight above the waist, while parasympathetic dominants had their weight below the waist. Based upon the relative
proportions between the upper and lower body, Page was able to
determine the extent of endocrine dysfunction. For objectivity, he
devised a series of measurements using a flexible tape and was
able to graph his results for each patient. He measured the lower
leg and lower arm. By dividing the sum of leg measurements by
the sum of those of the arm, he arrived at a ratio for each person.
Interestingly, he discovered that body proportion was in direct
proportion to dental decay. For those fortunate individuals with
perfect metabolism, there was immunity from any dental decay.
He cautioned, however, that for those beyond their twenties, the
measurements indicated past, not present, metabolism and
that some metabolisms could change to the opposite type over a
period of years. A patient in his forties might measure as a
parasympathetic but be a sympathetic dominant and vice versa.
His methodology here, eventually based upon 40,000 measurements, was later (1974) called the "Page Anthropometric Hypothesis," a blueprint for determining from the body type that
one has inherited a certain glandular condition.

Page found that a high phosphorus level in the blood was indicative of an absence of tooth decay and that a low level over a period of months would deplete the mineral structure of tooth dentine. He referred to radiocarbon studies that indicated that fat deposits were subject to constant "turnover" and stated that bones and teeth also gave up and took in calcium and phosphorus continuously even after primary calcification.

At an annual nutrition conference in the early 1980s in Atlanta, I was told that a good dose of sugar would throw your blood chemistry off for twenty-four hours. This was, to me, a shocking revelation. Apparently this was based on Page's work. Page did some human experiments that could make him quite unpopular with the sugar industry. On subjects for whom he had numerous blood tests, he found that nine pieces of chocolate (one-quarter pound) could throw the calcium-phosphorus ratio out of balance within two and one-half hours and "keep them below the margin of safety for immunity to dental decay for at least thirty-two hours." It was even worse than I thought. Page stated that alcohol and sugar addicts were deficient in posterior pituitary secretion and that too little calcium or too much phosphorus brought on nervous tension that was relieved by alcohol and sugar, which raised calcium and lowered phosphorus. Page's therapy involved a low sugar diet and minute doses of glandular extracts to stimulate weak endocrine glands.

Figure 41 and Appendix C summarize Page's two autonomic types: the sympathetic and the parasympathetic dominants, with a brief listing of their relationships to mineral balance and endocrine glands. A suite of the latter is dominant in each type. To Page, sugar, especially refined sugar, was the archvillain, disturbing the calcium-phosphorus balance more than any other single factor, so much so that he could use the blood levels of calcium-phosphorus to indicate your dietary misadventures. I don't know about you, but this work by Page is depressing since I seem to have inherited a "sweet tooth" from my father, and have accordingly lessened my contributions to the Hershey fortune. It is comforting to know, however, that an occasional candy or brownie binge will not destroy your teeth. It is how you eat on a day to day basis that really counts.

Page was aware of the remarkable fieldwork of Weston Price among the earth's people still living bodily and ecologically in the ecosystems of their environment. Page realized that there were two factors that shaped us, heredity and environment, and that food was the chief environmental factor affecting the body's

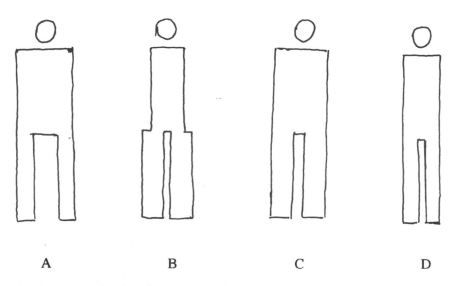

A   B   C   D

Figure 41.   Page's sympathetic dominant (A) (low calcium-high phosphorus) has weight in the upper body. His parasympathetic dominant
(B) (high calcium-low phosphorus) has weight mostly in legs. (Ideal calcium ratio = 2.5:1.) Two normal individuals (C, D) have weight equally
distributed. Page felt that since the endocrine glands control growth,
body proportion was a clue to body chemistry.

glands, hormones, and nervous system. He acknowledged that races
of people had adapted themselves to certain food requirements.

Page distinguished between short-gutted meat and fish eaters
which he called long-headed, blue-eyed Nordics, coastal dwellers
adapted to a larger intake of trace minerals, and the long-gutted,
grain and animal food eaters he called inland mid-Europeans with
dark hair and round heads that required a lesser amount of trace
minerals in their diet. Page recognized the vital effect that minerals (he actually said, "trace minerals") had on the endocrine glands,
which in turn controlled the calcium-phosphorus metabolism.

He stated that the readjustment of our genetic heritage of body
chemistry might take "thousands of generations" and that a general change in food intake in one or two hundred years "partakes of
the nature of a sudden disaster." Through his years of testing he
found that if the patient's immediate ancestors were from Europe
(where he considered nutrition better), the patient's response to
treatment or dietary change was faster than if several generations
in America had interposed themselves in a person's heritage.

CHAPTER NINETEEN

Do You Have a Pot Belly and a Thick Neck?

Elliot Abravanel, M.D.

In the forties and fifties I spent nearly five years knocking about in Japan, the Philippines, Borneo, Southeast Asia and South America. As I went about collecting animals or doing studies of them I was always struck by the uniformity of body size and shape and even facial structure in these various regions of the world. Like most men I suppose I paid more attention to the females, but I seldom saw people who were fat, tall, or "built funny." It is no wonder that our servicemen were so taken with the ladies of the Pacific Rim and Southeast Asia, for the girls were almost always uniformly petite and well formed, usually with small breasts. Couple this with a natural attitude towards bodily functions (including sex) and a superior personal hygiene, the combination was unsettling to say the least. Every time I would return to the United States, I would be astonished anew at the incredible variety of body types, especially among our females.

Pacific Rim diets were both limited and uniform in content. On my treks, I came to positively envy my guides' cuisine as they spread those delectable piles of steaming rice on banana leaves, while I snacked on field rations with stale, hard biscuits. What I didn't realize, of course, was that because of our mixed-up Caucasian heritage, I might not be able to be healthy on the "native" diet, which enabled my companions to work so tirelessly day in and day out.

The obvious physical characteristics of people have intrigued many writers, particularly people like Sheldon (1940) and Price

213

(1948). The effort to make some sense out of the polyglot of body shapes and sizes one sees when walking down the street led to the development of a classification of "body types." We've all looked in the mirror and (in admiration, disgust or just blah) at what we ourselves have been endowed with by Nature.

The next step was to try to relate body types to health or the absence thereof. A principal avenue of investigation seemed to be the metabolic "machinery" controlled by various glands of internal secretion. A breakthrough was to tie obvious physical characteristics to dominant endocrine glands (thyroid, adrenal, etc.) and the food that influenced them. One of the earliest to do this was the respected physician Henry Bieler (M.D.) who in 1965 published a book entitled *Food Is Your Best Medicine.*

Like Gittleman and others, Elliot Abravanel (1983; Abravanel and King, 1985) was inspired by the writings of Bieler. In treating patients who desired to lose weight, Abravanel was struck with the fact that two women patients on an identical diet (in this case high protein, low carbohydrate) reacted oppositely to each other. One lost weight and was full of energy, bright and bushy tailed. The other was not only losing weight but also was hungry, irritable and depressed to boot. Intrigued, he eventually concluded that these two women must have very different metabolisms.

From such experiences Abravanel developed a system which he called "metabolic body types," based on which of the four major endocrine glands was dominant: in men the pituitary, thyroid and adrenal and in women a fourth, the gonads (based on the ovaries) (Figure 42). This was a means of organizing and understanding what an individual knows about his or her own body. It is not difficult to learn Abravanel's system provided you answer some questions honestly and objectively while standing naked (or nearly so) in front of a full-length mirror.

For example, if you look like a candidate for a football squad, have a "beer belly" and a good steak with potatoes is your idea of eating, you are probably what Abravanel calls an "adrenal type." Your metabolism is dominated by the adrenal gland. Not only that, but you'll always try to eat whatever stimulates the adrenal glands so that you can use the hormones produced to "feel good." The key to health, Abravanel says, is to seek a more balanced metabolism by stimulating the other glands, such as by using dairy products to stimulate the pituitary gland. "Tough hombre" A-types may shrink from lapping up a cup of yogurt, but that may be the price of health.

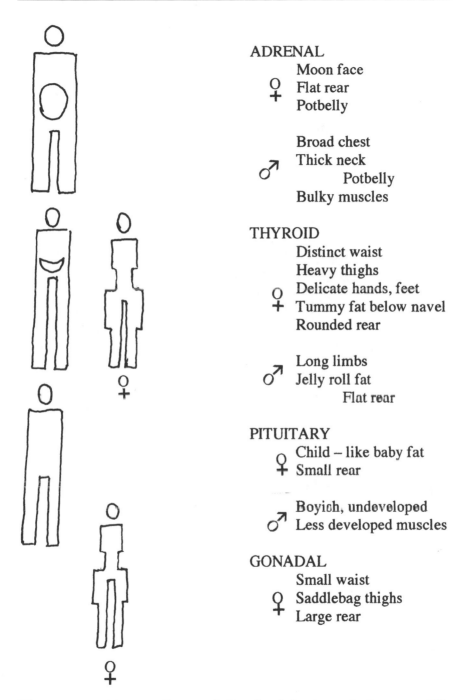

ADRENAL

    Moon face
♀ Flat rear
    Potbelly

    Broad chest
♂ Thick neck
        Potbelly
    Bulky muscles

THYROID

    Distinct waist
    Heavy thighs
♀ Delicate hands, feet
    Tummy fat below navel
    Rounded rear

    Long limbs
♂ Jelly roll fat
        Flat rear

PITUITARY

♀ Child – like baby fat
    Small rear

♂ Boyish, undeveloped
    Less developed muscles

GONADAL

    Small waist
♀ Saddlebag thighs
    Large rear

Figure 42. Abravanel's metabolic gland-dominant body types. His front and profile sketches of glandular body types is much more complementary in the later book (1985) than in the first (1983).

Thyroid types, especially when tired or under stress, want the quick, intense energy flush from consuming sweets, starches and caffeine, when an egg sandwich would stimulate their adrenals and give them steadier energy throughout the afternoon. Meanwhile, the Pituitary type should stimulate his adrenals with a hamburger rather than a pituitary-stimulating milkshake. Abravanel says that a billion Chinese are pituitary types.

Abravanel makes a point also emphasized by Barry Sears (1995) that foods should be considered drugs. As they do with drugs, people become "hooked" on certain foods that stimulate their dominant gland and make them "feel good," even to induce the brain to secrete the morphine-like endorphins, also sought by over-zealous joggers for a "runner's high." The way to break this dependency is to use foods that stimulate your less active glands, in which case food becomes almost a medicine.

Abravanel suggests both foods and supplements for each metabolic type to balance the metabolism. His first book (1983) barely considered supplements necessary; his second (1985) did. He now emphasizes the importance of trace minerals in controlling cravings and in balancing metabolisms. He also recommends various amino acids, glandular substances, exercises, stress reduction and accupressure. In developing his program, he was able to interact with thousands of students at the Skinny School Medical Clinics, weight control centers in southern California. The gist of what he has to say about his metabolic types is listed in Appendix D. Space does not permit listing all recommended supplements; most would be highly repetitive.

CHAPTER TWENTY

Are You a Closet Carnivore?

John Lawder, M.D.

John Lawder (1986) defined three basic biochemical types: fast, slow and mid-oxidizers. (Figure 43 and Appendix E.) The ideal intake ratios for each food type (carbohydrate, protein, fat) were as follows: fast 30-40-30; slow 60-20-20; mid 45-30-25. Lawder considered that everybody's metabolism fell somewhere on a bell-shaped curve, with 70 percent of people being mid-oxidizer omnivores, 15 percent being fast oxidizer carnivores and 15 percent slow oxidizer vegetarians. Only 2 percent, though, he considered to be "true" mid-oxidizers with perfectly balanced metabolisms. Most of us in the 70 percent mid-range would tend towards being somewhat fast or somewhat slow. The lack of clear distinctions, as would be the case for typical fast or slow oxidizers on each end of the bell curve, makes for confusion. How one eats, explained Lawder, also indicates what sort of disease they might have. He stated that for example, most cancers and heart attacks were suffered by mid-oxidizers with metabolisms on the slow side but who ate like fast oxidizers out of ignorance. Conversely, a fast mid-oxidizer eating too many simple carbohydrates would be plagued with weight problems, hypoglycemia, uncontrolled hunger and chronic fatigue.

Lawder considered carnivore types as fast oxidizers who tended to choose, or needed, foods that broke down more slowly, such as proteins or fats. Some of his carnivore types preferred raw ground beef straight from the refrigerator. Fast oxidizers tend to acidosis and apparently are afflicted with hypothyroidism, osteoporosis, calcium imbalance and hypoglycemia (low blood sugar) from the speed of their metabolism and the action of insulin. Fast

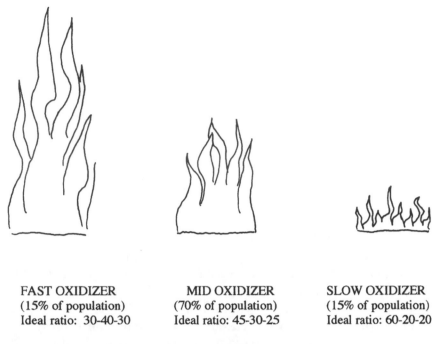

FAST OXIDIZER   MID OXIDIZER   SLOW OXIDIZER
(15% of population)   (70% of population)   (15% of population)
Ideal ratio: 30-40-30 Ideal ratio: 45-30-25 Ideal ratio: 60-20-20

Figure 43. Lawder's metabolic types with the percentage in each type and his "ideal" ratio of carbohydrates, proteins and fats. (Flame height equivalent to speed of oxidation).

oxidizers, he found, needed regular meals, protein-rich breakfasts, and more complex carbohydrates (instead of simple sugars) and should avoid large doses of vitamin C and B complex.

Lawder diverges from others in that he considered fast oxidizers to be under the dominance of the *parasympathetic* branch of the autonomic nervous system. His rationale was that stimuli from the parasympathetic nerves (to organs and glands) caused the gastrointestinal tract to digest and assimilate foods better and more rapidly.

In contrast, he considered the *slow oxidizer* to be sympathetic dominant, processing foods more slowly with reduced motility and stomach acid secretion and so forth. It is true that if you want your dinner to digest you don't leap out and do violent physical exercise or get angry or be stressed in other ways. We know that the body "shuts down" and may cut off the blood supply to systems not immediately needed to face the imminent problem of body motion and activity. Because the slow extraction rate of energy from foods, the slow oxidizer needs to eat a higher proportion of fast-burning foods (carbohydrates). Lawder opined that because of the reduced transit time of food passing through tubes of the digestive tract, the gut was more vulnerable to (have more time) form or absorb deleterious substances such as nitrites and MSG. Because of their poor ability to handle fats, he considered slow oxidizers prone to arteriosclerotic disease from elevated lipid levels and subject to diabetes, hypertension, glaucoma and anemia.

He pointed out that blacks, who are known to be more susceptible to hypertension (high blood pressure), came from a sympathetic-dominant area (African tropics) and are adapted to a diet of predominantly grains, with fruits and vegetables. Their bodies are ill-equipped to handle a large intake of meat. We used to take a black friend on our raccoon hunts. He would make my mouth water all night long talking about that pot of collard greens slowly simmering on the wood stove back home. The so-called "soul foods" may be founded on an underlying physiological need.

Lawder felt that slow oxidizers could forego breakfast and eat a substantial midday meal and a light supper. They would, in contrast with the fast oxidizer, need higher levels of the C and B vitamins.

There are two organizations that will determine your metabolic type by a computer analysis of a detailed questionnaire based upon John Lawder's work. Both seek to create a personalized nutrition program.

The SporTelesis program was initially developed by John Lawder in 1978 and appears quite similar to the one I took from Lawder in 1990. The SporTelesis program is available only through a licensed SporTelesis Fitness and Nutrition Center. If you take the program, they are contractually obligated to sell you the supplements provided by the company.

The Apex Fitness program also modeled after Lawder's work, offers standard and advanced programs but only through local gyms and health clubs. This includes a twelve-week individualized program with advice on exercise and nutrition, with weekly follow-ups. Supplements, exclusively sold by Apex are offered at a 10 percent discount. Following his tenure as Director of Fitness and Nutrition for Gold's Gym, Neal Spruce founded the Apex Fitness Group in 1995. He also holds the position as Director of Nutrition and Curriculum for the National Academy of Sports Medicine.

Beginning with the simple questionnaires developed by John Lawder and George Watson, Spruce has continued to refine and expand food preference questionnaires that enable a computer program to select the proper percentages of protein, fat and carbohydrate that define an individual's metabolic type. The program is based on Spruce's work with thousands of athletes and non-athletes. Currently, the Apex system of standard and advanced programs is marketed through a worldwide network of gyms.

The basis for assessing an individual's metabolic profile is a set of sixty questions that determines their preferred diet. This is compared to the following table that reveals percentages of diet components ranging from slow to fast oxidizers. (Spruce, 1997.)

	Slow	Medium Slow	Medium	Medium Fast	Fast
Carbohydrate	75	65	55	45	40
Protein	15	20	25	30	30
Fat	10	15	20	25	30

Spruce brings out another aspect of healing by diet—that taste preferences may figure importantly in the success of any diet. He recognizes the importance of both acquired and genetic preferences based upon a number of references. One (Falciglia and Norton, 1994) compares the diet of identical (monozygotic) twins with that of normal twins. Some researchers, testing with a bitter substance (phenylthiocarbamide, PTC), suggest a reason for a genetic aversion to certain foods, some of which contain PTC. Broccoli, strawberries and citrus are examples of suspect foods.

Using Lawder's approach and tests, Neal Spruce was able to change the diets of body builders (including his own) with remarkable success. By way of example, Spruce determined that one body builder, Mike Quinn, formerly ate high levels of carbohydrates but could not stay lean and even lost muscle. Quinn turned out to be a mid-fast oxidizer and after changing to a high protein-lower carbohydrate diet, was able to stay big and defined or "cut" (lower subcutaneous fat revealing the underlying muscles) on a carbohydrate-protein-fat ratio of 40-35-25. Another, Troy Zuccolotto, turned out to be a mid-slow type and thrived on a 55-25-20 ratio. According to Dobbins, Spruce went on to suggested that Arnold Schwarzenegger was a fast oxidizer, but that body builders like Bill Pearl and Andreas Cahling could maintain mass and definition without eating any meat at all and were essentially vegetarians.

Apparently, you can't use body type—one would think that all those stocky athletic mesomorphs would be fast oxidizers. Incidentally, Spruce worked with a woman athlete who was convinced that carbohydrates made her fat and was trying to survive on 75 percent protein intake. It turned out that she was an extremely slow oxidizer and needed a much higher proportion of carbohydrate. On her "new" diet she became "lean, defined and hard as a rock on about 1800 calories a day."

CHAPTER TWENTY-ONE

Do You Listen to Your Body or to Your Taste Buds?

Rudolf Wiley, Ph.D.

"Are you 40 going on 70, or are you 70 going on 40?"

—Emanuel Cheraskin, M.D.

Rudolf Wiley (1987, 1989) studied over 1,000 individuals over a twenty-year period. He found that they fell into one of three biochemical types: acid, alkaline and mixed. (Figure 44 and Appendix F), based upon their venous blood pH. He indicated that some are obligatory eaters of vegetarian-type diets and others are more carnivorous. He honored Watson's early work and witnessed the era of transition when many physicians turned to "holistic" protocols, along with many nutritionists and "alternative health care practitioners." Wiley was convinced that venous blood pH is the most accurate measure of human health and is superior to other blood tests and tests of saliva, urine and hair.

He found that normal pH was 7.46 (not 7.40) and, remarkably, that tiny variations of 0.01 were extremely significant in the diagnosis and prognosis of both mental and physical states. He would rate, for example, 7.49 as extremely alkaline and 7.40 as extremely acid. The highest (7.56) and the lowest (7.32) he ever observed were both inmates at mental institutions.

Wiley discovered that some individuals oscillate from one type (alkaline or acid) to the opposite over a twenty-four-hour period and some (principally women) over a twenty-eight day lunar

223

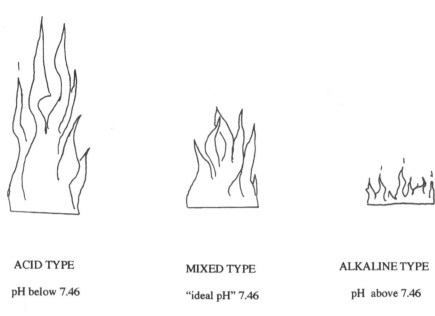

ACID TYPE

pH below 7.46

MIXED TYPE

"ideal pH" 7.46

ALKALINE TYPE

pH above 7.46

Figure 44. Wiley's metabolic types. Essentially similar to Watson (1972, 1979), including needed foods. Wiley found most diabetics to be the alkaline type. (Flame height equivalent to speed of oxidation.)

cycle. Some of his female consultees were extremely acid during the pre-menstrual period (day fifteen to day eighteen), but extremely alkaline from day one to day fourteen, in which case a cyclic diet switch would alleviate the problems.

Wiley claimed a success rate of 90 percent overall (55 percent complete recovery, 35 percent partial recovery, 10 percent no improvement) for his "bio-balance program"[21] as opposed to a 25 percent success rate for many well-known diets, including macrobiotics. (Wiley, 1989.)

Wiley agrees with most other "metabolic typers" that it is sheer folly to prescribe diets or supplements based on symptoms alone, without knowing the biochemical type. This constituted, in his opinion, nutritional Russian roulette. He indicated that the greatest threat to public health is the professional pitch for a "light" diet (low protein/fat high complex carbs, etc.), which he claims is appropriate only for alkaline biochemical types. He em-

---

[21] No longer available.

phasizes that the "light" diet (skinless chicken breasts, light meat, fish, salads, low-fat dairy, whole grains, fruits) is suitable only for a relatively small, extremely alkaline proportion of the population and could be harmful if not disastrous for mixed and acidic types. Acidic types need an opposing mirror-image diet to buffer the rapid burn-off of their blood sugar and dietary fat. Wiley inferred that some well-known diets were predicated on the author's own biochemical type and generally recommended for everybody, rather than recognizing that any diet can be applied with reasonable success only to *sub-groups* of individuals. In his opinion, macrobiotics may be good for some and bad for others. He remarked that he did not favor the "discharge of ugly toxins" theory acclaimed by Kelley, Rogers and others.

Wiley found that most females are genotypically acid dominant types, predicting that if most women went on the "light" diet suitable only for alkaline types, PMS and psychoneurotic disorders would reach epidemic proportions. He goes on to state that he is not saying that alkaline type women should eat a calcium-free diet but that "sunlight, vitamin D, folic acid, calcium-rich foods and anaerobic exercise (weights, not jogging, swimming or cycling) will do far more to reduce an alkaline woman's risk of incurring osteoporosis than will a high potency calcium supplement. . . ." Acidic females, he goes on to say, may need more supplemental calcium, but alkaline types should cautiously and gradually increase (250 mg/month) such a supplement (if needed), while sudden increases (250 to 1,500 mg/day) may resurrect pre-existing disease. Supplemental calcium is apparently unwarranted for alkaline females in general.

While the Tarahumara Indians make world-class marathon runs routinely on a very low protein, high complex carbohydrate diet, they do so after centuries of isolated adaptation. We are not so lucky. Take fasting as another example. While primitive man was adapted to periods of fasting, our indiscriminate breeding behavior across all ethnic and cultural boundaries has left us no clear genotypic categories either involving the type of diet or periods of no diet at all (fasting). According to Wiley, fasting works for alkaline and mixed types but can have an opposite effect on acidic types.

This author relates some convincing case histories. One consultee had spent 10 years in intensive psychotherapy. Placed on an appropriate diet, she lost her mental symptoms in one week.

Another who had been trying to live on the macrobiotic-vegetarian type diet, on switching to an acid-inducing diet, achieved her ideal weight for the first time in her adult life.

Wiley outlines (1989) two approaches to finding out your individual biochemical type. One is by the withdrawal of venous blood measured by a laboratory to the nearest hundredth (i.e., 7.41, not 7.4).[22] With a food-mood diary filled out for each test day and a "challenge" meal during that day, your type can be interpreted. The other approach is by trial and error (no blood sampling) and involves starting out with an alkaline diet and noting (in three days) your psychophysiological improvement or deterioration. If favorable, you stay on it; if not, switch to the acidic diet. If the response to it is very briefly positive but rapidly becomes unfavorable, one should switch to a "mixed" diet.[23] If you are so blessed as to be able to live healthily and happily on a mixed diet you can be thankful to both God and Nature.

Wiley (1999) states that the "listen to your body" school of thought is often wrong, being better described as "listen to your taste buds." According to him, 75 percent of men are alkaline and their idea of a great meal (steak and fried potatoes) is better suited for mixed metabolic types and *not* for them, explaining why many males end up with cardiovascular disease. Furthermore, Wiley says, the medical community's *light* diet is not light enough to assist alkaline males and far *too* light for the other 20 to 25 percent of the male population. Many women also claim that they are alkaline and fear that *heavy* eating will make them fat. Since, according to Wiley, 40 percent of women are non-alkaline at least part of the time, eating *light* is not the thing for them but will increase their psychological and stress-related disorders. These same women are also appalled at the very idea of devouring "a *heavy* regimen appropriate for acid or mixed types." Incidentally, all of Wiley's diabetics turned out to be alkaline and

---

[22] Ideally four blood samples are drawn over a course of twelve to sixteen hours on the test day. Venous plasma pH determined within two to three minutes of withdrawal.

[23] Meat, fish, or poultry at every meal; legumes, dairy and fruits sparingly, eggs, whole grains (at least once a day) and nuts, olive oil, butter, apples, pears, ice cream, cheese and select desserts such as ice cream, cheesecake and pastries.

are the only exception to the lack of correlation between symptom type and metabolic type.

Wiley emphasizes that the appropriate diet for acid (fast oxidizer) types is an alkalizing diet of high-purine proteins and fats with low carbohydrates and strongly advises that acid types eat protein at *every* meal. The nutritional regimen for alkaline (slow oxidizer) types is more or less a mirror image. He cautions that using foods based on their ash content (exemplified by Aihara's rankings, 1986), could cause serious metabolic damage.

Wiley offers a simple test for determining your biochemical type: in the morning sit down and have a cup of real coffee (with caffeine) and see how you feel. Apparently, to wake up and get started in the morning alkaline types need *at least* one cup. "Mixed metabolic types may typically feel a little tense or nervous after one cup of coffee and generally quite nervous after two or three cups," and acid types "cannot tolerate even one cup of coffee." Wiley's short true-false test to determine biochemical type follows.

Alkaline types (slow oxidizers) answer true to each statement; acid types (fast oxidizers) usually answer false to each. If you feel you could answer true or false to at least three out of six, then you are probably a mixed oxidizer. Unless you are certain of your type, Wiley feels that you should assume that you are alkaline. Most men and post-menopausal women are alkaline; women still menstruating would have a fifty-fifty chance. (After Wiley, 1991.) Permission courtesy of Rudolf Wiley (pers. comm.):

1. I need at least one cup of coffee every morning to wake me up and get started.

2. A glass of wine typically unwinds me and helps me relax.

3. The less I eat, the better I feel. In fact, I've tried fasting in the past and found that I've felt great.

4. After eating meat, fish or poultry for lunch (especially if it is fried as you'd find at a fast food drive-through or takeout), I find that I get sleepy and/or thirsty later during the day.

5. As far as sex is concerned, I can take it or leave it. Sex doesn't do much for me.

6. When I go to the dentist I usually don't need novocaine when I have my teeth drilled.

CHAPTER TWENTY-TWO

Can You Balance
Your Doshas?

Deepak Chopra, M.D.

"But at age 70, no two bodies are remotely alike. At that age, your body will be like no one else's in the world; its age changes will mirror your unique life."

—Deepak Chopra

No discussion of biological individuality would be complete without a look at Ayurveda. This 5,000-year-old Indian system that deals with mind body health was perhaps the first documented effort to classify humans as to body type. It is based on the premise that we are all born with a balanced blend of three body types called "doshas," and that we must try to maintain this balance throughout life. An imbalance is reflected by mental, behavioral or physical manifestations. I can do little more than try to summarize the detailed explanation given by Deepak Chopra in his book *Perfect Health*. The three body types are Vata, Pitta and Kapha. In their description, you can see similarities with other authors such as Abravanel (body types), Wiley, Bieler and Watson (metabolic types). Figure 45 and Appendix G attempt to summarize the attributes of Ayurveda's three main body types, condensed from the details given by Chopra (1991). According to Chopra, the Vata type has the poorest health of the three, having twice the medical complaints of Pitta types, while Pitta types have twice those of Kapha. Vatas are overly sensitive and react

229

negatively to loud noises, crowds and physical discomfort. Vata energy is thus exhausted by sudden shocks and grief and they readily exhibit "battle fatigue," all evidence of an overactive nervous system. Establishing regular habits seems to be the key to restoring and maintaining a Vata's health, i.e., restoring the relative amounts of Vata, Pitta and Kapha that the Vata-dominant type was born with.

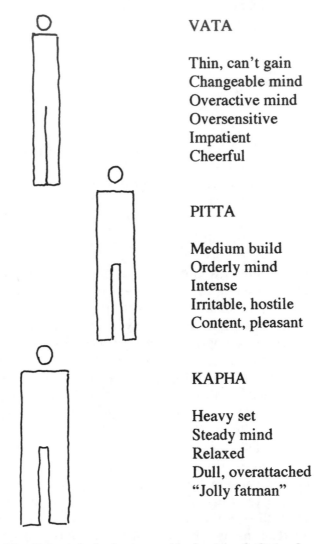

VATA

Thin, can't gain
Changeable mind
Overactive mind
Oversensitive
Impatient
Cheerful

PITTA

Medium build
Orderly mind
Intense
Irritable, hostile
Content, pleasant

KAPHA

Heavy set
Steady mind
Relaxed
Dull, overattached
"Jolly fatman"

Figure 45.   Principle body types (doshas) and their characteristics based upon the Ayurveda mind/body system of typing individuals. (After Chopra, 1991.)

The Pitta type, on the other hand, has generally good physical health, can eat anything (strong digestion) and, in the process, often forgets about the nutrient quality of foods. Pittas can stay in balance (stay at the "set point" of the three doshas at birth) if they can control their natural intensity and drive, the key being moderation which, for them, means slowing down.

Kapha types apparently take a long time to get "out of balance," remaining strong, healthy and content, but later years may find them as jolly fat men, quite insecure, overly possessive and reacting to various foods and aerial pollutants.

Balancing the three doshas within you seems to be accomplished by proper diet, exercise and establishing daily and seasonal routines, all sound health practices. In his 1991 book, Chopra has conveniently provided a way for you to test the proportion of the three body types, which you have inherited, by simply answering twenty questions for each body type. It will be interesting for you to compare your results with tests for metabolic types.

While there are only three main body types they can, according to Chopra, be combined in ten different ways to yield ten different body types. Each of us possesses all three but in different proportions (Figure 46). If you have one type that is much higher (possibly twice as high) than the others, then you are considered a "single dosha type," with the "dominant" type most obviously controlling your mind, body and behavior. A "two dosha type," which most people appear to be, would display qualities of their two leading types. The rare "three dosha type" would naturally have all three manifest themselves nearly equally to make you what you are.

The goal of Ayurveda is to enable you to reach a more ideal level of health. In contrast to Western medicine, which is concerned only with the physical and mental health, Ayurveda seeks to elevate *all* aspects of life to higher levels, including spiritual growth, personal relationships and social harmony. Some of Chopra's other books (1989, 1993) may be helpful in understanding the more esoteric benefits of this approach to health.

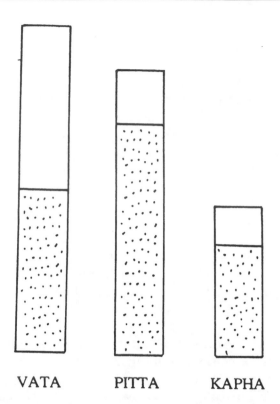

VATA   PITTA   KAPHA

Figure 46. Graphic representation of a hypothetical person's original balance of the three Ayurvedic body types at birth (shaded), contrasted with his types at adulthood (blank space). Here, the adult has too much Vata relative to Pitta, and this imbalance causes exaggerated mental, behavioral and physical symptoms from, in this case, an overly sensitive nervous system which was inherited. (After Chopra, 1991.)

CHAPTER TWENTY-THREE

Your Nutritional Protocol— A Hit Or Miss Gamble?

William Wolcott, D.C.

"The problem is that alternative medicine, like conventional medicine, lacks the technology necessary to effectively analyze and resolve the biochemical imbalances that are the underlying causes of chronic illness."

—William Wolcott

A modern and sophisticated concept of metabolic typing was developed by W. L. Wolcott and based upon the work of pioneers in the field, chiefly Roger Williams, George Watson, William Kelley, and the research of Francis Pottenger. The basic premises are relatively simply and make a lot of sense in light of our evolutionary heritage. The details of the methodology, however are not as easy to understand for Wolcott has developed and "fine-tuned" the concept of metabolic typing to what may be its ultimate complexity, possibly matching the genetic complexity resulting from the great American tradition of ethnic mixing.

Wolcott was heavily influenced by William Kelley. In fact, he worked as Kelley's clinical assistant for several years and in 1980 became Director of Kelley's International Health Institute, a position that he held for six years.

In the 1970's Kelley became the first researcher to classify people into metabolic categories based upon the autonomic nervous system. (Wolcott, 2000.) Kelley considered meat eaters to be under parasympathetic dominance while plant eaters were classed as sympathetic dominants. During his tenure with Kelley, Wolcott was puzzled as to why some people reacted exactly opposite to Kelley's clinical model based strictly on which autonomic nervous system branch appeared to control body chemistry. Struck with the fact that Watson's oxidative model contradicted Kelley's autonomic model, he realized that both might be right: that in some people an unbalanced autonomic system (over-controlled by either the sympathetic or parasympathetic branch) dictated proper nutrient requirements, while in others it was due to an imbalance within the oxidative system (either too fast or too slow). This led Wolcott to his major clinical breakthrough which he called the "Dominance Factor." In time he came to expand his clinical evaluations to include seven other physiological parameters he called "Fundamental Homeostatic Controls." Examples are categories called Catabolic/Anabolic, Electrolyte/Fluid, and Acid/Alkaline. He eventually founded an organization, Healthexcel, Inc., to market his concept of metabolic typing.

First, let's try a thumbnail summary of the Wolcott-Healthexcel approach. You may wish to occasionally glance at Figures 34 and 35.

How a given nutrient functions in your biochemistry appears to be dependent on whether the oxidative or the autonomic system is in control or "Dominant." About 1983, Wolcott advanced the somewhat startling hypothesis that any food can produce either an acid or an alkaline effect dependent on which of these two systems is dominant.

For example, by Wolcott's postulates, if your oxidative system is dominant over the autonomic system, fruits and vegetables will cause you to be acidic and proteins will alkalize you. Conversely, if you are autonomic dominant, fruits and vegetables cause alkalinity and proteins cause acidity, just the opposite effect. This is where the Wolcott hypothesis departs radically from the accepted convention. Prior to this it has been accepted that the same foods produce acid or alkaline effects on everybody, either determined from analysis of the ash on burning (Aihara, 1986) or by Rudolf Wiley's (1989) venous blood pH approach. The idea here is that the unique biochemistry of the individual determines a food's effect on blood pH, not that certain foods have an acidic or alkaline effect on the body. The outcome of all of this is that if you do not know your metabolic type, you cannot know whether the food or supplement has a good or bad impact on your body, i.e., makes you sick or worsens existing problems and possibly sets the stage for degenerative disease such as cardiovascular problems, diabetes or cancer.

For convenience, the two major controlling categories are listed in Figure 47 and Appendix H with reference to blood pH and what food groups are needed. In addition to knowing your metabolic type, the Wolcott-Heathexcel system requires knowledge of foods organized in three nutrient groups. For example, if you are in the oxidative dominant group and a fast acid oxidizer, you will need foods heavy in meat or fat (Group II Foods) to slow the oxidation rate, alkalize the blood and raise to normal your blood sugar. On the other hand, if you are a member of one of the autonomic sympathetic (acid) dominants you'll need vegetables and fruits (Group I Foods) to accomplish this same purpose.

Wolcott (1993) considers the *autonomic nervous system* to be the "master regulator" of metabolism and cites the basic work of William Kelley and Francis Pottenger. Wolcott believes that its structure and function are inherited but that its influence can be overcome. For example, if one is genetically thin by reason of autonomic dominance, disrupting the rate of oxidation may cause the individual to put on weight. Broadly speaking, the sympathetic branch favors more acidic, anaerobic and catabolic (energy using) conditions while the parasympathetic branch has the opposite effect (alkaline, aerobic, anabolic). Sympathetic dominants tend to acidosis, heartburn, insomnia, hypertension, high blood-sugar, high blood pressure, rapid heartbeat, emotional outburst and social withdrawal, while parasympathetic dominants have problems with alkalosis, excessive appetite, low motivation, loss of sex drive, allergies, respiratory and skin problems, chronic fatigue and depression.

Treatment of the *oxidative system* is based on the pioneering work of George Watson and Rudolf Wiley. The basic problem of both fast and slow oxidizers is their inability to efficiently use acetyl coenzyme A in the Krebs cycle (citric acid cycle), for opposite reasons (see Figure 33). Slow oxidizers who burn carbohydrates poorly tend to be alkaline and hypoactive with little appetite, depression, digestive troubles, calcium deposits, poor fat metabolism, lethargy and suppressed emotions while the fast oxidizers who "burn" carbohydrates rapidly are acid, hyperactive types with strong appetites and do well on heavy, fatty foods.

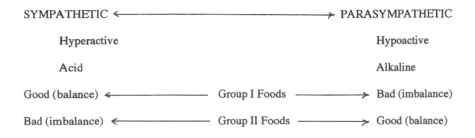

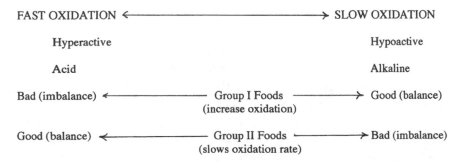

Figure 47.   The effect of two major food groups on blood pH and behavior (activity). Note that Group I Foods (favoring herbivory) and Group II Foods (favoring carnivory) appear to have opposite effects, depending on which system is dominant in your body. For example, Group I Foods stimulate the parasympathetic system unnecessarily since it is already alkaline and causing hypoactive behavior, but it helps counteract the acidity and hyperactivity of the sympathetic type, thus balancing the body chemistry. Some minerals have effects similar to the food groups. Potassium and magnesium act as do Group I Foods while calcium (and protein) act like Group II Foods. (Modified from Wolcott, 1998b.)

The third important homeostatic control, the *endocrine system,* contributes to the metabolic type more in the nature of "fine tuning." In discussing this system the author draws upon the work of Harrower (1939), Bieler (1965) and Abravanel (1983, 1985). While the endocrine system plays a critical role in relation to the autonomic system, it has a limited role in determining metabolic type. In "fine-tuning" metabolism, it is responsible for things like food cravings, weight gain, or why one sympathetic type puts fat on all over while another does so only in the mid-section, or as cellulite on the buttocks and thighs.

In summary, Wolcott has outlined six autonomic, six balanced and six parasympathetic types based upon interrelationships of the autonomic nervous system and the oxidative system, giving a total of eighteen metabolic types. Each of these eighteen types could also be under the dominance of any one of four endocrine glands; pituitary, adrenal, thyroid and gonad, giving a final total of seventy-two potential metabolic types. A series of tests and a lengthy questionnaire are needed to differentiate such complexity.

Weighing multiple factors on a test to arrive at your metabolic type is an "intricate, complex and formidable task" by hand, taking up to thirteen hours. Healthexcel uses computer technology to print out the results in what is called the "H.O.P.E. (Health Optimization Profile Evaluation) Report."

Wolcott comments on the geographical origin of the metabolic types, suggesting that sympathetic metabolizers developed in "warmer, more tropical climes" where they subsisted on diets with low fat, moderate protein and high carbohydrates, the vegetarian being the extreme example. Note that both the sympathetic and slow oxidizers need Group I Foods. I infer that the slow oxidizers developed in the same geographical area as the sympathetic dominants. The slow oxidizer, however, requires more protein. In what Wolcott calls the oxidative *dominant,* slow, sympathetic types, there are some unique needs distinct from sympathetic requirements In such a case both fat and calcium undesirably augment the oxidative slowdown. One way this works is that fats impede the natural calcium channel blocker, magnesium, allowing cellular levels of calcium to rise, in addition to providing unneeded acteyl-coenzyme A (see Figures 34 and 35).

Parasympathetic metabolizers, on the other hand, Wolcott feels, developed in colder climates and accordingly need a diet high in protein and fat and lower in carbohydrates. They don't do well on the simple carbohydrates of fruits and need root vegetables. They also need high purine proteins (as extolled by Benjamin Frank) in red meats and fatty fishes like salmon, tuna and sardines.

Wolcott (1993) also considers the influence of the dominant control system (autonomic or oxidative) on personality and behavior, stating that a sympathetic autonomic dominant generally has a "Class A" personality (aggressive, hyperactive and competitive), but if the sympathetic type is a slow oxidizer, they may be hypoactive and apathetic. But, he cautions, you cannot treat all Class A personalities as sympathetic dominants, since a fast oxidative dominant can also have a Class A personality. Thus the treatment of Class A can help some but make others worse: "For example, fruits tends to calm a sympathetic autonomic dominant, but tend to increase excitability in the fast oxidative dominant." (Wolcott, 1993.)

Apparently the fast oxidizer is also suited to colder climates since their dietary needs are similar to those of the parasympathetic dominants, so both are served by the Group II diet. Again, there are caveats. In what Wolcott calls the fast oxidative *dominant* parasympathetic types, phytate-rich grains (which most unsprouted grains are) bind up calcium which is "desperately needed by the fast oxidizer." He also states that, while parasympathetics can handle root vegetables and some grains, the fast oxidizer gets too high a rise in blood sugar from eating foods high in the glycemic index (parsnips, carrots, potatoes, wheat, etc.).

This is probably more detail than you might wish. It is included to lend credence to the idea that your metabolic type and ideal diet might require the kind of analysis provided by the Healthexcel program.

Wolcott also discusses ratios such as popularized by Barry Sears (1995) with the 40-30-30 ratio of the "Zonal Diet," but underscores the point that to enter "The Zone" requires more knowledge of your individual needs than is provided by a simple ratio of carbohydrate, protein, and fat. (Some people do not do well on the 40-30-30 diet.) The Healthexcel analysis does include your individualized ratio, which Wolcott (1998) views as a starting point. He emphasizes that, while it is important to know the ratios and percentages, it is also important to know what *kinds* of carbohydrates, proteins and fats should be present. He gives examples of his ratios: slow oxidizers should eat a high carbohydrate low protein/fat diet (60-25-15), fast oxidizers should consume another (30-40-30), while the mixed oxidizers need yet another (50-30-20). The problem is, as he states, that within slow oxidizers, there may be additional categories; slightly, moderately or extremely slow. Imposed on this are individualized Circadian rhythms and stress levels. He raises a good point that you should observe changes after every meal, carefully noting reactions involving appetite, satiety, sweet cravings, energy levels and mental and emotional well-being. This is sound advice for anyone striving to discover his or her metabolic type.

Recently this author has published the most definitive work to date on metabolic typing. (Wolcott, 2000.) He includes sixty-five questions to determine your metabolic type. In this book he describes only three metabolic types: Protein Type, Carbo Type and Mixed Type. In the Protein and Carbo Types either the Autonomic nervous system or the Oxidative System is in control, or better, in over-control. If you are the Protein Type and you are Autonomic Dominant, then your parasympathetic branch is over-controlling your biochemistry (an imbalance); if you are a Protein type and Oxidative Dominant, then fast oxidation is over-controlling your biochemistry (an imbalance). If, on the other hand, you are a Carbo Type and you are an Autonomic Dominant, then your sympathetic branch is over-controlling (an imbalance); if you are an Oxidative Dominant, then your slow oxidation is over-controlling and in an imbalanced state. The Mixed Type is neither a fast or slow oxidizer and has balanced autonomic nervous system control (see Figure 57 for food ratios).

The Protein Type needs a high-protein, high-fat diet. This strengthens the weaker sympathetic branch to achieve balance or it slows the oxidation rate. For this type, a high-carbohydrate, low-fat diet increases fat storage and may lead to catabolizing (cannabalizing) your muscle tissue for sufficient protein, as well as disturbing adrenal and thyroid function. In Carbo Types a high-protein, high-fat diet causes muscle tissue to be catabolized for desperately needed glucose fuel and also disturbs adrenal and thyroid function. Wolcott indicates that the 40-30-30 diet may catabolize muscle tissue for glucose in Carbo Types and for protein in Protein Types.

The central idea behind metabolic typing, as exemplified by Wolcott's thesis, is that which ever of the paired systems is in excess represents an "imbalance" and the opposite system needs to be stimulated to bring balance. This balanced state allows the body to normalize its biochemistry and correct degenerative diseases or fight invasions of alien organisms (viruses, bacteria).

As I have stated elsewhere, supplement formulas are a potpourri of ingredients thrown together, each of which has shown to have benefitted somebody, somewhere, sometime. Wolcott expands on this theme, stating that a generic "grab bag" protocol of nutrients succeeds only by chance and can actually worsen healthy problems. He gives the following two examples. A "shotgun" approach to high serum cholesterol includes niacin (B3). If you are a slow oxidizer (or sympathetic dominant), niacin will help normalize the dysfunctional cholesterol metabolism. Conversely, niacin given to fast oxidizers (or parasympathetic dominants) further disrupts and worsens the clinical condition (Figure 47).

Nutrients apparently work similarly in the Oxidative System. Here calcium inhibits fast oxidizers (normalized body chemistry) while magnesium exacerbates osteoporosis. These examples emphasize Wolcott's point that "standardized nutritional protocols are by definition hit or miss solutions."

Another important point that Wolcott makes is that poor eating may have pushed you into a certain metabolic type which he considers the "Functional Type." Stress, illness or nutrient deficiencies or excesses can also push you away from your actual genetic type. So the type you test out as today is not "cast in stone" to use Wolcott's words. The idea is to eventually learn the type you have inherited from your ancestors.

CHAPTER TWENTY-FOUR

Headaches are not Due to a Deficiency of Aspirin

Sherry Rogers, M.D.

Another physician who has dealt with biochemical individuality is Sherry Rogers. Her depiction of the "metabolic cross" (Figure 48) is helpful in understanding the relation of metabolic types, especially as they relate to healing diets. Note the extremes, alkaline or vegetarian (vegan) diets on the extreme left, acid carnivores on the extreme right and those with balanced (omnivore) diets in the center. Rogers relates the axes of the diagram to diets which heal, such as macrobiotics. According to her experience, as sick people normalize, they tend to shift toward the midline or more balanced diet.

Rogers, like Kelley, states that a person's biochemical type is not cast in stone but can vary with environment and state of health. Here we might recall that Lawder emphasizes that some 70 percent of people appear to be omnivores (mid-oxidizers). The experiences of Neal Spruce also bears this out. Some people, like the Eskimos, find bountiful health as carnivores and others are free of disease and have boundless energy on the other end of the spectrum, eating more like rabbits. I'll never forget the Gevaert family in Belgium. In their 60s their daughters were successfully treating terminal cancer patients with macrobiotics. At a macrobiotic restaurant in Paris, I met the Gevaert sisters, who were also on strict macro diets. They resembled refugees from Dachau but as thin as they were they were brimming with enthusiasm and energy which I couldn't understand at the time. (They were probably slow oxidizers.)

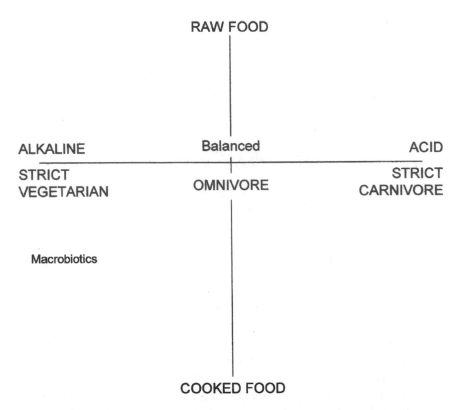

Figure 48.   The metabolic cross. The extreme left on the horizontal axis represents the alkalizing vegetarian (vegan) diet, the extreme right the acidifying carnivore diet. The macrobiotic diet, which has reversed many "incurable" cancers, is mostly a cooked diet. People eating on either end of the vertical axis may do so only temporarily while healing. Healing at opposite ends of the horizontal axis may also be temporary for most people (rough estimate only, perhaps 70%) but a permanent way of life for those specific metabolic types (rough estimate only, perhaps 30%) of the population. (Modified from Rogers, 1994, author of *Wellness Against All Odds,* Prestige Publishing, Syracuse, NY.)

It seems likely that most physicians see fewer of the more balanced omnivorous types and also fewer of those on either end of the spectrum who are eating right for their type. The great bulk of people with problems are probably trying to eat salads and greens because they think they are good for them when actually they are more carnivorous, and then there are the carnivores who cut down on the red meat and fat because of fears of cholesterol or other things they have read or heard about. Or, fearing clogged arteries, they have rushed to buy polyunsaturated fats, not realizing that their composition and rancidity promote cancer.

The vertical axis of Figure 48 represents the extremes of raw or cooked food. Some people, according to Rogers, do well on juice fasts and all raw foods but find this to be only a temporary healing phase. On the other extreme, Rogers describes patients in the terminal stages of cancer whose macrobiotic diet (grains, greens, beans, sea vegetables) had to be twice-cooked with double amounts of water until it was a soft and extremely digestible pablum like baby food.

To find out if you have a vegetarian or carnivorous metabolism, Rogers has a simple solution. If you don't have cancer, you eat at one end of the horizontal axis and if you get worse, you simply go in the opposite direction. In her experience, the majority of people heal on a macrobiotic diet for starters. This is essentially grains (50 to 60 percent), greens (20 to 30 percent), beans and sea veggies (5 to 10 percent) with seeds, roots and some fruits comprising the balance. She has three books (1988, 1991, 1992) that are essentially for the critically ill, dealing with macrobiotics.

Rogers briefly reviews the work of Max Gerson (M.D.) and William Kelley, both of whom led her to consider the importance of biochemical individuality in the treatment of disease, in this case cancer. Gerson developed a program of treating cancer with vegetable and fruit juices (up to thirteen times daily) that reminded Rogers of hydroponics (flooding an organism with high levels of nutrients and flushing away metabolic wastes). Gerson wrote a remarkable book (1958) on the success of his treatment, including fifty case histories complete with clinical diagnoses, biopsy reports, and prior history including X-rays. Gerson was a physician to Albert Sweitzer. His daughter currently runs a highly successful clinic in Tijuana, Mexico, based upon his therapy. As Rogers states, Kelley borrowed heavily from Gerson's program but came to realize that some people must be metabolically different since they could not tolerate Gerson's regimen. It was Kelley who discovered that a high meat and fat diet would cure some people of cancer, while the Gerson juice approach healed others. Thus the roots of metabolic typing came from dramatic dietary experimentation with cancer patients, hence the relevancy of cancer treatment to this story. Incidentally, Rogers recommends those with cancer and other unwell patients begin on the macrobiotic diet. In her book, *Tired or Toxic* (1990), she details thirty-two biochemical reasons why macrobiotics works in curing "incurable" diseases such as terminal cancers.

How this skilled and literate doctor got into all of this is a fascinating story. Even more than Gittleman, Sherry Rogers suffered and experimented on herself for many years. Her long history of personal illness led her to throw herself into search and research that took enormous motivation. In several of her books she very candidly and charmingly tells the story of her own search for health. Her face would break out if she ate certain foods. She'd cough and wheeze around dogs, barns, horses and carbon monoxide. If she touched a cat or horse and then her eyes, the whites would swell up violently beneath swollen lids. Wheat severely depressed her and foam mattresses or sleeping between permanent-press sheets caused her lost discs, collapsed vertebrae and arthritic bone spurs to flare up in agony. Natural gas, diesel fuel or glue would depress her terribly and make her cry. Before she studied with Michio Kushi, the guru of macrobiotics, a sip of wine gave her chest phlegm, hoarseness and asthma, and a dreadful facial eczema for several weeks, in addition to drenching night sweats. In 1976, she suffered atopic dermatitis, large red, painful cysts on her face that drained and merged into a lumpy mess. By trial and error she discovered fifty foods that she could not eat. After medical school, she had such terrible headaches that she thought she had a brain tumor. She also developed glaucoma from so many steroids and facial creams. To make a long story short, she was cured by injections of neutralizing doses of "bad" foods by Dr. Joseph B. Miller of Mobile, Alabama, and, in her words: "It was like being reborn." When she finally adopted a macrobiotic diet, the remainder of her troubles went away. For four years she traveled with a hot-plate in her suitcase and prepared simple meals in her hotel room. On the metabolic scale she rates herself as a modified vegan with occasional meat. She can now drink a whole bottle of wine without discomfort. When she was a child, there were four major food groups, dairy, grains, protein, fruits/vegetables. Years later, after a period on "health foods" (yogurt, granola, nuts, fruits) her continued ill health forced her to abandon the "four-food-group" philosophy and start over.

After reading six of her books, I came to deeply appreciate how her own personal story motivated her to learn, practice and teach others to find their own road to good health. The knowledge and zeal of this dynamic woman have to have an impact on the entire medical community, as society is now, more and more, seeking advice from physicians who have broadened their practice to include the philosophy and principles of what is now known as alternative or complementary medicine. No longer a stigma, it is leading to a deeper appreciation of all types of healing methods and of recognition that nature's own pharmacopeia has much more to offer. Sherry Rogers is playing a major role in this, along with such respected figures as Jonathan Wright, Andrew Weil and Deepak Chopra. Instead of letting the patient eat, drink and breathe whatever they want and then seek a pill for their symptoms, the new philosophy Rogers espouses will be to treasure the symptoms as nature's message that you need to heed in order to find the real culprit, the biochemical causes of the symptoms, and not to mask it with drugs. Pain is always a warning that should be informative. Rogers says to consider pain and other messages from your internal biochemistry as warnings from Nature that has served vertebrate life very well indeed for millions of years. If God did set all this marvelous and almost incomprehensible cellular machinery in motion, why should we violate natural laws that were set into place long ago for our welfare? The medical establishment must be respected as brilliant diagnosticians and master surgeons. Personally, I have enormous respect for physicians and barely missed going to medical school myself. At the first hint of something I don't understand, I race for the nearest physician or specialist. But thanks to people like Sherry Rogers with the zeal and humility to learn all they possibly can, the rules of medicine can and may change. Cancer, as she says, is not a chemotherapy deficiency any more than a headache is due to a lack of aspirin. Rogers feels that ultimately it is the patient who will play the major role in recovery and that physicians are merely his consultants.

In our quest to identify our own personal nutrition needs and to lessen the confusion it might be wise to consider being tested for allergies caused by the air we breathe or the food and water we ingest. In light of what Rogers has written, rather than attribute our health problems to eating wrongly for our metabolic type, we just could be reacting to the carpets in our home or some of the common foods we crave.

To return to the topic of nutritional types, Rogers discusses general guidelines for both vegetarian and carnivorous diets as well as guidelines for what she calls "transitional" vegetarians and carnivores; transitional because the tenure of most individuals in one realm or the other may be either an abrupt change (you get worse) or a gradual one (to a more balanced diet). Her food recommendations are essentially similar to those of other researchers reported herein. She agrees that the basis for individualized nutrition lies in the chemistry of energy syntheses. She considers a number of factors which modify or bear upon the metabolic pathways: genetics, hormone levels, nutrient levels, climate, heavy metals and so on.

She says that, if a carnivore places himself on a macrobiotic or vegetarian diet there are clues that tell when he should go in the opposite direction: it stopped working or he stopped feeling good, or was overcome with cramps, lost too much weight, developed a loathing for greens or an intolerance for grains. Conversely, if a vegetarian is on a carnivorous or fast oxidizer diet he may start to crave greens or salads.

Because of her exhaustive work with the toxic effects of the human environment, Rogers explains that the carnivore or "acid-loving" person has damaged and leaky cell membranes from years of nutrient deficiencies, hydrogenated oils from French fries and exposure to toxic chemicals. His cells lose proteins (vasoactive peptides) that control body swelling and the person starts reacting to everything. Calcium leaks back into the cell and the acid carnivore diet apparently keeps it outside of the cell where it belongs. The "alkaline loving" vegan or macro, on the other hand according to Rogers, has tight cell membranes and needs diets high in magnesium and potassium to offset the excess calcium. Gerson's diet, incidentally, is one of high potassium (from vegetable juices) and low sodium, and hence would work for vegetarians, but not for carnivores.

The data that Rogers presents in her books (especially 1990, 1996) about the threat of environmental toxins and the detoxification system of the body are right in line with the thinking of Henry Bieler, Max Gerson, William Kelley and others. Bieler's thoughts of healing the liver first, which will subsequently normalize the endocrine glands, bears repeating. Bieler's "therapeutic antidote" diet shares many similarities with those of other healers who came later. In fact, Rogers reiterates that knowledge of the detoxification system is ushering in a possible revolution in medicine, antiquating our current classification system of diseases and opening a new era of ultimate wellness.

You may or may not wish to study Figure 49 (based on Rogers' writings), which may help those readers who wonder what the detox system is and where it operates. The diagram shows not only the locations of key cell components but is intended to emphasize exactly where a deficiency of certain vitamins and minerals cripples the cell's job of coping with free radicals and the toxins from our environment, or, if a liver cell, with the breakdown products of cancer and other diseased tissues. We talk so glibly and abstractly about this and that vitamin or mineral and most of us don't have the slightest idea exactly how and where it works.

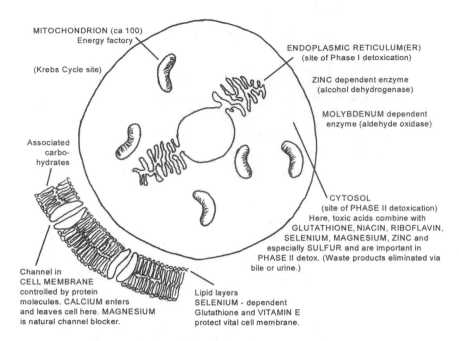

MITOCHONDRION (ca 100)
Energy factory

(Krebs Cycle site)

ENDOPLASMIC RETICULUM(ER)
(site of Phase I detoxication)

ZINC dependent enzyme
(alcohol dehydrogenase)

MOLYBDENUM dependent
enzyme (aldehyde oxidase)

Associated
carbo-
hydrates

CYTOSOL
(site of PHASE II detoxication)
Here, toxic acids combine with
GLUTATHIONE, NIACIN, RIBOFLAVIN,
SELENIUM, MAGNESIUM, ZINC and
especially SULFUR and are important in
PHASE II detox. (Waste products eliminated via
bile or urine.)

Channel in
CELL MEMBRANE
controlled by protein
molecules. CALCIUM enters
and leaves cell here. MAGNESIUM
is natural channel blocker.

Lipid layers
SELENIUM - dependent
Glutathione and VITAMIN E
protect vital cell membrane.

Figure 49. Diagrammatic structure of a typical animal cell, showing organelles (like mitochondria) suspended in a semi-fluid matrix (cytosol). Cell membrane grossly enlarged to show important structure. Note protein controlled "gates" or channels by which substances such as calcium enter and leave the cell. Main purpose of this figure is to show where a few nutrients perform their vital functions. The very important detoxication phases are indicated. Note that a deficiency of zinc or molybdenum will cripple detox Phase I while Phase II is retarded by deficiency of other vitamins and minerals, particularly selenium needed by the anti-oxidant glutathione. Since the cruciferous vegetables (cabbage, kale, broccoli, etc.) and onions supply sulfur, you can see their importance in keeping Phase II detoxication operating and helping to prevent such diseases as cancer.

CHAPTER TWENTY-FIVE

It's All a Matter of Homiostasis

Guy Schenker, D.C.

A somewhat different and more clinically oriented approach to biochemical individuality is that of Guy Schenker. With an impressive grasp of nutritional dynamics his contributions are the antithesis of allopathic medicine, being patient-specific rather than disease-specific. Schenker has developed a series of objective tests to define and guide nutrition therapy for the nutritionally-oriented clinician. Intended to be done by professionals, the tests are rapid, non-invasive, and require no laboratory analysis.

Instead of attempting to determine a person's biochemical type and then treating that type, Schenker has chosen to incorporate some of the classical metabolic types (notably fast and slow oxidizers, sympathetics and parasympathetics) into five major physiologic systems which supposedly cover most of the causes of ill health. To extract order from the many thousands of biochemical reactions in the human body, Schenker identifies five fundamental control systems, calling them the "five fundamental balances": water/electrolyte balance, anaerobic/dysaerobic balance, glucogenic/ketogenic balance, sympathetic/parasympathetic balance and acid/alkaline balance.

Schenker recognizes that in a healthy body there is no such thing as a "steady state"; everything cycles back and forth to maintain a reasonable homeostasis. Simply stated, your blood sugar can and does go up and down, above and below a "normal" value, depending on the foods you eat and their impact on the controlling hormones such as insulin and glucagon. With this in

249

mind, each of Schenker's five metabolic balance control systems can shift out of balance in two opposite ways, i.e., you can be either acid or alkaline. Thus ten states of imbalance are possible. The five major balances are very briefly described below.

The quantity and ratio of the electrolytes, sodium and potassium, and the amount of water needed to handle excess electrolytes by the kidneys are the subject of the fundamental water/electrolyte balance. As a practical aside to this, according to Schenker, the so-called sports drinks actually contribute to dehydration and need to be diluted with from two to five times their volume in water to prevent the damaging effect of electrolyte stress. In both electrolyte overload and insufficiency there is an inefficient use of oxygen coupled with an inefficient movement of nutrients into and waste products out of cells.

The anerobic/dysaerobic balance is apparently based on the research of Rivici (1961). The anaerobic individual, as defined by Schenker, doesn't produce energy normally with the aid of oxygen, but gets it from fermentation, a process requiring little or no oxygen from the lungs. In contrast, the dysaerobic patient has normal oxidation out of control that, instead of providing energy, furnishes free radicals. Both types are said to have lipid imbalances, either too little or too much fatty acids and/or sterols.

Schenker's glucogenic/ketogenic balance system is based on the fast and slow oxidizer types developed by George Watson. Both glucogenic and ketogenic types do not derive sufficient energy from oxidation, having lost their ability to use either fats (Krebs cycle) or carbohydrates (beta oxidation cycle) pathways for energy production. Glucogenic patients are said to have extreme sensitivity to insulin while ketogenic patients are relatively insensitive to insulin (which apparently sets off a chain reaction of biochemical and endocrine disorders). Both imbalances here should diminish intake of refined sugars and starch-dominant meals. The glucogenic imbalance type should eat like a fast oxidizer (high-purine proteins), while the ketogenic imbalance type should eat the proteins recommended for a slow oxidizer. Schenker apparently does not emphasize the high complex carbohydrate diet usually recommended for the slow oxidizer.

As we have seen, the autonomic nervous system is often used in defining metabolic types. Schenker states that either of the two branches (sympathetic or parasympathetic) can be "stuck" in a state of overactivity. He states that the calcium-potassium ratio determines the effect of the two branches on target organs. The overly parasympathetic dominant is advised to eat more protein/fat and the overly sympathetic type more vegetables. This diverges from general recommendations (Appendix O).

The reader may more readily identify with the acid/alkaline balance that is affected by the other four balances, i.e., if you're either acid or alkaline you'll need to increase water intake, usually with selected electrolytes. Foods contribute here: a too-alkaline person may be consuming too much potassium, magnesium, or calcium or an excess of carbohydrates like fruits and juices, or they may be deficient in protein and fat with respect to carbohydrates.

Schenker's organization, "Nutri-Spec" provides physicians and other health professionals with a manual (Schenker 1995) and a source of special supplements to address the problems involving the five balance systems. In each of the ten imbalances a client is instructed to take a very specific combination of vitamins, minerals and amino acids available from the Nutri-Spec company. A patient taking the tests from a qualified health practitioner will be asked to return for re-testing the first and third week after taking the supplements. If the imbalances have been corrected, and quite often they will be, the patient can stop taking the special supplements. It is important that recommended dietary changes be continued.

For a lay person, it is detailed and complex. Recognizing the metabolic differences of individuals via such patterns of biochemical imbalance is a unique and apparently successful approach to discerning the genetic or acquired metabolic problems of individuals. Time may reveal it as a novel and workable practical approach for the non-allopathic health professional and may help our own personal path through the physiological jungle.

Although understanding Schenker's approach is detailed and complex, the tests themselves are simple, rapid and noninvasive, dealing with such things as saliva, urine, pulse rate and so on. A breath-holding test, for example, may give a clue as to the acidity of the blood. I took the tests with John Glaccum (D.C.) of Lilburn, Georgia, who told me that the Nutri-Spec system has been powerful and effective with his patients. Locating a practitioner near you may be a problem. I suggest calling the Nutri-Spec Company.

CHAPTER TWENTY-SIX

500,000 Hair Analyses Can Tell You Something

David Watts, Ph.D.

Like Kristal, Wolcott, and others, David Watts drew upon the early work of Roger Williams, Melvin Page and George Watson. Based upon close to 500,000 mineral analyses of human hair tissue Watts found that these tests revealed metabolic characteristics that correlated well with early investigators. Storage of minerals in hair tissue is more reliable than levels in blood or scrum.

Watts has identified eight distinctive metabolic categories that describe biochemical individuality. Each has a set of characteristic endocrine glands, members of which (adrenal, pituitary) function with one or the other of the systems. For example, a hard-driving type A personality will draw a sustainable blast of epinephrine (adrenaline) from the central core (medulla) of the adrenal gland, as well as a continuing supply of several steroids from the outer rind (cortex) of the gland. He thus qualifies as a sympathetic type characterized by the dominance of the action-promoting hormonal outputs of epinephrine so useful in fight or flight situations, whether the office floor, internecine strife at home, or the battlefields of war.

Out of all this Watts has defined two basic types, each with four subtypes. People generally fall into these large categories, one identified as sympathetic dominant, fast oxidizers and the other parasympathetic slow oxidizers. According to Watts, 20 percent of us are afflicted with fast metabolism and 80 percent with slow metabolism. Appendix I summarizes this information. It is admittedly complex but neither is the road to health smooth with no bumps. You can see that fast metabolizers have acid tissues, are low in the sedative minerals (Ca, Mg). They are "type A's," usually workaholics and hyperactive. They may be late for appointments and their body is apple-shaped. On the other hand, slow metabolizers tend to be well-organized, methodical, may need rest and have been known to dwell overly on the past. Unlike the fast oxidizers they tolerate protein poorly and tend toward vegetarianism, according to Watts. Their bodies are pear-shaped.

Watts classifies glands as anabolic and catabolic as first outlined by Melvin Page. The fast metabolizer appears to have a dominance of catabolic glands (Figure 50). In his aggressive driving behavior he is using up his resources. The slow oxidizer is considered anabolic and tends to conserve energy. The endocrine glands work by increasing or decreasing absorption and re-absorption by the kidneys or by decreasing or increasing absorption by the intestines, to achieve the all-important balance (called "homeostasis") of minerals in the bloodstream.

Consider calcium, commonly prescribed for osteoporosis. A Cornell study of the eating habits of 6,500 Chinese concluded that osteoporosis occurs most often in countries where calcium intake is highest and where dairy products are used excessively. Many factors, excessive adrenal cortical hormone levels (causing increased calcium and protein loss from bone matrix), overactive thyroid and estrogen deficiency (increased calcium re-absorption from bone) are at play here. Too much calcium can, remarkably, cause osteoporosis, where calcium extracted from the bone reservoir will float around in the bloodstream and deposit in certain vulnerable tissues especially when magnesium, phosphorus, zinc and copper are lacking. Excess vitamin A, by antagonizing vitamin D or synergizing zinc, may prevent calcium utilization. While calcium supplements may work for Type I osteoporosis, Type II, with an overactive parathyroid gland, has too much calcium circulating and will not be helped by supplements. In fact, in a Mayo study, calcium supplements tripled the risk of non-spinal fractures in osteoporitic women. (Watts, 1991.)

Figure 51 diagrams the completely different mineral relationships in two diabetic patients of opposite types relative to the autonomic nervous system. (Watts, 1999.) In the sympathetic type, note the higher levels of the stimulative minerals sodium and potassium, with potassium higher than sodium. This illustrates what may happen with increased corticoid secretion by the adrenal glands of the fast oxidizer.

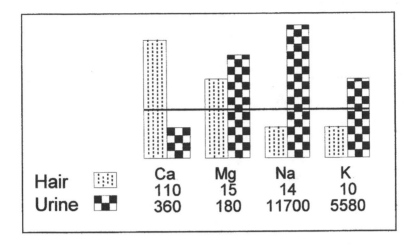

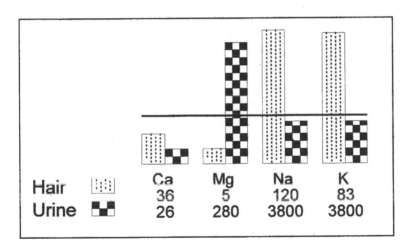

Figure 50. Contrast of slow and fast metabolizers based on tissue (hair) mineral analysis, with urinary excretion rates (mg/24 hrs.). In the slow oxidizer (top graph, parasympathetic dominant) the under-active adrenal glands allow increased urinary losses of sodium and potassium, leading to low tissue levels of these important electrolytes. In addition, calcium (especially) and magnesium are elevated. In the fast oxidizer (bottom graph, sympathetic dominant), the overactive adrenals decrease urinary loss of sodium and potassium, leading to higher tissue levels, while calcium and magnesium are characteristically low. (From Watts, 1999b.)

In contrast, the diabetes of the parasympathetic type may be due to insulin resistance (sufficient insulin but ineffective in lowering blood sugar). Contributing to this are the high calcium relative to magnesium and the high copper, which may raise calcium levels, increase parathyroid secretion and enhance vitamin D activity. Figure 51 emphasizes the main premise of those who classify metabolisms: that you must treat the patient, not the disease.

There is a danger in megadosing yourself with some supplement that you've read about. While there can be an initial favorable result, an induced deficiency of another nutrient may result. Excessive vitamin E decreases vitamin A as well as magnesium, while too much vitamin A may eventually produce a vitamin D deficiency. It would be more advisable to simply reduce vitamin E. Rather than gulping more calcium pills, Watts contends that it is far better to use things that increase calcium availability (synergists) such as vitamin D, or copper or to reduce those that decrease availability (antagonists) such as vitamin A and potassium (Appendix J). One should also limit foods with phytic acids, such as unfermented grains and foods high in oxalic acid (like spinach), which render food calcium unavailable. (Watts, 1990.)

Of interest here is that the susceptibility to disease-causing organisms is also related to metabolic type. Viruses tend to induce parasympathetic activity, and slow metabolic (parasympathetic type) types appear to be more susceptible to virus infections. (Watts, 1989.) Parasympathetic types have high calcium levels as you recall and it seems that certain viruses, such as the Epstein-Barr virus, have calcium-dependent enzymes. Theoretically, things that increase tissue calcium retention like vitamin D, copper, insulin, estrogen and parathyroid hormone invite viral infection. Conversely, things which lower tissue calcium concentrations like vitamin C and A, pantothenic acid, niacin, vitamin B6, zinc, magnesium, iron and phosphorus, should aid in preventing or suppressing viral disease. The under activity of our endocrine glands such as the thyroid can produce depression and extreme fatigue. Chronic viral infections could lead to thyroid and adrenal insufficiency. Thus Watts postulates that this might explain the chronic fatigue syndrome (CFS) which he thinks is not coincidentally tied in with our fervor for calcium supplementation, since calcium has similar effects on these endocrine glands.

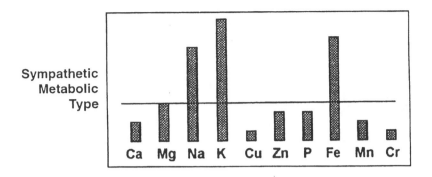

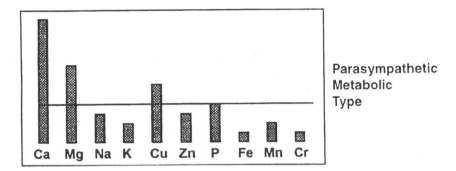

Figure 51. The levels of metals in the hair of two diabetic patients with different metabolic types, based upon the two divisions of the autonomic nervous system. In the sympathetic type, diabetes is indicated by high sodium-potassium levels and the low sodium-potassium ratio, which lowers calcium, probably due to overactive adrenal glands in this fast oxidizer type. Note also the high iron and low copper in this type. This can cause damage to insulin-secreting cells in the pancreas. Apparently, adult onset diabetes can also occur from having ineffective insulin (insulin resistance) as well as having too little insulin. This is usually brought about by dietary abuse. In the parasympathetic patient, insulin resistance may be the primary cause of high blood sugar. In this individual, note the high calcium and its ratio with magnesium which may contribute to insulin resistance. The high copper also promotes insulin resistance as well as weight gain. The cause and treatment of these two patients is completely different and is further proof that you must treat the patient, not the disease. (From Watts, 1999b.)

A psychologist, Richard Malter (Ph.D.), has been very successful in relating tissue mineral (hair) analysis to behavioral problems. He has worked closely with David Watts and uses Watt's metabolic types, mineral ratios and correlation of tissue mineral analysis with neuroendocrine function. In perusing the synopsis of his paper (Appendix K, Malter, 1994) one is struck with how important mineral balance is to human health and behavior, even in children as young as one and one-half years of age. Metabolic typing as done by David Watts is largely based on tissue hair analysis, and it is also part of Wolcott's Healthexcel programs.

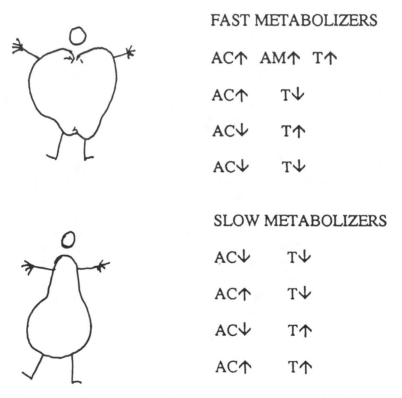

FAST METABOLIZERS

AC↑ AM↑ T↑

AC↑   T↓

AC↓   T↑

AC↓   T↓

SLOW METABOLIZERS

AC↓   T↓

AC↑   T↓

AC↓   T↑

AC↑   T↑

Figure 52.   Watt's metabolic categories, based mainly on tissue mineral (hair) analysis. The acid, apple-shaped fast metabolizers are low in the sedative minerals (calcium, etc.) and high in stimulatory minerals like potassium, just the opposite of the pear-shaped slow oxidizers. Abbreviations for glands: AC (adrenal cortex); AM (adrenal medulla); T (thyroid). Up arrow means increase, down arrow decrease.

CHAPTER TWENTY-SEVEN

A Litany for Lectans

James D'Adamo, N.D.
Peter D'Adamo, N.D.

To body and metabolic types we can add a third possible measure of biochemical individuality, the blood type. Obviously you can classify people into four groups based at least on their blood types (O, A, B, AB). One of the first attempts to differentiate people based on their blood type was proposed by a Japanese, Masahiko Nomi, said to have studied empirical evidence of this for thirty years and to have written forty-two books. This led to theories that one's personality was affected by one's blood type, "officially" called Blood Type Personality Analysis (BTPA). The Japanese society, according to Nomi and Besher (1983) have applied what they have learned "with great success." These authors indicate that, for example, " . . . people with O Type blood are high achievers, very goal-oriented and likely to become leaders in business"; Type A people are assumed to be deep thinkers, Type B's are highly creative and Type AB's are excellent problem-solvers. Because of these presumed relationships it is said that Japanese firms advertise and hire specific blood types for specific jobs. A Japanese brewery conducted a survey among 2,464 beer drinkers and is said to have found differences relating to blood types. One company even manufactures blood-type specific condoms. I have not seen actual data confirming all of this. Nomi lists the qualities and weaknesses of each blood type, their performance at work, in love and romance, marriage and sexual compatibility. For example, " . . . Japanese believe that if you want wild sex you should go out with O-type women." (Nomi, 1983.)

259

A naturopath, James D'Adamo (1989) said that he found evidence (not cited) that certain diseases were more common to one blood group, such as higher frequency for uterine cancer in Type A's. He began to look at diets and noticed that Type A's thrived on vegetarian diets, while Type O's "found it impossible" (to eat this way). James D'Adamo listed the characteristics of individuals with each blood type. He said that the road to health for Type O's was through exercise and that they were capable of running "up to fourteen miles every day." Type A's, on the other hand, were born with creativity and intellectual prowess and required but light exercise. He also discussed menus and supplement combinations for each blood type.

The somewhat novel concept that each of the four blood types would also need different diets was pioneered by the D'Adamo family. Based on thirty years of observations by his father, Peter D'Adamo, also a naturopathic physician, spent fifteen years exploring the connection between blood type, food and disease. His recent book (D'Adamo and Whitney, 1996) offers a dietary approach to health based upon blood type, which he holds is "a more reliable measure of your identity than race, culture or geography." He also attempts to relate the origin of blood types to human evolution. D'Adamo claims that the predominantly carnivorous hunter-gatherers (he calls "the hunter") had Type O blood and that Type A (he calls "the cultivator") blood was the result of a mutation brought about by the major change to a grain and livestock diet between 25,000 and 15,000 B.C. He suggests that, because Type A was more resistant to infections characteristic of denser populations, it was ideally suited to urban industrialized societies and indicated that survivors of plagues like cholera and smallpox "show a predominance of Type A over O." Blood Type B (which he calls "the Nomad"), D'Adamo claims, originated in the Himalayan highlands of Pakistan and India between 15,000 and 10,000 B.C., presumably carried by Mongolian peoples into southeast Asia, which became agriculturally based. Another branch of the pastoral nomad with Type B blood reached eastern Europe; Germans and Australians have a high incidence of this blood type. It is claimed that the interruption of the Bering land bridge stopped the flow of Type B, leaving the Native Americans mostly Type O. The rare Type AB (called "The Enigma") D'Adamo thinks was a late mutation not earlier than 900 A.D. and the result of intermingling of Types A and B, as may have happened when "Barbarian hordes" bred with the Roman Empire. The AB's immune system, according to D'Adamo, makes them more resistant to allergies and autoimmune diseases but predisposes them to certain cancers.

D'Adamo provides dietary plans for each blood type (Appendix L). His recommendations stem from his conviction that our immune and digestive systems still favor the foods eaten by ancestors with the same blood type. His support for this relies on the reaction of proteins called "lectins," which, when absorbed into the circulation from certain foods we eat cause red blood cells to agglutinate, or clump together. Widely distributed (from 1 to 5 percent) in many foods, only D'Adamo claims they enter the blood stream, "where they react with and destroy red and white blood cells." They are reputed to also inflame the intestinal mucosae.

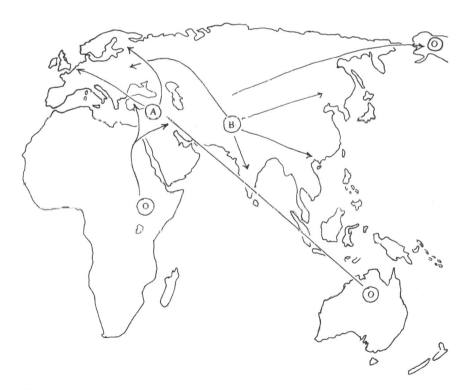

Figure 53. Origin and movements of blood Types O, A and B according to Peter D'Adamo. He claims that these blood types are less than 25,000 years old, and that blood Type AB is less than 1,000 years old. (Modified from D'Adamo and Whitney, 1996.)

The key to D'Adamo's dietary recommendations is that some lectins are harmful to a specific blood type but may be beneficial to the cells of another. He bases his beliefs on watching isolated lectins agglutinate blood cells under the microscope (in vitro). He claims that a simple urine test (the Indican Scale) can detect the presence of unwanted lectins in the body on the basis that improperly metabolized proteins produce toxic byproducts called *indols,* which the test measures. He gives an example of a Type A eating a cured food, bologna, after which the effects of the nitrites are magnified to ninety times in Type A's, making them particularly susceptible to stomach cancer.

According to Sharon (1977), it has been known for years that lectins found in such widely divergent species as lima beans and snails could distinguish between human blood types, stimulate white blood cells to reproduce and identify malignant cells. A soybean lectin can apparently agglutinate malignant cells within thirty minutes. It was also known, as early as 1950, that the lectin of a common herb, wintergreen (*Gaultheria spp.*) could liquefy human tumor cells. Lectins work by binding to the branched chains of sugar molecules that extend from the surface of cell membranes. The different kinds of sugar molecules apparently cause the differing responses among blood groups. Sharon (1977) proposed that plant lectins protect plants against plant pathogens during germination and early seedling growth, based on the fact that a wheat germ lectin inhibits the growth of certain attacking fungi which contain chitin in their cell walls.

Prior to his 1996 book, Peter D'Adamo published a series of articles (1990, 1991, 1993) reviewing lectins and their dietary effects. I'll try to summarize some of this information. (He offers references on request.) Lectins are abundant in legumes (1.5 to 3.0 percent of total protein in soy and jack beans). The second most abundant source seems to be seafood, especially eels, shellfish, halibut and flounder. The high lectin content of soy beans products was suggested as a reason for the positive effects of a macrobiotic diet in combating cancer. According to D'Adamo, the destructive effects of wheat gluten lectin in coeliac disease apparently works by increasing gut permeability to large allergenic molecules. He claims that soybean lectin can destroy intestinal villae. Certain sugars (galactose, lactose) inhibit this destruction, whereas glucose and sucrose worsen it.

Approximately 1 to 5 percent of ingested dietary lectins are said to be absorbed into the bloodstream, clumping both red and white cells, and have been implicated in anemic Third World people who eat a lectin-rich grain and bean diet.

Bacteria, it seems, use their surface lectins (with immunosuppressive ability) to bind to the sugars of epithelial cell membranes in the gut, thus becoming infective. It is thought that the effectiveness of cranberry juice in urinary tract infections is due to its mannose sugars which preempt the binding sites of the bacteria's lectin-like outer covering. D'Adamo states that wheat germ lectin agglutinates the bacteria that cause gonorrhea. Lectins in tomato, cantaloupe and wheat are said to be effective against infections by *Staphylococcus aureans* and S. *mutans*. Some lectins stimulate mitogenesis (reproduction by cell division) of white blood cells. The lectins of pokeweed, when eaten, stimulate both B and T cell lymphocytes. (D'Adamo, 1993.)

Many lectins are fortunately destroyed by cooking, which is why most grains and beans are edible, but heat does not apparently destroy all lectins. Wheat germ agglutinens are heat-sensitive but other wheat gluten lectins "resist autoclaving" (110 degrees celsius for thirty minutes). Of 100 food plants with active lectins, seven (apple, carrot, wheat bran, canned corn, pumpkin seeds, banana and wheat flour) were autoclave resistant according to D'Adamo. High lectin activity was noted in roasted peanuts, corn flakes, Rice Krispies and Kellogg's Special K. Fortunately, presoaking beans results in the complete loss of lectin activity, lending credence to Fallon's admonition to always soak beans well before cooking (and throw away the soak water). According to D'Adamo, a high fiber diet is a high lectin diet and fiber-rich foods are an important cause of allergies, stimulating mast cells to release histamine.

D'Adamo has numerous instructions for eating. Since Type O's originated in Africa, he claims that they should be encouraged to eat lean red meats and game over lamb or chicken. Seafood, especially cold water fish, he recommends for Type O's of Asian and Eurasian descent. Africans, he says, should eliminate dairy and eggs. He is apparently assuming that most Afro-Americans are not descendants of the north African pastoral peoples who used dairy products extensively. Figure 66 attempts to summarize attributes of the major blood types (from D'Adamo, 1996).

CHAPTER TWENTY-EIGHT

Been There—Ate That

Ann Louise Gittleman, M.S., N.D.

In the forefront of nutritional guidance today is Ann Louise Gittleman, a resident of Bozeman, Montana. She recognizes that we are on the brink of a new diet paradigm—the personalizing of nutritional needs. She is one of the few authors to have written a book specifically addressing nutrition individualized by metabolic type. Former Director of Nutrition at the Pritikin Longevity Center, Gittleman proposed a natural weight loss diet which she termed "Beyond Pritikin" (1988). In a later book (1996) this prolific author described the experiences that led her to recognize two principal metabolic types which she called fast burner and slow burner. She was able to make valuable evaluations of current diet plans and fads, from calorie-restricted diets to high protein-low carbohydrate diets, low protein-high carbohydrate diets, through macrobiotics and juice diets, realizing that some people did well, others poorly, on each of these diets, attesting that we indeed have individualized metabolisms.

Like many of us, Gittleman, in her personal life, tried out with almost religious fervor diet regimes that were currently in vogue. Although we seize on to every scrap of data that science can offer, many of us have had to operate on a trial and error basis. Gittleman (1996) was refreshingly candid in recounting her dietary misadventures. In the 1970s she (along with 12.4 million other Americans) became a vegetarian, believing that there were even moral and spiritual reasons for avoiding meat and most animal products and "that fruits, vegetables, seeds and nuts were man's natural foods. . . . " She drank green juices, felt that cooking destroyed enzymes and, in her own words, was "a walking example of a health nut." She could recite in her sleep, she said, all the physical attributes of the human animal such as length of intestine and size of teeth that supported beliefs that man was a vegetarian.

Finally, in her senior year, when her hair fell out, her skin erupted and she was wasting away in obvious ill health, she sought a nutritionally oriented physician who started her eating animal protein. It took her four and one-half years to regain her health after she started eating meat. Her acne scars still remind her of the "severe imbalance I had imposed on my body." Later, she met James Templeton who had cured himself of fourth-stage cancer with a macrobiotic diet. It so impressed her that she decided to pursue a macrobiotic regime into which she plunged with characteristic thoroughness but, again, it was not her cup of tea. Gaining weight, feeling sluggish in midmorning and midday, craving sweets, constantly snacking on rice cakes, crackers and popcorn, she realized through her relationship with Templeton that she was a fast burner and must have substantial amounts of meat in her diet.

Gittleman concentrates on two metabolic types, slow and fast burners (Figure 54 and Appendix M). She has seen so few examples of "balanced burners" that she does not treat this category. Her clients by and large almost always burned off carbohydrates too quickly or not quickly enough. Somewhat innovatively, Gittleman also considered blood types and other aspects of ancestry. She refers to both the work of James D'Adamo (1989) and his son Peter as well as Toshitaka Nomi (1983), for information from blood types that might modify the needs of the basic metabolic type, but was emphatic in saying that metabolic type was the premier issue in regaining health through nutrition. As an example of how blood types might work, her associate James Templeton was "primitive" blood Type O, which normally would do well on meat. But, being a slow burner, he had to choose eating a little more low-fat meat (chicken, fish) and adding high amounts of essential fatty acids from cold water fish because he was of northern European origin. Gittleman points out that skin, eye, hair color and even personality may be outward evidence of the internal need for certain dietary regimes. This underscores an important point that I have tried to make elsewhere, that your metabolic requirements are determined by genes derived from living for long periods of time in specific regional ecosystems.

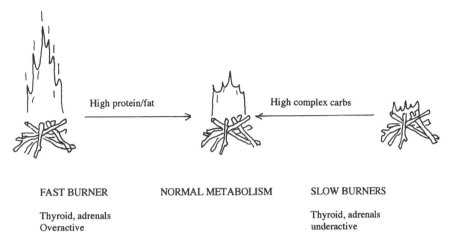

FAST BURNER   NORMAL METABOLISM   SLOW BURNERS

Thyroid, adrenals   Thyroid, adrenals
Overactive   underactive

Figure 54. Gittleman's metabolic types. To dampen and normalize flame (speed of oxidation) eat high protein/low fat (red meat, oily fish, organs, full fat dairy) and calcium. To increase and normalize flame, ad high complex carbohydrates (sweet potatoes, peas, corn, squash) and potassium. According to Gittleman, Atkins and Scarsdale diets address fast burners while Weight Watchers, Pritikin and Ornish offer variations of the slow burner diet.

With all the emphasis today on weight loss regimes, it would be well to briefly review some salient points that Gittleman clarifies. Many of her female clients have gained weight on the popular low fat high carbohydrate diet, which includes things like "fat-free" yogurt, health cookies and fruit juices. Unless you critically read the label on a "health food" cookie package, you may not realize that the manufacturer has increased the sugar content so that the sweeter taste masks the lack of fat, which is what makes a cookie "good." They *never* taste as good as a "normal" cookie and you may eat more of them to "make up for it." And so, as Gittleman is quick to say, weight gain results from too many calories, whether from sugar or fat.

I used to read to my classes from their biology text that, if you just ate properly, you'd get everything you needed from your food. The list was intimidating: meats, so many servings of yellow and orange and red vegetables, so many servings of greens, cooked and raw, bowls of whole grain cereals, so many slices of whole grain breads and glasses of milk and so on. By the time I had finished reading, most of the class was either laughing or tittering.

We all realized that nobody, but nobody, eats in this fashion in this modern society. Further depressing news is that a supermarket tomato might not really be a tomato anymore. In this vein Gittleman reiterates that federal guidelines of the Eating Right Food Pyramid that say you need to eat six to eleven servings a day of complex carbohydrates, three to five of vegetables (also carbohydrates) and two to four of fruit (also carbohydrate). She intimates that very few people could eat this quantity of food, let alone the fact that, for many metabolic types, the diet is overloaded with carbohydrates.

As Gittleman points out, sugars from pasta, bread, and one might add, high glycemic vegetables like carrots and parsnips, if not immediately used in exercise or by storage in the liver as glycogen, go directly to body fat as the final storage. The high carbohydrate diet produces a lot of insulin which not only sends sugars from carbohydrates to storage depots but prevents the hormone glucagon from unlocking body fat cells so that you can get rid of what you already have. Caffeine also stimulates insulin production. Furthermore, one of our principal carbohydrate sources, grains, has an associated factor, gluten, to which people from large parts of the world are not adapted. This "gluten intolerance" causes glandular disorders and malabsorption of nutrients. An interesting aspect of calorie-restrictive diets addressed by Gittleman harks back to our hunter-gatherer heritage. Since man didn't always have three squares a day, if you cut calories too low, thinking that you are going to lose weight you set up a metabolic roadblock that will defeat your best efforts. The body can sense low caloric intake and if it does, it goes into starvation mode. Less thyroid is secreted, thus lowering the metabolic rate. Apparently, enzymes that prepare fat for storage are increased up to twenty-five times. Apropos of this, Gittleman elucidates an amazing phenomenon: that eating three meals a day burns up to 10 percent more calories than if you only eat two meals a day. Breakfast skippers beware because you've already just fasted all night long, so why are you prolonging your fast until the noon meal? When Gittleman speaks of "yo-yo" dieting, she proffers some information that may confuse a devotee of Page's body type methodology: yo-yo dieting may actually change your body type from a pear to an apple, i.e., redistributing fat from hips and thighs to the belly.

As with food, it is important to note that exercise should be tailored to metabolic type: slow burners need to stimulate their metabolic rate with strenuous exercises such as running, cycling and aerobics. Fast burners, on the other hand, need to tone their body and burn fat but take it easy on their already overactive glands. Gittleman suggests for them, yoga, tai chi, swimming, peaceful walks, gardening and undemanding bike rides. So before you start huffing and puffing, listen up.

CHAPTER TWENTY-NINE

"Sleek" Types Need To Eat Protein And Lift Weights

Jay Cooper, M.S.

After twenty years of coaching thousands of clients in "wellness centers" and going through a health crisis himself, Jay Cooper discovered, as others have, that some of his clients thrived on a vegetarian diet while others needed more protein and fat. Eventually, leaning on early workers like Sheldon, Bieler and Rubin (1952), who addressed body shapes, endocrine glands, and personalities, he decided that most of his clients fell into three (four for women) "mind-body" categories. His book (1999) is yet another verification that identifying our individual physical and metabolic types is the optimum way to health. Cooper's observations confirm Bieler's thesis that while all our endocrine glands are active in each of us, one tends to dominate.

By using questionnaires about body shape, area of fat gain, food preferences and personality, Cooper's readers can place themselves into "strong" categories, like "warrior" (adrenal dominant), "nurturer" (ovary dominant) or "sleek" categories like "communicator" (thyroid dominant) and "visionary" (pituitary dominant). Appendix N is a synopsis of some characteristics of the four types. Cooper's basic approach using glandular types, food cravings and needs, and fat distribution is almost identical to that of Abravanal (Figure 46), except that Abravanel postulated that pituitary types required the highest protein intake of all. Cooper conveniently groups the types that need more protein (thyroid, pituitary), in contrast with the types that need more carbohydrates. And, in an important contribution, Cooper relates exercise and energy patterns to the anatomic and glandular types. He believes that the energy patterns of the four types correspond to the Ayurvedic doshas Pitta, Vata, and Kapha (see Chopra).

Regarding diets, he found, as others have, that you crave certain foods that stimulate your dominant gland but that you should avoid these and consume those foods that stimulate the other glands to bring the body more in balance, and in accordance with the size and shape dictated by your genetics.

Mesomorphic adrenal types (who comprised about 50 percent of Cooper's male clientele) should limit protein and fat and should eat a plant-based vegetarian type diet, while ectomorphic "sleek" types need more protein. Cooper says that in the thyroid-driven ectomorph, cold and raw foods can actually hinder metabolic function.

Cooper believes that your body weight will adjust to your genetic "ideal" if you eat the right foods and get the right amount of what he calls "body motion" (exercise). He claims that many obese people have inadvertently reset their "body fat thermostat" at higher levels by prolonged devotion to both improper foods and the living room couch. He states that the low-carbohydrate, high-protein diets will not work for the "strong" types while the "sleek" types have trouble with the low-protein fat, high-carbohydrate diet.

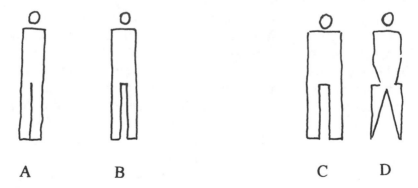

A   B   C   D

Figure 55. Cooper claims his "sleek" types (A, B) have moderate to fast metabolisms, need protein rich diets and warm, cooked foods. His slow metabolizers, the "strong" types (C, D) are more traditionally vegetarian and can take raw, cold foods. Sleek types need strength (muscle building) exercise which strong types should avoid, opting instead for aerobic forms.

Regarding "body motion," Cooper concludes that all body types need twenty-five to sixty minutes of rhythmic exercise three to six times per week to keep body chemistry balanced. He emphasizes that, to be aerobically effective, body motion needs to be in a certain range dependent on your body type, in percentages calculated from your maximum heart rate (standard formula for maximum heart rate: 220 minus your age). Already strong adrenal types should avoid strength training in favor of aerobics while the sleek types need strength training with resistance equipment. Cooper, who was a runner himself, feels that it is important that those (strong types especially) who need aerobics should push themselves into what he calls the "flow zone," where the release of analgesic brain chemicals (beta endorphins and enkephalins) will give a euphoria (runner's high) which will not only last for several hours but inspire you to look forward to your workouts.

His comments on the physical degeneration of the Pima Indians, an example of how people must return to their original life style to regain health, supports the theme I have pursued in the first half of the book. Particularly interesting were his statements that our ancestors who lived in warm climates had longer digestive tracts for subsistence on plant foods, while those from "harsh" (colder?) climates had shorter guts for processing animal foods. This accords with theories I have discussed elsewhere. You might think, however, that the stocky, cold-adapted Ice Age humans of northern Europe were short-gutted adrenal types tending toward carnivory. I suppose it could be argued that, since the dawn of the agricultural revolution, some of these same physical types could have acquired longer guts to process the increasing amount of plant foods.

CHAPTER THIRTY

Are You "Clean" or "Lean?"

Kenneth Baum
With Richard Trubo

One of the latest to use a metabolic classification is Kenneth Baum, President of the Biodynamics Institute. Baum was a former staff member of the Elite Training Institute in Los Angeles, a training center for the U.S. Olympic Team.

The subtitle of his recent book (Baum and Trubo, 2000) is "The Personalized Program for Weight Loss." The book includes a self-test which he claims considers the autonomic nervous system and the oxidative system, as well as body and blood type. His twenty-six questions are supposed to place the reader in one of five types: Super-Clean and Clean (assumed to be fast oxidizers), Lean and Super-Lean (assumed to be slow oxidizers) and Mixed. According to Baum his Clean categories (burn red meat "cleanly") are sympathetic dominants, while his "lean" categories have parasympathetic dominance.

For the "clean" types he recommends foods typically prescribed for fast oxidizers: red meats, dark poultry, wild game, slowly metabolized grains and foods low in the Glycemic Index. Conversely, his low fat "Asian type" diet for "lean" types should use lean meats, low fat dairy and foods high in the Glycemic Index. Baum gives lists of foods, ranking them in three categories (preferred, sometimes, seldom) according to how often they should be eaten.

His sample menus appear to be excellent guides to types and kinds of foods to fit each diet. The text is quite readable and simple. Baum discussed exercise with emphasis on a program he has developed called the seven "no-sweat energy movements" for conditioning the body. He includes a chapter on the value of proper breathing involving the diaphragm.

Before adopting his eating program, Baum advises keeping a three-day food diary noting one, feelings (tired or rundown and rundown or great on a scale of one to five), following a "normal" meal.

His company, (Biodynamics Institute) offers publications, audio tapes, videos, supplements and other products.

CHAPTER THIRTY-ONE

Pigeon-Holing Individuals

Consensus

"One simply can't take 'a day off' from sound nutrition. Whether or not one likes it, the heart beats on, the liver, kidneys and nervous system keep functioning, and their requirements simply can't be postponed."

—George Watson

Most of the authors discussed in prior pages agree that there are three major types of people which, for convenience, are classified by the rate at which they burn, or oxidize, food. We call them fast, slow and mixed oxidizers (they could just as well be called "burners" or "metabolizers"). Most of the authors are in agreement with the synopsis in Appendix O, which does not list the "mixed" category because it is simply a mix of fast and slow. This figure also lists the dominant endocrine glands which either speed up or slow down metabolism or cause specific reactions in the body characteristic of anabolic (building up) or catabolic (tearing down) activity.

Where Metabolic Typists Differ

While most of the authors cited ascribe acid or alkaline states to their metabolic types, only one, Wiley, describes his types under these headings. In fact, his entire book (1989) is based on a presumed acid-alkaline solution to the "food-mood-health puzzle."

His work, as you may recall, is based upon four blood plasma pH samples before and after eating a "test" meal.

Two of the workers cited lean heavily on body type or what you look like, nude or nearly so, in front of a mirror, front, side, and rear views. For those who have the intestinal fortitude to face such an honest appraisal of themselves, it can be, ultimately, a rewarding experience. Page (1949), of course, wrote books about this approach to metabolic typing, illustrated with revealing (but not titillating) photographs. You may remember that he found sympathetic dominants to be heavy below the belt. The opinions of this remarkable dentist was based on some 40,000 actual measurements. In addition, as you recall, some 20,000 blood tests enabled Page to positively relate the condition of your teeth to the ratio of calcium and phosphorus in your blood. Along with Kelley, Kristal, and Wolcott, Page used the autonomic nervous system to categorize his metabolic types. His sympathetic type was obviously a fast oxidizer, his parasympathetic a slow one.

Lawder (1986) offered a reasonable explanation of his own position. He considered his sympathetic types as slow oxidizers but, in addition, he put his catabolic "speed up" glands in the slow oxidizer category. His rationale for placing fast oxidizing carnivores as parasympathetic dominants was, he reasoned, that the parasympathetic system stimulated the gastrointestinal tract so that digestion and absorption was "sped up" and thus food was oxidized more rapidly than in the sympathetic vegetarians. I am not sure how he equated this with the fact that the glands functional with the sympathetic system (thyroid, adrenal medulla) normally cause the oxidative "fires" to burn more brightly in cells and tissues, while at the same time adrenaline suppresses the organs of digestion and assimilation. This dilemma can apparently be resolved by assuming that the autonomic system may, in some people, be independent of the oxidative system. This means that, in Appendix O, both slow and fast oxidizer types can have either branch of the autonomic system overactive.

Wolcott, who followed in Kelley's footsteps, apparently discovered this anomaly when he found that some acid sympathetic types could become healthy by eating fruits and vegetables, thereby alkalizing their systems, and surprisingly, that there were parasympathetic types who must acidify their bodies by eating meals heavy with meat and fat. To accommodate this eventuality, Wolcott created two major systems, either Autonomic or Oxidative Dominant.

To those who find all this a bit bewildering, let me recount the statement of a beneficiary of fifty years of experience with food and endocrine glands, Henry Bieler, who said that we are all a combination of glandular types *but* that one type gland always appeared to be dominant at least by his empirical clinical records. Even more comforting is John Lawder's advice that we are all somewhere on a bell curve, one side or the other of the 2 percent of those lucky people with perfect metabolisms. Is it possible to discern one's metabolic type? We can do it through questionnaires, simple tests on body fluids and even by the old tried and true method, trial and error. And, with that, we are ready for the final chapter, practical and economical ways to go about discovering a personal nutrition for yourself.

CHAPTER THIRTY-TWO

End of the Journey— Redefining Ourselves

"This is the vision of true healthcare that Metabolic Typing offers on the eve of the millennium, a vision that puts health and well-being front and center, while giving individuals the tools that allow them to take full responsibility for their own health."

—Harold Kristal

In the introductory chapter of Part II we theorized that, while we still have many of the adaptations of the hunter-gatherers of Paleolithic times, secondary adaptations may have been imposed since the Neolithic revolution began 10,000 years ago. While we still find people adapted to high protein/fat-low carbohydrate diets (Subarctic, Asiatic steppes) others have had to adapt to high carbohydrate-low protein/fat diets (Central America, Andes, Southeast Asia). Regional differences may exist even in Europe, grading from the Mediterranean climate zone to Scandinavia and northern Russia. " . . . Scottish, Welsh, Celtic, Irish, Danish, Scandinavian, and Northern Coastal Indian peoples all display an inherited need for more essential fats in their diet than other populations." (Gittleman, 1996.) Most people of European origin seem to be, or should be, somewhere in the middle between the carnivore and vegetarian extremes. Modern transportation has resulted in a mixture of body types with more subtle physiological adaptations to locally available foods. Metabolic typing seeks to make sense out of this modern ethnic mix.

Let's assume that you are less than happy with your health. Perhaps you are often sick, have headaches, can't sleep, can't reach your optimum weight or have little or no sex life. It could be your unfortunate choice of a job or mate, or maybe you don't get enough exercise or sleep. On the other hand, it just could be due to the air you breathe, the fluids you drink or the food you eat, as Emanuel Cheraskin was fond of saying.

In the ecological niche that describes an animal, food looms large. In fact, the whole life style and anatomy of most animals seems to be adapted to food-getting. Beyond weaning, water was the only fluid for most mammals; barring volcanic catastrophes, air has been more or less pristine until the Industrial Age. Today we are concocting a variety of beverages and food refinements unknown in the multimillion-year history of primate life. Now isolated by civilization from the hard but efficient rules imposed by nature we must, using all the knowledge at our command, make our own rules for survival.

First things first. Before you attempt to take various tests to determine your metabolic individuality try to trace your lineage back as far as possible. There's a rule in science; don't look for unknowns until you've exhausted the knowns. Your genealogy is a known, your metabolism may be unknown. Your family tree may give you an idea of where your people came from and what types of food they were adapted to. Previous chapters on agriculture, traditional diets, and genetics should be helpful. For example, people from southern Europe (Mediterranean area) can be expected to be adapted to more grains, fruits, legumes, leafy vegetables, light fish, olive and almond oils. Those from cold northern European climates would be adapted to eat root vegetables, oily fish, meat and perhaps some heavy breads. If of Asiatic or African origin your background is probably agricultural, although it *could* be pastoral, from the more remote, isolated regions of the continents.

Begin by asking questions of all your older relatives. One can contact family history centers. There are 3,500 around the world (fourteen in metro Atlanta). Or, with access to a computer you can tap various online databases. The largest is the "Family Search" web site (www.familysearch.org) involving a billion people in 110 countries. The Mormon Church has one of the largest family history libraries and a web site with 400 million entries going back as far as ten generations. There is even a book (*Genealogy Online for Dummies* by April Helm, co-author). Another vital aspect of your history is your grandparents. Here's why. It would be desirable to "weed out" symptoms and diseases due to *inherited* conditions *before* you try to determine which environmental causes (food being one) are responsible. It makes no sense to spend money determining your metabolic type *if* you have inherited conditions that interfere with or control your metabolism.

A predisposition to food allergy can be inherited. (Gerrard *et al.*, 1976.) If both parents are allergic to certain foods, 67 percent of the children may be allergic, 33 percent if only one parent has the allergy. (Taub, 1978.) An Australian team, Chris Reading (M.D.) and Ross Meillon (1984) found that powerful vitamin-mineral supplements had little or no effect on many of their 2,000 cases of diseases caused by inherited defects in absorption or utilization of foods.

Your genetics may suggest a classic food allergy such as to dairy products or grains. If you cannot glean such information from a "family tree" a food allergy test might help. You may be seriously or mildly allergic. I had an aunt who became violently ill if she ate anything with a trace of egg in it. Ironically, strong cravings may signal an allergic response. It is thought that food allergies place an adverse load on immune defenses, reducing our ability to respond to new and chronic infections, interfering with recovery and repair processes and even provoking autoimmune diseases.

Food Allergies

We know that food allergies can originate by the pathologic invasion of our bloodstream by undigested food molecules which act as allergens. But suppose we become allergic to a food by eating it day after day? Could it mean that it was not available to our ancestors in the region where they lived, or had it not been eaten long enough by them to establish adaptation to it? I have seen no data that suggest that people of southeast Asia become allergic to rice by eating it three times a day all their lives, or that New Guineans develop allergies to yams and taro. It seems reasonable to believe that where ethnic or regional foods have been eaten for centuries if not millennia, those who developed allergies would have been weeded out long ago. Even if this is unfounded theory, it would appear wise to learn as much as we can about our ethnic and regional background and be cautious of the

too frequent consumption of a food that was not in long association with our ancestors.

If such an overview is correct, each of us may be adapted to
eat frequently or daily only those foods available to our ancestors. If they came from two regions each with different basic diets
then, theoretically, the offspring could subsist on either or both
of the two different menus. Unless we learn what our ancestors
ate, are we doomed to eat a continuously variable diet, rotating
each food every few days? Except for things like milk, eggs and
wheat, this may be what has happened to develop our present
eating habits, our closest thing to a "national cuisine."

In Part I the genetic distribution of celiac disease was discussed. Additional data suggest its importance. In seventeen
studies conducted in nine countries, celiac disease occurred in
1 to 8 percent of the people tested. (Cronin and Shanahan, 1997.)
In another study, 12 percent of healthy blood donors had antibodies against wheat gluten. (Hadjivassiliou *et al.*, 1996.) It may
even be of unrecognized importance in neurological disease; of
fifty-three patients with nervous system disorders, 57 percent
tested positive for anti-gliadin (from wheat gluten) antibodies.
(Fowkes, 1998b.) Fowkes states that, if further confirmed, this
allergic response to wheat proteins could be "one of the biggest
health problems that modern man routinely faces."

Intolerance to certain foods such as grains can apparently
induce a "craving." It is known that food allergies produce an in-
flammatory response and a shift to a more acid blood pH. "Perceived by the brain as a sharpening of attention and focus, this
pleasurable association creates the psychological force for repeating the experiment." (Fowkes, 1998a.)

The gastro-intestinal tract is said to have the largest and most
immune-reactive surface of the body, being larger than a tennis
court. In fact, it has been stated that immune reactions in the gut-
associated lymphoid tissue comprise 50 percent of the body's immune system response and is the principal site for antibody
production. (Bland, 1998.) Incompletely digested proteins are
recognized by the immune system as foreign substances and antibodies are formed against them by immunoglobulins (usually IgE
and IgG). Allergic reactions in the mast cells of the gut wall then
make the intestinal wall more permeable ("leaky gut" syndrome).

The IgG antibody test is a convenient way to test for problems
with intestinal permeability. Here is a simple explanation provided by Richard Lord, Ph.D. (pers. comm.) of MetaMetrix Inc.:

The term "leaky gut" is used to describe a degeneration of the physical barrier of cells that separate your internal tissues from the mass of food and microbial products in the lumen (inside) of the small intestine. In addition to the physical barrier there is another barrier made of antibodies. The antibodies are secreted by a large collection of special immune cells that are in the walls of the intestines. They detect any foreign materials that gain entry through the physical barrier and bind with them, forming complexes that can be removed.

By definition, then, someone with a leaky gut has greater amounts of undigested food molecules passing through the physical barrier and forming the immune complexes. Of the many classes of antibodies made by the immune system, the specific ones that respond most dramatically to the food challenge from the gut are called IgG1 and IgG4. Laboratory testing can show when you have increased levels of these antibodies. Since they are only present when there is a leaky gut problem, they are the most definitive test for the condition, showing not only the degree of "leakiness" by the number of high levels to individual foods, but also identifying which foods are the main offenders.

Of course, the foods that are eaten most often tend to be the ones that show high levels. The way to overcome the condition is to increase the intake of nutrients that help heal the gut while rotating the offending foods out of the diet. Fortunately, for most people, the gut has very great ability to regenerate, so this type of immune response need not be long lasting, as with classical allergies that are caused in an entirely different way.

More than one-third of foods tested or as few as three to fifteen IgG4 reactions may indicate an intestinal permeability syndrome and may require the total elimination of *all* reacting foods for one month, coupled with nutritional support such as glutamine, pantothenic acid and zinc, or you can eliminate the three to six most reactive foods and not eat the others that you react to oftener than once every four days. (MetaMetrix, 2000.) Richard Lord reports (pers. comm.) that physicians are getting consistent results in healing up the gut.

The best discussion of the Leaky Gut Syndrome, or LGS, is found in the recent book *No More Heartburn* by Sherry Rogers (2000). Doctor Rogers begins by stating that if the colon or gut is not healthy then the rest of the body won't be either. In addition to the unnatural passage of large protein molecules into the blood, Rogers indicates that an inflamed intestinal lining (from celiac disease or Candida) allows bacteria and yeast to pass through the intestinal barrier and, carried by the blood stream, set up infection elsewhere such as in the prostate, sinuses or gums. To diagnose LGS Rogers suggests the Intestinal Permeability Test (done on a urine sample). The next step is to find the cause of the leaky gut. This is done with a Comprehensive Digestive Stool Analysis (CDSA).[24] Step two (in an eight-phase test and treatment list in her book) is to remove the cause, be it a food allergy or an overgrowth of Klebsiella, Candida or other organism.

Rogers has a do-it-yourself test for a leaky gut. Simply ingest L-Glutamine (five grams twice a day one or two hours before or after meals) for a month and if your gut symptoms diminish, you have had and successfully treated a leaky gut condition.

In conclusion, according to Rogers, things that inflame the gut and lead to LGS are "uninvited" bacteria, such as Clostridia (and presumably the protozoan Giardia) and yeasts (such as Candida); alcohol, food additives, and, worst of all she says, are drugs like aspirin and NSAIDS such as Motrin, Aleve, and Advil. "NSAIDS are a major cause of LGS because they so viciously inflame the intestinal lining, causing a widening of the spaces between cells and sometimes even hemorrhaging." Additional threats are food allergies, lactase deficiency and celiac disease.

One of the most devastating effects of a leaky gut is that it sets the stage for generating antibodies that can attack your own tissues (autoimmune disease). (Rogers, 1999.)

For food allergy (or intestinal permeability) tests your physician or health practitioner orders a kit from the laboratory making the tests. Equipped with a physician's request your blood is drawn at a local clinic or lab that ships it by air express the same day. For food allergies, a number of labs do the ELISA test (Enzyme Linked Immunosorbent Assay). Some do the ELISA-EIA (Enzyme Immunoassay). The ELISA Assay tests for immunoglobulins IgE and IgG, using the reaction of antibodies in your blood serum to antigens in select samples of food coated on a plate. In theory here's how it works: Once antibodies have been formed any future ingestion of that particular food creates an allergic response manifested in various parts of the body. Within minutes IgE antibodies cause immediate reactions such as

---

[24] Both tests are offered by Great Smokies Diagnostic Laboratory, 63 Zillicoa Street, Asheville, NC, 28801-1074.

asthma, hives, headaches, itching mouth or even anaphylactic shock. The level of these antibodies in the blood may drop within weeks but quickly return if the same offending food is eaten again. Such foods may need to be avoided for life.

IgG antibodies, however, create responses delayed for hours, even days, after ingestion of a given food. Symptoms, often chronic, may be joint and muscle pain, headaches or fatigue. It takes three to nine months for the IgG antibody level to drop significantly and reactive foods need to be eaten frequently over weeks and months to bring back the allergic response. Following a three to six month's abstinence, foods can be eaten on a rotation basis of once every four days and seldom need to be avoided for life. (GSDL, 1999.)

Various criticisms have been voiced about the reliability of ELISA-EIA tests. (Gaby, 1995; Miller, 1998.) One conclusion was that the responsibility should rest with the physician. In some cases, the "elimination diet" has been successfully substituted.

A different type of test is the ELISA-ACT that involves exposing lymphocytes (white blood cells) to surfaces coated with potential antigenic foods. This procedure measures changes (functional lymphocyte response) in all types of white blood cells to reactive antibodies (IgG, IgM and IgA), immune complexes and cell-mediated reactions.

A third type of allergy food test is the ALCAT. It measures volumetric shifts in the various white blood cells upon incubation with antigens. An interesting side light is the laboratory's statement that, based on clinical studies, as many as 98 percent of participants lost weight or improved body composition by eliminating reactive foods from their diet. In one study, females who had "leveled off" on their weight loss program once more began losing weight, "especially a preponderance of fat from their thighs." Their brochures endorse the theory that after eating an offending food, blood levels of the "feel good" neurotransmitter serotonin go down, causing people to crave foods high in the glycemic index, such as simple sugars and refined flours. They reiterate the oft-cited refrain that the very foods we crave most may be the ones that cause our problems.

I took all three tests (ELISA-EIA, ELISA-ACT, and ALCAT). Unfortunately, for me at least, each test generated a completely different set of foods giving allergic reactions. If you do take a laboratory food allergy test the most sensible solution would seem to be to eliminate the foods with the strongest reactions one by one and see if, after three or four days, you feel better. Most labs suggest that you eliminate strong reactors for six months, moderate or weak reactors for three. After three to six months, you can add back the objectionable foods one by one and see if any symptoms reoccur. Ideally, health care professionals should order food allergy tests before and after adding supplements to your daily diet.

There is a theory that just because we can't detect any adverse reaction to a particular food, it does not mean that there is no effect. The immune system may be weakened- something you can't "feel." (Golub, 1987; Sell, 1987; Jaffe, 1989.) If this is true what could be more critical than the reaction of your immune system to disease organisms and cancer cells? There is a current belief that some cells are more or less continuously becoming cancerous in the normal individual, but are rapidly destroyed by killer white blood cells, and that cancer is basically the result of a weakened immune system. Using coffee as an example: White blood cells may react strongly not only to caffeine, but to other substances in the coffee bean itself. If one over-indulges in coffee, it might keep the immune system suppressed long enough to be dangerous.

Tissue Mineral Analysis

This test is usually done on a hair sample and is especially helpful in documenting the levels of potentially harmful metals in your body, such as lead, mercury, cadmium, iron and aluminum. High levels might indicate a need to have your drinking water analyzed. Your county agent will help. Analyzing common foods is much more expensive but can be done through the Cooperative Extension Service of most universities.

Elevated heavy metals, such as mercury from root canals and dental amalgams are reported as a probable cause of "leaky gut" syndrome (and nutrient loss), thus leading to autoimmune disease, fortunately correctable if you can eliminate the toxins or their origin. (Rogers, 1999.)

Several reliable organizations do tissue mineral analyses. To remove excess metals from your body, you may want to consider chelation therapy. Though expensive, it has the added benefit of reducing the chances of atherosclerosis by removing the metal calcium from plaques in blood vessel walls. Consult the Watts chapter, especially Figure 51, which contrasts tissue metal levels in two diabetic patients with different metabolic (autonomic system) types.

Hazardous Chemicals

You will certainly want to monitor your intake of potentially hazardous chemicals to be found in our environment and our foods. The importance of eliminating toxic substances from our diet was highlighted by Dr. Sherry Rogers. In your review of what toxic chemicals you might be getting in your diet you need to also be aware of hormone-disrupting chemicals, which work their changes largely through interfering in the reproductive biology of animals. These have been brought to our attention by Theo Colborn and her associates (Colborn *et al.*, 1997) in a startling book *Our Stolen Future.*

Many hormone-disrupting chemicals mimic natural hormones in the human body such as estrogen. (Excessive estrogen is implicated in breast cancer.) Many plants have evolved things like estrogen mimics that suppress the fertility of animals that eat them. These substances lurk in many of our favorite herbs and vegetables such as parsley, garlic, wheat, soy, potatoes, carrots, apples and cherries. Colborn indicates that we have evolved defenses against many of the phytoestrogens in common plants (such as soybeans) but not against synthetic estrogens that leach out of such things as PVC pipe and polycarbonate containers. Here is an eye-opening example: plastic coats the inside of about 85 percent of food cans in the United States. Among twenty brands tested, about one half contained the contaminant Bisphenol-A (a synthetic estrogen mimic). Stunningly high concentrations were found in peas, artichokes and corn. In some instances, canned foods contained twenty-seven times more than enough synthetic estrogen to make breast cancer cells proliferate.

Parasites

You must also be able to rule out parasites gotten from travel, pets or other sources. It has been noted by a CDC survey that one out of every six people has one or more species of parasites, living as unwanted guests in their bodies. One estimate by a physician concluded that as many as 25 percent of the inhabitants of metropolitan New York City were infected. (Gittleman, 1993.) In her book, *Guess What Came to Dinner*, this author emphasizes the importance "of an in-depth personal history that examines both present and past travel, lifestyle, and dietary patterns. . . ."

Determining Your Personal Nutrition or Metabolic Type

Suppose you can find nothing significant in your genetic background or revealed by food allergy or hair analysis, and your physician finds no medical reasons for anything wrong. You have eliminated sources of toxins in your environment that you have breathed, drunk or eaten. Yet you still feel un-well or can't achieve a reasonable weight for your body type. You sense that something must be wrong. You are probably ready to try to determine what many authors call your metabolic type.

This is not an exact science for it deals with enormous individual and genetic variation. We're apparently just as different inside as we are outside, given our mixed-up heritage and widely divergent life styles. By various tests and test diets we can come closer and closer to how we react to the world at a cellular level. Keep in mind that some authors in Part II, such as Watson and Gittleman, may classify individual metabolisms in terms of the oxidation rate (fast or slow). Others such as Wiley, concentrate on pH (acidity or alkalinity). Still others like Page and Kelley use the autonomic nervous system for the major categories. It is important to remember that Wolcott's clinical experience suggests that one can speak equally in terms of either the autonomic nervous system or the oxidation rate being in control (or better, in overcontrol, creating an imbalance).

Test-Guided Nutrition

In addition to tests that detect hidden food sensitivities, heavy metal and parasites, there are other tests collectively called "Test-Guided Nutrition" which allows detection of hormonal and metabolic disorders often central to determining your individual metabolism. These are non-invasive tests of saliva and urine. In a section that follows ("Getting Help") several of the organizations cited may use simple tests of this type. Your physician or health advisor may, however, wish you to take other, more expensive lab tests, such as the intestinal permeability test (for "leaky gut") mentioned elsewhere.

In the chapter on Genetics the emergency role of the hormone adrenaline was discussed. It produces body changes essential to survival when we are faced with danger, but its continual low-output secretion (via sympathetic nerves and adrenal medulla) can constitute a chronic stress leading to ill health. Another stress hormone, cortisol, is produced by the outer rind of the adrenals and can be equally damaging, especially when blood levels are permanently elevated by near-constant stress. Chronic cortisol secretion can be brought about by numerous aspects of our modern artificial environment: commuting in traffic, work deadlines, debt worries, too much noise, crowds, over-exercising (especially in women), allergens and toxins.

As with adrenaline, during the occasional emergency in natural environments, cortisol provided for support by increasing energy (sometimes at the cost of protein breakdown) and temporarily suppressing non-essential functions, such as inflammation in a wound (immune system action). Unfortunately its continued secretion drops DHEA (the "mother of all hormones") levels, thus accelerating aging and diminishing hormones derived from DHEA such as the sex hormones. The chronic stress of modern city life can produce a "state of siege," eventually exhausting the adrenal gland and setting the stage for serious medical conditions. There is thus an essential test called the "functional adrenal stress profile" (on saliva) which reveals daily fluctuations in your levels of both cortisol and DHEA. It is offered by a number of labs.

Another series of tests (on urine) that are very relevant are collectively called a "metabolic assessment profile." There are three or more tests. One, an "oxidative stress test" determines the degree of danger from free radicals to which your cells are exposed. Tests on efficiency of digestion are also important (as well as the intestinal permeability tests). Another test deals with the ability of your liver to detoxify pollutants. Your physician or health care provider can arrange for these tests from various labs or, sometimes, from a single source.

Getting Help

If you don't wish to drastically change your diet as an experiment or for whatever reason and you still wish to persist there are organizations that will help you, for a price of course. One, Healthexcel, will analyze your metabolism (see section on Wolcott-Healthexcel). The easiest way to use their program is through an "alternative" physician or other health-care practitioner. After a preliminary consultation you will be asked to fill out a lengthy questionnaire and do a two-day diet test at home. You may need to visit a health-care practitioner for some simple tests involving things like blood pressure, pulse, respiration rate, breath-hold time, blood glucose, urine and saliva pH tests. Alternatively, you could purchase the testing equipment for home use. These data, coupled with your other at-home tests and questionnaire will be analyzed by Healthexcel computers and the report will reveal your metabolic type, your carbohydrate-protein-fat ratio, customized diet and supplement regimes. Some follow-up testing to monitor your progress may be in order.

Harold Kristal, a friend and former student of Wolcott, has developed a Personalized Metabolic Self-Test Kit that you can use at home, with enough supplies for two complete tests on yourself (not on two different people). The test kit includes equipment such as a blood glucose meter and supplies, a self-test chart and a questionnaire. The test requires approximately three hours, plus "down time" between the various tests. From a "mini-glucose challenge" test Kristal can infer the relative acidity or alkalinity of the blood (on either side of pH 7.46); fast oxidizers (and sympathetic dominants) have more acid blood while slow oxidizers (and parasympathetic dominants) have more alkaline blood. Slow oxidizers (and sympathetics) tend to feel better after this test; fast oxidizers (and parasympathetics) tend to feel worse. (Kristal, 2000.) Results affect other tests on saliva and urine (pH, respiratory rate, breath holding ability, etc. Reaction to a potassium-rich preparation helps determine the autonomic type. (Kristal and Haig, 2000.) After submitting the test results, chart and questionnaire clients receive a "Personalized Metabolic Typing Report" and a diet plan. Additional analyses and refill supplies are extra. Both the Healthexcel and Kristal tests use some of the same techniques, as does Guy Schenker's Nutri-Spec.

The testing method for these organizations and some of Schenker's analyses are based in part on the work of Emmanuel

Rivici that what food or supplement may be alkalizing to one may be acidifying to another.[25] It would seem that the simple lab tests that accompany these evaluations tell the researcher whether your system is too acid or too alkaline, on either side of a "normal" urine pH of 6.0. It is a type of biofeedback—the proper dietary and supplement changes are designed to correct any imbalance. Retesting may be necessary. Rivici apparently spent over fifty years investigating the relation of such metabolic imbalances to disease.

In the section on John Lawder, two organizations that have derived their metabolic typing background from Lawder's work are discussed. Indeed, as Figure 57 shows, their carbohydrate-protein-fat ratios are quite similar. Both require that you join a gym or health club and they offer varying degrees of personalized service. *SporTelesis* requires their licensees to sell you, or try to, their line of supplements. *Apex Fitness* will give you a discount on their exclusive line of products. Both offer a computer-derived profile of your metabolic type based on a detailed questionnaire and may recommend appropriate diets and exercises. Through the questionnaire, both groups address your lifestyle, genetics, eating habits, activity levels, work schedule and body type. Bone structure and percentage of fat may figure in. For details, see the section on John Lawder. If you want to combine physical workouts and/or body building, weight management and individualized nutrition, this may be the route to go for you.

Naturally such programs and testing involves costs but they are reasonable. At the same time, realize that a good supplement program may cost you between 100 and 150 dollars a month, assuming you don't eat a perfect diet (Who does?). At this point let me say most emphatically that such costs are inconsequential compared to the big bucks you might otherwise spend on illness, prescription drugs and hospitalization, apart from loss of valuable time and feeling rotten.

Since there are many fine laboratories scattered around the world, it would be unfair to list just those that have come to the author's attention, thus specific labs and clinics are not

---

[25] In general, meat, nuts, most grains, corn, tomatoes, vinegar, intensive exercise, surgery, asthma and antibiotics are acidifying (catabolic) while beans, eggs, refined flour, millet, vegetables, fruits, seaweed, chocolate and the "additives" (sugar, dairy, alcohol, caffeine, nicotine, salt) exercise, meditation and sleep are alkalizing (anabolic). (Johnson, 1988.)

footnoted. Also, addresses and phone numbers have a way of changing. Some organizations that can help determine your metabolic type have already been discussed. Addresses and phone numbers are thus not listed.

Instead, the Center for Aging Control (CAC) (5575 South Semoran Boulevard, Orlando, FL 32822, web site at www.center-foragingcontrol.com) has agreed to act as a "clearing house" to provide up-to-date addresses and phone numbers of reputable organizations and products, as well as noting books and other references, available to you on receipt of your letter or on-line message. The CAC may also be able to help locate a local health practitioner close to where you live for assistance with things as blood (pressure, glucose tolerance, intestinal permeability, food sensitivity, etc.), urine and saliva tests, and cancer therapies.

In addition, the CAC may be able to provide updates on progress in the field of metabolic typing, as well as other advances in human nutrition.

Self-Testing

There are also several very simple do-it-yourself type tests involving your reaction to various ingested, easily obtainable substances. One, offered by Rudolf Wiley, involves a simple cup of coffee.

Wiley now feels that the lab work to determine plasma pH is probably too difficult for the average person. He suggests using the simple coffee test to determine your metabolic type. (Wiley, pers. comm.) To do this test, refrain from drinking coffee for seven to ten days, then drink a full cup of "real," non-decaffeinated coffee, and see how you feel. Alkaline (slow oxidizer) types should feel good, acid (fast oxidizer) types will have difficulty tolerating one cup and mixed types may "feel a little tense or nervous" after one cup (and very nervous after two or three). During the pretest period it might be wise to refrain from, or limit your intake of, caffeinated soft drinks, chocolate (which contains caffeine) and, of course, green or black tea. Most men, post-menopausal women and diabetics appear to be alkaline. You may wish to re-read the chapter on Wiley. After you have done the coffee test, take Wiley's short quiz (Chapter 21). Simple tests by Kelley involve the vitamin niacin on an empty stomach, or vitamin C (see chapter on Kelley). Try these tests at home along with answering the simple questionnaires. Something else you can do at home is to stand naked or in a bathing suit in front of a full length mirror or a sympathetic friend, and assess your physical type using the write-ups on Page and especially Abravanel and Cooper. Your own appearance may give you a welcome clue.

A psychochemical odor test ("sniff test") was developed and heavily relied upon by George Watson. Personally, I found it very difficult to distinguish the odor categories, perhaps because I'm close to a mid-oxidizer.

An inexpensive solution, at least for extreme fast and slow oxidizers, may be to imitate one of Watson's early tests with students, by simply crushing a 100 mg tablet (or emptying a capsule) of thiamine in a small plastic vial (capped), and smelling it from time to time. Refer to the chapter on Watson for analyzing your reactions to the odor.

A do-it-yourself workbook has been published. (Johnson, 1988.) It involves home-testing your urine pH (2), which is supposed to fluctuate between acid (catabolic, peaking at 4 p.m.) readings by day and alkaline (anabolic) readings at night (peaking in early morning). Theoretically, you feel better or worse in either extreme acid or alkaline state, the object being to search for a pH "comfort range." One is cautioned to be aware that environmental (processed foods, rancid fats, noise and other stress), mental, emotional and physical factors also affect "feelings." There are indications that many of the signs of aging are tied to an anabolic imbalance. (Johnson, 1988.)

Finally, to organize your approach to finding a personal nutrition try to follow the nine suggestions in "Steps to determine your metabolic type." One of these steps refers to a list of "characteristics of the three metabolic types" at the end of this section. Gleaned from the various authors of Part II, it also lists self-tests and reactions that may help you decide in which direction your metabolism leans.

I found Wolcott's simple one-page "fine tuning mini-quiz" (2000, p. 265) contrasting the right and wrong protein/carbohydrate ratios, to be especially helpful. One of the problems of the longer quizzes offered by various authors is that they ask you how you feel after eating a meat and fat-rich meal. A lot of us, myself included, can't remember how we felt in the past after

cating a certain type of meal. Before trying to answer questionnaires, it would be wise to keep good notes for several days on the
general meal type such as a high protein/fat, low carbohydrate
meal (or the opposite) and monitor yourself afterward. Also observe how often you get hungry or "need" snacks or coffee, tea or
caffeinated drinks like colas or Mountain Dew. As Barry Sears
points out, if you eat the correct balance of carbohydrate, protein
and fat at a meal, you should not be hungry for at least four
hours. If you have to sneak a snack, watch out, your previous
meal may not have been balanced.

The easiest simple test would be to eat two entirely different
breakfasts and observing your energy and feelings for the four or
five hours prior to lunch. For example, one morning eat a pro-
tein/fat rich breakfast that should include some or all of the following: eggs, sausage, bacon, fried potatoes, cheese omelet.

If, for four or five hours afterwards, you feel good and energetic, your metabolism is probably being dominated by either fast
oxidization or parasympathetic nervous control. On another
morning, limit your breakfast to fruits and cereals with skim or
low-fat milk and perhaps coffee. The slow oxidizer and the sympathetic dominant should feel good on this, while the fast oxidizer (and parasympathetic) should feel lousy. No marked
feelings or energy gain or loss either way suggests a Mixed Type.

Finding Your "Ratio"

The basic nutrients needed by metabolic types are often defined
as a ratio of carbohydrate to proteins to fat.

In trying to find your ideal ratio of carbohydrate, protein and
fat, you can be comforted by the fact that you lie somewhere
along a bell curve (Figure 56). Compare your ratio with Lawder's
"ideal" ratio and those of Wolcott and Sears (Figure 57). Expect
surprises, as Spruce found with his bodybuilders—not all mus-
cular mesomorphs will benefit from the same diet. Figure 58 presents more or less "ideal" ratios for fast and slow oxidizers, along
with the general consensus regarding kinds of foods in each category. You might find it interesting to compare these ratios with
those percentages in Figure 59 depicting the USDA food guide
pyramid, which would seem to favor very slow oxidizers (carbohydrate 77 percent, protein 17 percent). You may wish to refer

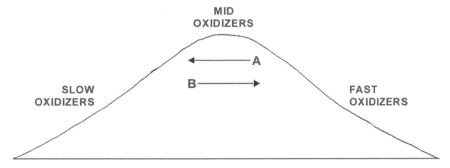

Figure 56.   An approximated bell curve with 70% of people as mid-oxidizers, according to John Lawder. If mid-oxidizers on the slow side (B) eat too far in the direction of the arrow, they may suffer from heart problems and cancer, while those on the fast side (A) who eat too far in the opposite direction may suffer weight problems, hypoglycemia, chronic fatigue and uncontrolled hunger (see section on Lawder). Lawder claims only 2% of people are perfectly balanced mid-oxidizers. To discover our metabolic type, the rest of us have to take simple tests, pay for analyses by organizations or simply eat strongly in one direction for several days and see how we feel. Rudolf Wiley contends that most (75%) males and all diabetics are alkaline (slow oxidizers). He found most women to be genotypically acidic (fast oxidizers). Some women, however, apparently oscillate over their lunar cycles, being alkaline (day 1 to 14) and then acid (day 15 to 28). A few individuals (male and female) seem to cycle over a twenty-four-hour period, according to Wiley. Compare with Rogers' metabolic cross (Fig. 48).

back to the three food pyramids pictured in the section on traditional diets.

To test where you fall on Lawder's bell curve you can always resort to the trial and error approach, eating more like a fast or more like a slow oxidizer, as along the horizontal axis of Sherry Rogers' "metabolic cross" (Figure 48). Use Appendix O as a general guide, plus trying to verify yourself in the write-ups and summaries (Appendices A-N).

Finally, if you can't get reasonably close to a believable ratio (your metabolic type), or you are too busy to do-it-yourself, then the thing to do is to seek outside help from organizations which specialize in assessing your metabolic type. This is especially necessary if you wish to learn which glands and branches of the autonomic nervous system are dominant.

	FAST	MID	SLOW
Lawder's "ideal" ratios	30-40-30	45-30-25	60-20-20
SporTelesis ratios	30-40-30	55-25-20	75-15-10
Spruce ratios	40-30-30	55-25-20	75-15-10
Healthexcel (Wolcott) ratios	30-40-30	50-30-20	60-25-15
Sears "Zonal" ratios	40-30-30		
Eaton, Shostak and Konner ratios Preagricultural people average		45-30-22.5	
Range		40-50; 25-35; 20-25	
Suggested modern ratio			60-20-20
Jaffe (Healing diet for stressed individuals with subnormal gut physiology), i.e., disordered microbial ecology; impaired protein digestion, etc.		55-20-25	
Rogers' ratios Carnivore	30-40-30		
Omnivore		50-30-20	
Vegan			75-15-15
Raw Vegan			80-10-10

Figure 57. Comparisons of some carbohydrate-protein-fat ratios grouped (approximately) under oxidative type. (From Lawder, 1986; Healthexcel, 1998; Sears, 1995; Spruce, 1997; Eaton, Shostak and Konner, 1988; Jaffe, 1989; SporTelesis, 1999; Wolcott, 2000; and Rogers, 2000.

In seeking help an initial step is to locate a sympathetic physician or other health care professional. You will need their assistance in authorizing lab work and in analyzing food allergy and tissue mineral problems. They must also diagnose any medical conditions before you look for the more subtle signals induced by your diet.

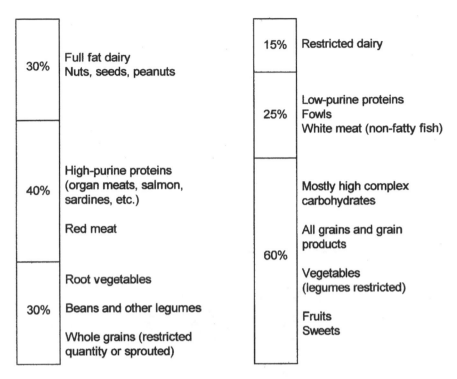

Figure 58. "Food columns" comparing recommended ratios (in %) and types of carbohydrates, proteins and fats for fast (left) and slow (right) oxidizers. Amounts of each type of food are not indicated. Note that kinds of foods vary between columns; for example, quite different protein sources are indicated for fast and slow oxidizers. While nuts and seeds have good protein they are listed here largely as fat sources. (Ratios from Lawder, 1986 and Healthexcel, 1998.)

Why We Eat Like We Do

Here we face some challenging questions. Do people choose what they should eat or what they want to eat? How are "cravings" for certain foods explained? Have some of us lost the ability to select the "right" foods or do we ignore our body's subtle signals and opt for a quick energy fix?

Most researchers seem to duck these questions and simply tell you how to eat based upon the two routes by which cells are energized. A few, such as Abravanel and Cooper, in addition to saying what you should eat, also list foods you crave but should not eat.

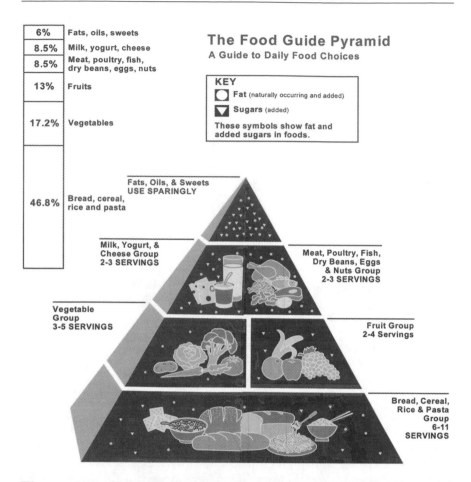

Figure 59. The USDA food pyramid guide to *daily* food choices, and a "food column" derived from it, showing the approximate percentages of foods. Carbohydrates total 77% (not including sweets) and protein 17% (fatty nuts are included with protein). Cheese, often 40% fat, is not listed in the fat group. (Pyramid courtesy Center for Nutrition Policy and Promotion. 1996. USDA. Home and Garden Bulletin 252.)

Lawder and Watson are examples of workers who believed that the individual would, if given a chance, eat the foods appropriate for their metabolic type. Lawder felt that fast oxidizers would choose fatty and protein-rich foods such as bacon, pork chops, olives, eggs, nuts, luncheon meats and steak whereas slow oxidizers would rarely desire these foods. He thought that fast oxidizers would also want three meals a day and between-meal and late evening snacks. Slow oxidizers would go for the quick energy fix of bread and jam rather than bread with cheese.

Watson, using a questionnaire supported by psychochemical data and blood tests, revealed that fast oxidizers would want meats and fatty things, heavy breakfasts, had energy let-downs after eating sweets, had to snack frequently and reacted badly to coffee. His slow oxidizers, on the other hand, loved salads, preferred a sweetened dry cereal with milk for breakfast or could skip it altogether and did well on coffee. Wiley agreed with most of these preferences.

While individuals can have legitimate desires for certain foods Watson, on a cautionary note, said that people can and do choose foods that are bad for them, and that "liking" it is not necessarily grounds for eating it. Taste can be a poor basis for choice, according to Watson. Wiley concurs, stating that "listening to your taste buds" can spell disaster. You need not be the hapless victim of your taste buds, conditioned since childhood by the sensitive primate tongue designed for the sweet tastes of tropical fruits. Remarkably, some of these taste preferences or "hedonic reactions" may be inherited, including desire for the taste of broccoli, orange juice, chicken, hamburger, strawberry, green beans, cottage cheese and bacon. (Falciglia and Norton, 1994.) For whatever reason, what you like may be deleterious to your health. Because you've eaten "that way" all your life, changes will be tough. Like somebody said about progress: "Progress was once OK, it's just gone on too long." In addition, your new dietary course may be fraught with social peril. You will be called, as Bieler was, a "health nut" or "dietary kook," and subject to the ridicule of friends.

Lawder and Watson may be right but it seems possible that many of us simply eat things that give us a "quick fix" or energy boost. In this we indulge these cravings hourly if necessary, but in 99 percent of our prehistory we had to eat what the environment provided at that time of year—snacks and stimulating beverages were not available the year around or throughout the day (and night).

Perhaps our "cravings" or "tastes" for certain foods may or may not be what our metabolism needs. Looking again at Figures 34 and 35 we see that there are two routes by which food energizes a cell, the principal (fast) and slow routes. "Principal" does not mean the best route. Both routes must be utilized to create a balanced and sustainable flow of energy. If Abravanel and Cooper are correct, could some fast oxidizers "crave" a quick energy boost by frequently eating simple or refined carbohydrate snacks and caffeinated beverages? Do slow oxidizers (Figure 34) have the opposite problem, getting a "quick fix" of energy by devouring proteins and fats?

As mentioned earlier, there are inherited taste preferences to consider, along with possible preferences acquired, often when sweets and chocolate helped fuel the ceaseless activity of childhood. These things aside, there are several things that work in our favor. One is that so-called "addictions" or "cravings" may really reflect our need for additional energy. These may subside when you "eat right" for your metabolic type. Our insatiable desire for repetitive snacks of simple carbohydrates and caffeine-laced beverages may be reduced or eliminated by the steady energy flow induced by eating sufficient proteins and fats along with appropriate carbohydrates. Rogers (2000) offers an easy test for food addiction. If you suspect a certain food just stop eating it for from four to eight days. Then, while sitting, take your pulse. Then eat the food and take your pulse every ten minutes for one hour while still sitting. A consistent pulse rise of ten beats or more per minute (or other symptoms) indicates that your body is "unhappy" with that particular food.

In the same book, Rogers proposes a similar solution to verify your food allergies. To test for a lactase deficiency, for example, stop eating dairy products in any form for one week. Then, for one day, consume everything you can think of that might contain dairy, such as ice cream, sour cream, cheese and cream sauces. According to Rogers, your gut will, within forty-eight hours, inform you of a problem. Gas, bloating, diarrhea and other discomfort suggest an allergic reaction to an offending food.

Fortunately, an appetite "control" is built into the human brain. This involves several neurotransmitter substances like serotonin. (There are so many of these messenger neuropeptides that the brain can be likened to a giant gland.) If you eat too much carbohydrate the brain signals you not to want it, thus reducing consumption. Conversely, too much protein in the diet causes the brain to send a message to eat more carbohydrate. (Wurtman, 1982.) This is a mechanism that apparently worked for early man and still helps some children balance their diet after having eaten too much sweets or protein. Unfortunately, unlike our Paleolithic forebears, modern man can get refined and concentrated carbohydrates daily and the year around. Carbohydrates are known to be "addicting" by stimulating the pleasure centers of the brain and temporarily raising both blood sugar and brain serotonin levels (serotonin is the "feel good" hormone). Then when blood sugar and serotonin levels drop, withdrawal symptoms set in and include the craving for more carbohydrate food. (Fowkes, 1998a.)

All this is not lost on the industries that package foods and operate fast-food drive-ins. They capitalize on presenting things that taste good. This is especially obvious in the use of sugar and salt, especially when combined with fat. Products containing sugar and fat (doughnuts) and salt and fat (french fries, potato chips) are especially "tasty."

I have not found critiques of many of the specific diets prescribed by the numerous authors in the field of nutrition. The few that have surfaced suggest caution, especially if the author touts a diet that everybody should follow. Some of the diets apparently work well enough for some people who naturally suggest it to their friends and think it will work for them as well, not realizing that it may apply only to those whose genetics and metabolism are similar to theirs.

Another confusing aspect is that many of the health advisors, in addition to their own special recommendations, also prescribe general practices that would promote good health in anyone regardless of their individual metabolism: lessening stress, stopping smoking, eliminating soft drinks and excessive alcohol, and "adequate" supplements. So how can the patient tell whether his improvement was due to his advisor's specific advice, or because they made all these other good changes in their lifestyle?

Sears' (1995) low calorie diet, with its "ideal" ratio of carbohydrate (4 g) to fat (3 g) may not work for everyone. Klaper (1999) considers that low carbohydrate diets put the body into a constant state of ketosis and fears that they would lead many to suffer from "damaged vital organs and more lethal degenerative diseases," but he does admit that some people can benefit by "eating less carbohydrates, more protein, etc." Sears, however, indicates that his diet avoids ketosis and promotes health, provided you can stay in the "zone" where carbohydrate-protein ratios are kept between 4:2.5 and 4:4.

Several tables are included to assist your efforts to eat wisely for your own individual metabolism. Appendix P tries to summarize the food recommendations of most of the authors in Part II.

Bear in mind that many of the tests and questionnaires by these authors address the oxidation rate (the Oxidative Dominant system of Wolcott) as the main metabolic control. All nutritional types need to be particularly careful to distinguish the kind of carbohydrate you eat. All must restrict processed complex carbohydrates since white flour products (even made from whole-grain flour), exploded rice cakes and many dry cereals act in the body the same as the obvious sugars made from cane, beets, corn, fruits or milk, which are called "simple carbohydrates." Overindulgent eating of them can lead to health problems. As much as feasible, stick with the complex carbohydrates found in whole grain foods (slow cooking oatmeal, steamed whole grains), legumes, potatoes and red, yellow and green vegetables. Remember, slow oxidizers may crave simple carbohydrates to give themselves quick energy.

Proteins are more easily identified. Figure 60 will help you identify the sources of those special proteins that are purine-rich, which fast oxidizers need to eat and slow oxidizers need to downplay. In addition to foods shown in Figure 60, other foods are good

	RNA		RNA
Canned Sardines	590	Fresh Salmon	289
Pinto beans	485	Great Northern beans	284
Lentils	484	Beef Liver	268
Chicken liver	402	Oysters	239
Garbanzo beans	356	Fresh Mackerel	203
Fresh Sardines	343	Fresh Squid	100
Black-eyed peas	306	Canned Salmon	26
Small white beans	305	Canned Tuna	5
Lima beans	293		

Figure 60. This figure, compiled from Benjamin Frank (1976), ranks foods according to their content of ribonucleic acid (RNA). (To get RNA content, purines are multiplied by 3.5.) This listing helps explain why beans, largely ignored today, were so important to the health of western cowpunchers and seafarers.

This figure also explains why the protein-rich legumes (beans, peas) are excluded from the diet of slow oxidizers. Frank was puzzled why, with the remarkable exception of sardines, canned fish was so much lower in RNA than fresh fish.

sources of the RNA provided by purine-rich proteins: Meat extract, nuts, dark-meat poultry, spinach, oatmeal, asparagus, mushrooms and onions. Beets in all forms including borscht, are excellent in that they induce cellular RNA synthesis. (Frank, 1976.) Since the nucleic acids of purine-rich proteins speed up the production of energy at the cellular level, Frank considers them essential in an anti-aging program. His no-aging diet, however, is best suited for those individuals on the fast-oxidizing side of the population. Frank advises them to eat proteins largely from aquatic ecosystems (sardines four times a week, salmon once, invertebrates once and other fish once a week) and once or twice a week to have calf's liver, beets, legumes, and once a day eat one of the other vegetables mentioned above. He cautions to drink plenty of fluids. Vegetarians he advised to eat from the following at least four times a week: collards, cauliflower, turnip greens, spinach and soy bean sprouts.

Another important metabolic factor is how rapidly carbohydrates raise blood sugar and insulin. Carbohydrates high on a scale called the Glycemic Index (GI) raise blood sugar and insulin to high levels rapidly; those low on the scale yield energy slowly and continuously over a longer period of time. While slow oxidizers can use foods high on the GI to boost their energy levels, fast oxidizers must avoid them. Low to moderate GI foods yield sustained energy and are things like legumes, yams, some pastas, tortillas, old-fashioned oatmeal, yogurt, many fruits and dairy products. Foods high in the GI are processed cereals such as (regrettably) corn flakes and all the puffed and crunchy oat and rice cereals; exploded grain products (rice cakes, krispies, puffed grains), baking, red skin and "new" white potatoes, oat bran, whole wheat and white breads (even made from whole-meal flour), "instant" oatmeal, maize and popcorn, pastries, candies and soft drinks. Remarkably, several vegetables (carrots, parsnips) are very high on the Glycemic Index. Sweet potatoes[26]

---

[26] In the U.S. we often call "our" sweet potato *(Ipomoea sp.)* "yams." Chiefly from Central America, they have spread throughout Polynesia. The true edible yam *(Dioscorea sp.)* is from Africa and Eastern Asia and was a staple crop, before rice, in much of Southeast Asia and the Western Pacific. (Some species are steroid sources.) Both tubers range from moderate through high on the GI, depending on the data source, a possible result of confusing the two quite different plants.

seem to vary from moderate to high. It seems that the *type* or variety of rice or white potato makes a big difference. It has been found that rices low in amylose (such as Calrose) are high, while the "sweet" of "sticky" rice served in Asian restaurants has no amylose at all and is highest in the GI. (Miller *et al.,* 1992, 1996.) The position of white potatoes on the GI scale is apparently determined by their starch content. Baking potatoes (Idaho) are highest, medium-starch potatoes (Peruvian Blue, Yukon Gold) and low-starch potatoes (Fingerling, Pontiac) have lower values.

A few words about sugars. Most simple sugars, such as honey or table sugar, are rapidly absorbed and are high on the Glycemic Index. Fruit sugar or fructose, while low on the Glycemic Index, is more slowly absorbed than the other simple sugars. Fructose, however, can boost triglyceride formation in the liver, increase "bad" LDL cholesterol, and can be dangerous for those who consume a lot of fruit and fruit juices. (Gittleman, 1996.) It also elevates uric acid levels in the blood, leading to gout. Read the label on any sweet commercial product or soft drink and especially curtail or avoid those containing "high-fructose corn syrup." Because fruit sugar is "natural," most people believe it can be consumed freely. Because of its sensitivity to sugars of any kind (including alcohol) immune system function may be cut in half by one glass of fruit juice. Even if we avoid the juice and eat fruit there is a caveat: most commercial fruits have been bred for a higher content of sugar and juice than the fruits eaten during most of our ancestry, or like bananas, citrus and pineapple, they are either imports and/or made available the year around by modern transportation.

Finally, after learning how we should eat, we may need to modify our intake of supplements. Figure 61 lists different kinds of vitamins and minerals required by each of the two major metabolic types. As we have learned, most of us are in the mid-oxidizer range, but lean to one side or the other of the curve (Figure 56). Accordingly, we may have to lighten or increase specific supplements to achieve optimum health and life span.

Steps To Determine Your Metabolic Type–Chapter Summary

Provided you have no obvious hereditary or allergy problems of consequence, or problems with yeast infections, heavy metals or

FAST OXIDIZERS	SLOW OXIDIZERS
A **(1)**	A **(1) (2)**
E **(5)**	B 1 (thiamine)
B 12	B 2 (riboflavin)
Pantothenic acid	B 3 (niacin)
Inositol	B 6 (pyridoxine)
Choline	Folic acid (B vitamin)
Niacinamide (form of B3)	PABA
C **(4)**	C **(4)**
Calcium	D **(3)**
Phosphorus **(5)**	Magnesium **(5)**
Zinc	Manganese **(5)**
Iodine	Potassium
	Iron **(6)**

1. Kelley and Watson consider vitamin A for both fast and slow oxidizers.
2. Watts says vitamin A is stimulative; Watson suggests the palmitate form for fast oxidizers and the fish liver form for slow oxidizers.
3. Watts believes that vitamin D sedates the thyroid gland.
4. Vitamin C is often recommended for both fast and slow oxidizers although Kelley and Wiley list it with slow oxidizers.
5. Watts considers phosphorus, vitamin E and manganese as stimulative for slow oxidizers and magnesium and copper as sedatives for fast oxidizers.
6. Considered necessary by Watts and Gittleman.

Figure 61. Consensus (from Part II) of which vitamins and minerals are appropriate for fast and slow oxidizers. Endnotes list some conflicting opinions. In general, slow oxidizers need supplements that increase the metabolic rate, as do many of the B-Complex vitamins and potassium. There seems to be no consensus on copper, chromium or iron. See Fig. 34 and 35 in "Feeling Good" for where certain of these vitamins participate in the cells' energy reactions.

other toxins or parasites (an intestinal permeability test would be very helpful) you can:

A. Seek professional help from the organizations discussed above for a reasonable fee, or . . .

B. Take the following steps yourself at little or no cost:
    1. Do the coffee and niacin tests.
    2. Try to identify yourself with one of the nutritional types in the Characteristics of Nutritional Types at the end of this chapter.
    3. Carry a small notebook for one week and note down how you feel after meals, especially protein/fat rich and carbohydrate—rich ones.
    4. Try the two breakfasts as suggested in this chapter.
    5. If you have a clue as to what your personal nutritional type might be, try to determine what ratio of carbohydrate-protein-fat makes you feel good or, conversely, eliminates or curtails sub-clinical problems such as headaches, depression or fatigue. Use Appendix P as a general food guide.
    6. Eliminate foods high in the Glycemic Index and start reading grocery store labels for things like hydrogenated vegetable oils, high-fructose corn syrup and MSG-containing additives.
    7. If you are a fast oxidizer, try increasing purine-rich proteins (Figure 60), and see how you feel.
    8. Try adjusting your supplement intake (allow several weeks or a month or more) and see if you feel differently.[27]
    9. If you are eating for a nutritional type ascertained by lab or other tests, with negative results, switch to a completely opposite diet.

---

[27] Depending on the individual and the extent of their deficiency, even supplements do not guarantee speedy healing. In the 1950s, Dolores Tyner, a nurse, was in an Orlando, Florida hospital with heart and kidney problems. Through a friend she began an intensive supplement program. She told me that nothing happened for months. Then she started to heal and her medical problems vanished, her hair turned brown again, and her friends no longer recognized her as the same person. She was so impressed that she quit nursing and opened a health food store.

CHARACTERISTICS OF NUTRITIONAL TYPES

FAST OXIDIZER (Acid type)

Very tense or nervous after cup of regular coffee on empty stomach.

Skin turns red, hot and itchy after 50 mg of niacin on empty stomach.

Odor of thiamine powder strong, sharp and unpleasant at 10mg but only gassy or prickly sensations at 100 mg. (Mood goes from good to depression.)

Likes bacon, salami, oily nuts, steaks.

Prefers bread with cheese to bread with jam.

Desires heavy breakfasts (meat, eggs, hash browns, pancakes swimming in butter).

Feels drop in energy (after delay of at least thirty minutes to one hour) after eating a candy bar or fat-free sweet dessert.

Needs to eat every three to four hours.

Likes between-meal and evening snacks.

Finds many sweet foods too sweet.

High levels of most B vitamins cause energy loss or depression.

Finds many sour foods objectionable.

Likes plenty of mayonnaise on sandwiches.

Prefers bacon cheeseburgers to regular kind.

Prefers warm, cooked heavy foods to cold, raw light "rabbit" foods.

Dotes on potatoes, especially with gravies, or french fries.

Insufficient protein/fat may cause cravings for sweets, flour-based foods and caffeine.

Can eat chips straight.

SLOW OXIDIZER (Alkaline type)

Feels good after a cup of regular coffee on empty stomach.

No effect with 50 mg of niacin on empty stomach.

Odor of thiamine powder featureless at 10 mg, but sweet and pleasant at 100 mg. (Mood goes from low to high.)

Does not normally desire bacon, salami, oily nuts, steaks.

Prefers bread with jam to bread with cheese.

Prefers sweet, dry cereal with milk for breakfast.

Loves salads and light, cold, raw "rabbit" foods.

Feels energetic for several hours after eating a candy bar or fat-free sweet dessert.

Normally does not eat between meals.

Can tolerate very sweet foods.

High levels of B vitamins increase energy and positive outlook.

Likes mustard and sour foods (pickles, grapefruit juice, etc.).

May prefer salad dressing to mayonnaise.

Prefers hamburgers with lettuce, tomato and onion, not cheese and bacon.

Does well on pastas and refined whole grain foods.

Insufficient carbohydrates may cause cravings for meat, fat, salt and alcohol.

Usually prefers chips dipped in salsa.

MID OXIDIZER

A little tense or nervous after regular coffee on an empty stomach.

Feels warmer with some facial color after 50 mg niacin on empty stomach.

Can eat either a light or heavy breakfast or combination.

Prefers a balance of cold, raw and hot, cooked foods.

Does well on a variety of meats, whole grain products, fruits and vegetables.

Other food preferences intermediate between those of fast and slow oxidizers.

May eat one group of foods for awhile, then switch to another.

In conclusion, I return to the theme that one of the most profound and epic stories in human history were changes that took place when we began to stop hunting and gathering the diversity of foods from natural ecosystems. For Europeans and their descendents this was followed by soil-based cultures where we grew or raised specialized foods of our choice, eventually completely abandoning our personal relationship with nature to purchase entire meals from commercial outlets. Coupled with this has been the increase in quantity but decline in quality of many foods available in the supermarkets of today. Both hunter-gatherers living in harmony with natural laws and sustainable agriculturalists were forced by necessity to eat properly—in advantaged nations it is up to us.

Early man used his intellect and skills to gather foods that fueled his survival. I like to think that he was not so much "primitive" as he was beautifully "adapted" to his environment. As an opportunistic omnivore, early man's diet changed only with the slow pace of ecological change in the plants and animals he lived with. In the "advanced" cultures of today we are no longer guided by natural environments to eat just the things that we evolved to eat. Instead, faced with an unlimited supply of all types and quantities of foods, we are left with only our intellect to guide us through a healthy lifespan.

This book has mostly dealt with eating to prevent disease, presumably in healthy people. Unfortunately, once you get to know them, most middle aged and over people are either ill, have just recovered from an illness or operation, or have health problems. So it is only fair to close this chapter by emphasizing that not only can proper eating cure or heal, but it may be necessary to heal before you can learn to eat properly. This consideration of healing makes the contributions of Sherry Rogers and Andrew Weil even more relevant.

Healing is obviously required for those who are sick, or are breathing or ingesting toxins. They are in no condition to experiment with drastic changes in diet or supplements without medical supervision. Another "wild card" here is that your present metabolism may change depending on how sick you are, or on factors such as stress, toxicity and nutritional status. We have been informed of this by the writings of Bieler, Kelley, Rogers and others. Healing often involves restoring liver function and eliminating toxins, as well as dealing with a leaky gut. It is a matter to be worked out with a sympathetic physician and may involve lab work with tests for intestinal permeability,

CDSA, minerals and toxic metals (RBC mineral test) and fatty acids. (Rogers, 2000.)

In our search for a personal nutrition I suspect that most of us will opt for some type of trial and error self-testing to determine our "ideal" carbohydrate-protein-fat ratios. We may even be able to ascertain the presence of some inherited defects in metabolizing grains and dairy products by the "stop and start" and "pulse rate" tests. And, if we really want to take the bull by the horns we can eat exclusively like a vegetarian or a carnivore for enough days to elicit definite "feelings" or other reactions. Using Rogers' "metabolic cross" (Figure 48) is part of such a do-it-yourself approach to health. To maximize healing Rogers makes a compelling case for sick and even cancerous individuals to use the metabolic cross. She emphasizes, however, that while macrobiotics seems to work best for many, eating either the vegetarian or carnivorous diets may well be only temporary for most of us.

While a drastic change towards vegetarianism or carnivory may have immediate beneficial results in healing, it could take longer. Since some of us have unique metabolisms, we may need patience. Some individuals may be quite slow to recover especially after decades of improper diet. Recall that Ann Louise Gittleman took over four years to completely regain her health after including meat in her diet, following years of vegetarianism.

Our gastronomic adventures, using the metabolic cross or other self-testing devices can have a lasting benefit because it pushes omnivorous types towards a more and more nutritionally balanced diet. As we heal, most of us will be able to enjoy a greater variety of foods more nearly like our natural environments once provided. Then we can aspire to fulfill the scriptural commendation that we might eat from every living thing that dwells upon the earth, as we once did in the forests and savannas of our origin.

Epilogue

Hopefully, most people realize that adaptation to environment is the principal requirement for the survival for all living things, including humans. Wild animals eat only what nature provides. Since ten thousand years ago, many humans have increasingly eaten what man provides. This is particularly culpable for supermarket-dependent city dwellers, where nutrition is not determined by collective wisdom but by corporate morality and the commercialization of foods.

Even given 10,000 years of adaptation, a large number of humans are still not able to cope with the dominance of grains, refined carbohydrates and the concentrated calories that modern marketing presents, nor the all-pervasive vegetable oils, additives, toxins and endocrine inhibitors that accompany them. It is with selecting from such an enormous choice of concentrated foods, along with the accompanying desire for a "good life," that places so heavy a burden not only on the body but on the organic wealth so carefully accumulated for millennia by the earth's ecosystems.

While some cultures, using sustainable agriculture, have reversed a normally irreplaceable loss of fertility, world consumer demand may destroy the way of life for many of them. The self-regulatory adjustment of life to its environment, inherent in the structure and function of natural ecosystems, has been designed and tested through eons of time and cannot be substituted for by technology.

Either we humbly accept the tenets of ecology that spell out how the interrelationship of life and non-life work or we condemn much of mankind to the inglorious prospect of widespread famine, disease and social conflict. For better or for worse we, as large-brained primates from prehistoric times, have developed a technology that is transforming the world through power, avarice and ignorance.

Reay Tannahill aptly puts it "What self-preservation and the quest for food had done during millions of years of evolution had been to transform a particular family of apes into two-legged super-animals. What the next 7,000 years were to do—the years of the Neolithic Revolution, when the new super-animals learned how to cultivate plants and tame their fellow animals—was to set them off on an independent course that was to change the face of the earth and the life of almost everything upon it."

During our tenure in the original natural environments we collectively call Eden, natural selection made sure that our species was generally similar externally and internally. Our lifestyles and foods were in strict conformance with the laws of nature, and had evolved to prevent degenerative disease. Our spontaneous healing system, so well described by Andrew Weil (see Chapter 12) was strong.

For some cultures, the post-Eden years ended the exacting control by natural selection. For the densely populated areas of Eurasia "new" lifestyles and foods conformed less and less to the rules laid down in Eden, resulting in the accumulation of anatomical and physiological changes in the genetics of the human species. The body's ability to prevent degenerative disease was thus compromised, as well as the spontaneity of healing once disease had begun. Genetic deterioration would have been most rapid in isolated populations with much inbreeding.

If these regional groups became genetically mixed by reason of migration or rapid transportation, it would seem that the search for a lifestyle and nutrition for our species would be less effective than a similar search for each individual. Today, certain rules for healthful living can certainly apply to all of us, but effectively preventing degenerative disease, as well as activating the spontaneous healing system may require lifestyle and nutritional changes tailored more to the unique person that is each of us. Thus, the suggested course for many in the genetic melting pot of the developed nations would be to try to select one's own individual path through the jungles of modern lifestyles and foodstuffs.

The measures suggested in the last chapter are good, basic steps in guiding this journey towards perennial health. Our own efforts, either through self-testing or through organizations discussed in the last chapter, would be greatly benefited by a network of practitioners skilled in preventive or holistic health methods devoted to individual lifestyles and nutrition that could provide the guideposts in our own personal search. If the past is any indication of the future, conventional medicine, excellent as it is, may not be able to meet such a need in time. Ideally, we may require a nation-wide system of health surveillance clinics that can determine all your individual autonomic, endocrine and oxidative peculiarities, in essence your metabolic profile. Placed on a "smart card," this information would print out for physicians, nutritional advisors, hospital kitchens, home computers and even supermarkets. Everyone then would know the correct foods to eat at that stage in their lives, including the proper ratios of carbohydrates, proteins and fats and other life-style indications suitable for your own physiology, such as the proper exercise, stress tolerance and even social compatibility.

Equipped with knowledge of your own personal nutritional needs, and your own awareness of the medical history of self and family, hopefully assisted by our rapidly advancing knowledge of the human genome, you will know exactly what it takes to adapt to your present environment which, after all, is what health and survival is all about.

To put this in true perspective with the operations of the planetary life-support systems, it would be extremely valuable to have models of sustainable agriculture of the type successful for each type soil and climate, be it a tiny home garden or a large organic farm. These could be visited as "living museums" how man and nature can subsist together indefinitely in a balanced state we could call "ecolibrium."

Let's face it. While modern agriculture is, to a degree, imitative of nature, it is now exploitative, especially of soils and water. It decimates not only soil organisms essential for recycling organic matter, but it uses up existing organic matter and certain minerals. This makes the soil more and more dependent on man-made chemical fertilizers, pesticides and herbicides. If university-based agricultural services could get away from the support of chemical-based commercial farming and cooperate with university ecologists, the infrastructure is already in place to present truly sustainable agriculture. Until that happens, perhaps permaculture specialists and successful organic farms based upon the principle of recycling nutrients and wastes among plants, animals and soil, could lead the way. At the very least, museums and zoological parks could provide a network of living or non-living exhibits of enormous educational benefit, either emphasizing an idealized local nature-based food production unit or presenting models of widely different systems, such as the Aigamo Method, the Sri Lankan rice paddies, or the doorway gardens of Indonesia.

The search for personal health could then be based on a more widespread knowledge of fundamental principles dealing with how plants, animals and environments must interact together to produce lasting health and prosperity. Such information is desperately needed to counterbalance public infatuation with technology and the possible downside of their dependence on it, as well as on modern drugs and gene-based therapies to correct the maladies we shouldn't have acquired in the first place. The technology of energy-conservation and information exchange can, of course, benefit the world. Information exchange, along with the news media, can be especially valuable in making the public aware of the fundamental life-support systems that underlie our divergent economies and cultures seeking any kind of permanence.

There is another aspect of this. Such programs and exhibits highlighting sustainable living and perennial health can be immensely valuable in helping the people of developed nations understand what is happening to the large number of subsistence-based and less-advantaged peoples of the earth. Their way of life, which has had to be more or less sustainable, is being destroyed by commercial interests of the developed nations, whether under pressure of debt repayment or due to the octopus-like influence of the International Growth Society (IGS).

The IGS was defined by the Norwegian ecophilosopher Sigmund Kvaloy, and is based on the accelerated growth and production of industrial articles and methods, and both the resources and markets of the entire planet are grist for its mill. (LaChapelle, 1988.) We are vulnerable to its influence because of its immediate, large economic benefits from which the costs of the free resources of the earth are, unfortunately, not subtracted. As LaChapelle quotes, we are the first humans "in the history of the world to totally inhabit a commodity culture." Instead of every day being an endorphin-producing adventure as with our predecessors in Eden, many of us are now trapped in a relatively boring and monotonous existence in man-made ecosystems fueled entirely from finite sources of soil fertility, the water cycle or stored carbon compounds, whose underground reserves are legacies of the ancient past. Eating has become a rewarding addiction and drug use provides substitutes for stimuli lacking in modern life.

Identifying such an overview is apparently the first step in a return to the way living was and should be. The ultimate solution to the "one world" control by the Industrial Growth Society is to begin to live a close relationship in ecolibrium with the land and life forms where we are, guided by the ecology of our bioregion. "We," here, meaning all the peoples of the earth.

Lit Cited

Abrams, H. Leon. 1987. "A preference for animal protein and fat: A cross-cultural survey." Chap. 8 IN Marvin Harris and Eric Ross (Eds.) *Food and evolution,* Temple University Press, Philadelphia, PA.

Abravanel, Elliott. 1983. *Dr. Abravanel's body type diet and lifetime nutrition plan.* Bantam Books, New York, London.

Abravanel, Elliot and Elizabeth King. 1985. *Dr. Abravanel's body type program for health, fitness and nutrition.* Bantam Books, New York, London.

Aebi, Hugo, J. Von Wartburg and S. R. Wyss. 1981. "The role of enzyme polymorphisms and enzyme variants in the evolutionary process." Chap. 13 IN Walcher and Kretchmer (Eds.) 1981. *Food, nutrition and evolution.* Masson Publishers, USA, New York.

Aihara, Herman. 1986. *Acid and alkaline.* George Ohsawa Macrobiotic Foundation, Oroville, CA.

Alley, Richard and Michael Bender. 1998. "Greenland ice cores: frozen in time." *Scientific American,* February, pp. 66–71.

Albrecht, William. 1947. "Soil fertility as a pattern of possible deficiencies." Journal of the American Academy Applied Nutrition, Spring issue, p. 283. IN *The Albrecht Papers,* Vol. I, Charles Walters (Ed.) 1996. Acres USA, Metairie, LA.

Albrecht, William. 1975, 1989, 1992. IN Charles Walters (Ed.) *The Albrecht Papers,* Vols. I-IV, Acres USA, Metairie, LA.

AMTL Corporation. 1999. "Physician's guide for using and interpreting the ALCAT test." American Medical Testing Laboratory, Hollywood, FL.

Atkins, Robert. 1998. "Health revelations," Vol. VI, No. 11 (November), p. 2. Agora Health Publishing, Baltimore, MD.

Atkins, Robert. 1999. "Health revelations," Vol. VII, No. 9 (December) Agora Health Publishing, Baltimore, MD.

Bailey, Covert. 1994. *Smart exercise.* Houghton-Mifflin Co., New York.

Baum, Kenneth and Richard Trubo. 2000. *Metabolize.* G. P. Putnam's Sons, New York.

Bear, Firman, Stephen Toth and Arthur Prince. 1949. "Variation in mineral composition of vegetables." Proceedings, Soil Science Society of America, Vol. 13. New Jersey Agriculcural Experiment Station, Rutgers University.

Beiler, Henry. 1965. *Food is your best medicine.* Random House, New York.

Bland, Jeffry. 1998. "The use of complementary medicine for healthy aging." Alternative Therapies, Vol. 4, No. 4.

Brothwell, Don and P. Brothwell. 1969. *Food in antiquity.* Frederick A. Praeger, New York.

Brown, Kathryn. 2000. "The human genome business today." Scientific American, July. pp. 50–55.

BSCS. 1968. *BSCS Biology: an ecological approach.* Kendall/Hunter Publishing Co., Dubuque, IA.

Bunyard, Peter. 1980. "Terraced agriculture in the Middle East." The Ecologist, Vol. 10, Nos. 8–9.

Burkitt, D. P., A. R. P. Walker and N. S. Painter. 1972. "Effect of dietary fiber on stools and transit times and its role in the causation of disease." The Lancet 2, pp. 1408–1411.

Byrnes, Stephen. 1999. "The myths of vegetarianism." The Ecologist, Vol. 29, No. 4, pp. 260–263. July.

Calder, Ritchie. 1961. *After the seventh day. The world man created.* Simon and Schuster, New York.

Campbell, H. J. 1973. *The pleasure areas. A new theory of behavior.* Delacorte Press, New York.

Cannon, Walter. 1932. *The wisdom of the body.* W. W. Norton and Co., New York.

Capra, Fritjof. 1996. *The web of life.* Anchor Books, Doubleday, New York.

Cassata, Carla. 1996. "What's your dietary profile?" Let's Live. April, p. 57.

Charney, Dennis. 1999. "The infinite mind—fears and phobias." PBS, May 3, Lichtenstein Creative Media.

Chopra, Deepak. 1989. *Quantum healing.* Bantam Books, New York.

Chopra, Deepak. 1991. *Perfect health. The complete mind/body guide.* Harmony Books. New York.

Chopra Deepak. 1993. *Ageless body, timeless mind.* Harmony Books. New York.

Claiborne, Robert. 1970. *Climate, man and history.* W. W. Norton and Co., New York.

Clancy, Katherine. 1986. "The role of sustainable agriculture in improving the safety and quality of the food supply." American Journal of Alternative Agriculture 1, pp. 11–18.

Clark, John. 1956. *Hunza, lost kingdom of the Himalayas.* Funk and Wagnalls, New York.

Cleave, T. L. 1973. *The saccharine disease.* Keats Publishing Company. New Canaan, CT.

Cochran, Gregory and Paul Ewald. 1999. "High-risk defenses." Natural History, February, pp. 40–43.

Cohen, Mark. 1977. *The food crisis in prehistory.* Yale University Press, London. New Haven, CT.

Cohen, Mark, 1987. "The significance of long-term changes in human diet and food economy." Chap. 10 IN Marvin Harris and Eric Ross (Eds.) *Food and evolution.* Temple University Press, Philadelphia, PA.

Cohen, Mark. 1989. *Health and the rise of civilization.* Yale University Press, New Haven, CT.

Colborn, Theo, Dianne Dumanoski and John Myers. 1997. *Our stolen future.* Plume (Dutton Signet), Division of Penguin Books, New York.

Coleby, Pat. 1997. "The copper-zinc connection." Acres USA. June, pp. 24–25.

Cook, O. F. 1916. "Staircase farms of the ancients." National Geographic Magazine, May, pp. 474–534.

Cooper, Jay with Katherine Lance. 1999. *The body code.* Pocket Books, New York.

Cronin, C. C. and F. Shanahan, 1997. "Insulin-dependent diabetes mellitus and coeliac disease." The Lancet 349, pp. 1096–1097, 12 April.

Cryer, P. E. and K. S. Polonsky. 1998. "Glucose homeostasis and hypoglycemia." Chap. 20, pp. 931–971 IN Williams *Textbook of Endocrinology,* W. B. Saunders Co., Philadelphia, PA.

Cummings, Claire. 1999. "Entertainment foods." The Ecologist, Vol. 28, No. 1, pp. 16–19.

D'Adamo, James. 1989. *The D'Adamo diet.* McGraw-Hill Ryerson. Montreal.

D'Adamo, Peter. 1990. "Gut ecosystem dynamics III." Townsend Letter for Doctors. August-September.

D'Adamo, Peter. 1991. "Gut ecosystem dynamics I." Townsend Letter for Doctors. April.

D'Adamo, Peter. 1993. "Gut ecosystem dynamics—special characteristics: lectins and mitogens." Townsend Letter for Doctors. November.

D'Adamo, Peter with Catherine Whitney. 1996. *Eat right for your type.* G. P. Putnam's Sons, New York.

Davies, David. 1975. *The centenarians of the Andes.* Anchor Books, Garden City, NY.

De la Peña. 1983. *The psychobiology of cancer.* Praeger Publishers, New York.

Diamond, Jared. 1992. *The third chimpanzee.* Harper-Collins Publishing Inc., New York.

Diamond, Jared. 1997. *Guns, germs and steel.* W. W. Norton and Co., New York.

Diamond, Jared. 1997. "Mr. Wallace's line." Discover Magazine, August, pp.76–83.

Douglass, William. 1985. *The milk of human kindness is not pasteurized.* Last Laugh Publishers, Marietta, GA.

Dubos, René. 1965. *Man adapting.* Yale University Press, Ltd., London.

Eaton, Boyd and Melvin Konner. 1985. "Paleolithic nutrition: a consideration of its nature and current implications." New England Journal of Medicine, No. 312, pp. 283–289.

Eaton, Boyd, Melvin Konner and Margorie Shostak. 1988. "Stone agers in the fast lane: chronic degenerative diseases in evolutionary perspective." American Journal of Medicine, 84, pp.739–749.

Eaton, Boyd, Marjorie Shostak and Melvin Konner. 1988. *The paleolithic prescription.* Harper and Row, New York.

Eck, Paul. 1988. Interview IN "The secret of youth." The Lafayette Institute for Basic Research, Charlottesville, VA.

Eckstein, Eleanor. 1980. *Food, people and nutrition.* Avi Publishing Co., Westport, CT.

Enig, Mary. 1993. "Trans fatty acids—an update." Nutrition Quarterly, Vol. 17, No. 4, pp. 79–95.

Enig, Mary. 1995. "Trans fatty acids in the food supply: a comprehensive report covering 60 years of research." (2nd Ed.). Enig Associates, Silver Springs, MD.

Ezzell, Carol. 2000. "Beyond the human genome." Scientific American, July. pp. 64–69.

Falciglia, G. A. and P. A. Norton. 1994. "Evidence for a genetic influenced preference for some foods." Journal of American Dietetic Association, 94, pp. 154–158.

Fallon, Sally, Pat Connally and Mary Enig. 1995. *Nourishing traditions.* ProMotion Publishing, San Diego, CA.

Fallon, Sally and Mary Enig. 1995. "Soy products or dairy products? Not so fast . . . " Health Freedom News, September, pp. 12–20.

Fallon, Sally and Mary Enig. 1996. "Americans: then and now." Health Journal, Price-Pottenger Nutrition Foundation, Vol. 20, No. 4, pp. 1–3.

Fallon, Sally and Mary Enig. 1996. "An additional note to the fat controversy: an historical approach." Health Journal, Price-Pottenger Nutrition Foundation, Vol. 20, No. 4, pp. 4–6.

Fallon, Sally and Mary Enig. 1997. "The cave man diet." Health Journal, Price-Pottenger Nutrition Foundation, Vol. 21, No. 2.

Fallon, Sally. 1999. "Nasty, brutish and short?" The Ecologist, Vol. 29, No. 1, pp. 20–27.

Firth, Peta. 1999. "Leaving a bad taste." Scientific American, May, pp. 34–35.

Fowkes, Steven. 1998a. "Insulin resistance." Smart Life News, Vol. 6, No. 7, pp. 1–5.

Fowkes, Steven. 1998b. "Food allergy and neuro degenerative disease." Smart Life News, Vol. 6, No. 9, pp. 1–4.

Frank, Benjamin. 1975. *Nucleic acid therapy of aging and degenerative disease.* 3rd Edition. Lisbon: Fiquima.

Frank, Benjamin. 1976. *Doctor Frank's no-aging diet.* The Dial Press, New York.

Franke, Richard. 1987. "The effects of colonialism and neocolonialism on the gastronomic patterns of the third world." Chap. 19 IN Marvin Harris and Eric Ross. *Food and evolution.* Temple University Press, Philadelphia, PA.

Freeman, Peter and Thomas Fricke. 1984. "The success of Javanese multi-storied gardens." The Ecologist, Vol. 14, No. 4.

Friend, Gil. 1983. "The potential for sustainable agriculture." IN Dietrich Knorr. (Ed.), *Sustainable food systems,* pp. 28–47, Avi Publishing, Westport, CT.

Fukuoka, Masanobu. 1978. *The one-straw revolution.* Rodale Press, Emmaus, PA.

Gallinger, Shirley and Sherry Rogers. 1992. *Macro mellow recipes for macrobiotic cooking.* Prestige Publishers, Syracuse, NY.

Gerrard, J. W., C. G. Ko and P. Vickers. 1976. "The familial incidence of allergic disease." Ann. All. 36:10.

Gerson, Max. 1958. *A cancer therapy, results of fifty cases.* Whittier Books, Inc., New York.

Gerwing, Jeffrey, Pamela Lockwood and Christopher Uhl. 1999. "Acorn foraging as a means to explore human energetics and forge connections to local forests." Bulletin of the Ecological Society of America, April, pp. 117–120.

Gibbs, Wayt. 1998. *Natural-born guinea pigs.* Scientific American, February, p. 24.

Gilman, A. G., T. W. Rall, A. S. Nies and P. Taylor. (Eds.) 1990. *The pharmacological basis of therapeutics.* 8th Ed., Pergamon Press, New York.

Gittleman, Ann Louise. 1988. *Beyond Pritikin.* Bantam Doubleday, Dell Publishing Group, New York.

Gittleman, Ann Louise. 1993. *Guess what came to dinner?* Avery Publishing Group, Garden City, NY.

Gittleman, Ann Louise with James Templeton and Candelora Versace. 1996. *Your body knows best.* Pocket Books, Simon and Schuster, Inc., New York.

Glantz, Kalman and John Pearce. 1989. *Exiles from Eden.* W. W. Norton and Co., New York.

Goldsmith, Edward. 1982. "Traditional agriculture in Sri Lanka." The Ecologist, Vol. 12, No. 5.

Goldsmith, Edward, Nicholas Hildyard, Patrick McCully, and Peter Bunyard. 1990. *Imperiled planet.* MIT Press, Cambridge, MA.

Goldsmith, Edward. 1998. "Learning to live with nature: the lessons of traditional irrigation." The Ecologist, Vol. 28, No. 3.

Golub, E. S. 1987. *Immunology: a synthesis.* Sinauer Assoc., Inc., Sunderland, MA.

Good, Kenneth. 1987. "Limiting factors in amazonian ecology." Chap. 16 IN Marvin Harris and Eric Ross (Eds.) *Food and evolution.* Temple University Press, Philadelphia PA.

Gore, Rick. 1996. "Neanderthals." National Geographic, January, pp. 2–35.

Gore, Rick. 1997. "Tracking the first of our kind." National Geographic, September, pp. 92–99.

Gray, G. W. 1941. *The advancing front of medicine.* Whittlesey House, New York and London.

Gross, John, Zuwang Wang, and Bruce Wunder. 1985. "Effects of food quality and energy needs: changes in gut morphology and capacity of *Microtus ochrogaster.*" Journal of Mammals, Vol. 66, No. 4, pp. 661–667.

GSDL. 1999. *Functional assessment resource manual.* Great Smokies Diagnostic Laboratory, Asheville, NC.

Gussow, Joan. 1987. "Is organic food more nutritious?" New Jersey Organic News, Vol. 11, No. 3, Summer.

Hadjivassiliou, Gibson, G. A. B. Davies-Jones *et al.* 1996. "Does cryptic gluten sensitivity play a part in neurological illness?" The Lancet, 347, pp. 369–371, 10 February.

Hamaker, J. D. and D. A. Weaver. 1982. *The survival of civilization.* Hamaker-Weaver Publishers, Michigan and California.

Hamilton, William, III. 1987. "Omnivorous primate diet and human over consumption of meat." Chap. 4 IN Marvin Harris and Eric Ross (Eds.) *Food and evolution.* Temple University Press, Philadelphia, PA.

Harris, David. 1987. "Aboriginal subsistence in a tropical rainforest environment: food procurement, cannibalism and population regulation in northeastern Australia." Chap. 14 IN Harris, M. and E. B. Ross (Eds.) *Food and evolution.* Temple University Press, Philadelphia, PA.

IIarris, Marvin. 1985. *The sacred cow and the abominable pig. Riddles of food and culture.* Simon and Schuster, New York.

Harris, Marvin. 1987. "Foodways: Historical overview and theoretical prolegomenon." Chap. 2 IN Marvin Harris and Eric Ross (Eds.) *Food and evolution.* Temple University Press, Philadelphia, PA.

Harrower, Henry. 1939. *An endocrine handbook.* The Harrower Laboratory, Inc., Glendale, CA.

Hayden, Brian. 1981. "Subsistence and ecological adaptations of modern hunter-gatherers." Chap. 10 IN Harding, R. and G. Teleki (Eds.) *Omnivorous Primates,* Columbia University Press, New York.

Healthexcel. 1998. "The diet coin." Healthexcel, Inc., Winthrop, WA.

Health Studies Collegium. 1997. *Information handbook.* Serammune Physician's Laboratory, Sterling, VA.

Healthview Interview. 1977. "The Healthview Newsletter." No. 12. Charlottesville, VA.

Ho, Mae-Wan. 1999. "One bird—ten thousand treasures." The Ecologist, Vol. 29, No. 6, pp. 339–340.

Hornick, Sharon. 1992. "Factors affecting the nutritional quality of crops." American Journal of Alternative Agriculture, Vol. 7, Nos. 1–2.

Howell, Edward. 1985. *Enzyme nutrition.* Avery Publishing Group, Wayne, NJ.

Hrdy, Sarah. 1999. "Body fat and birth control." Natural History, October.

Jaffe, Russell. 1989. "Improved immune function using specific nutrient supplementation and ELISA/ACT 'immunologic fingerprint' to detect late phase responses ex vivo." Journal of American College of Nutrition, Vol. 8, No. 5, p. 424.

Jaffe, Russell. 1989. "Immune defense and repair systems in biologic medicine I: autoimmunity. Clinical relevance of biological response modifiers in diagnosis, treatment and testing." Bulletin 179, Health Studies Collegium, Sterling, VA.

Jensen, Bernard and Mark Anderson. 1990. *Empty harvest.* Avery Publishing Group. Garden City Park, NY. (Available Price-Pottenger Nutritional Foundation.)

Johnson, Jan. 1988. *Metabolic balancing organizational workbook.* Bottomline Books, Palo Alto, CA.

Katz, Solomon. 1987. "Fava bean consumption: a case for the co-evolution of genes and culture." Chap. 5 IN Harris, M. and E. B. Ross (Eds.) *Food and evolution.* Temple University Press, Philadelphia, PA.

Kelley, William D. 1997. *One answer to cancer. A do it yourself booklet.* Sterling Press, Cancer Coalition, Mineral Wells, TX.

Kelley, William D. 1999. *One answer to cancer with cancer cure.* College of Metabolic Medicine. Republished by The Road to Health, Walnut Creek, CA.

Klaper, Michael, 1999. "Challenge to the plant-based diet of the 90's: 'The Zone' and 'Blood Type' diet fads." Institute of Nutrition Education and Research. *http://www.vegsource.com/Klaper/diet.HTM*.

Knorr, Dietrich and Hartmut Vogtmann. 1983. "Quality and quality determination of ecologically grown foods." Chap. 14 IN Knorr, D. (Ed.) *Sustainable food systems.* Avi Publishing Co., Inc., Westport, CT.

Koonig, L. J., J. A. Nienaber and H. J. Mersmann. 1983. "Effects of plane of nutrition on organ size and fasting heat production in genetically obese and lean pigs." American Institute of Nutrition, pp. 1626–1631.

Krause, Carol. 1995. *How healthy is your family tree?* Fireside Books, Simon and Schuster, New York.

Kristal, Harold. 1998. "The death of allopathic nutrition." Address to Society for Orthomolecular Health-Medicine, March 1. Healthexcel, Inc., Winthrop, WA.

Kristal, Harold and James Haig. 2000. "Understanding the testing procedures of metabolic typing." Metabolic News, Vol. 2, No. 1, p. 4. Personalized Metabolic Nutrition, Corte Madera, CA.

Kristal, Harold. 2000. "Soy reconsidered." Metabolic News, Vol. 2., No. 2. Personalized Metabolic Nutrition, Corte Madera, CA.

Kunzig, Robert. 1997. "Atapuerca. The face of an ancestral child." Discover Magazine, December, pp. 88–101.

LaChapelle, Dolores. 1988. *Sacred land, sacred sex, rapture of the deep.* Kivaki Press, Durango, CO.

Lairon, D., E. Termine, S. Gautier, M. Trouilloud, H. LaFont and J. C. Hauton. 1986. "Effects of organic and mineral fertilizations on the content of vegetables in minerals, vitamin C and nitrates." IN Vogtmann H., E. Boehncke and I. Frike (R. Eds.) *The importance of biological agriculture in a world of diminishing resources.* Proceed. 5th IFOAM, International Scientific Conference at University of Kassel (Germany), Verlagsgruppe, Witzenhausen.

Lamb, D. S. 1893. American Journal of Medical Science, 105:633.

Lawder, John. 1986. *I.N. Diet—the individualized nutritional plan.* John Lawder, M.D., Inc., Torrance, CA.

Leaf, Alexander. 1973. "Every day is a gift when you are over 100." National Geographic, January.

Leakey, Meave. 1995. "The farthest horizon." National Geographic, September, pp. 38–51.

Leonard, Jonathan. 1973. *The first farmers—The emergence of man series.* Time-Life Books, New York.

Lieberman, Leslie Sue. 1987. "Biocultural consequences of animals versus plants as sources of fats, proteins and other nutrients." Chap. 9 IN Marvin Harris and Eric Ross (Eds.) *Food and evolution.* Temple University Press, Philadelphia, PA.

Liener, Irvin. 1986. "Nutritional significance of lectins in the diet." Chap. 10 IN *The Lectins—properties, functions and applications in biology and medicine.* Academic Press, New York.

Life Extension. 2000. "Custom cancer care: an interview with Dr. Robert Nagourney." January. Life Extension Foundation, Hollywood, FL.

MacLean, Paul. 1973. *A triune concept of the brain and behavior.* University of Toronto Press, Toronto, Canada.

MacLeod, L. B. 1965. "Effects of nitrogen and potassium on the yield and chemical composition of alfalfa, bromegrass, orchard grass, and timothy grown as pure species." Agron. J., 57, pp. 261–266.

Malter, Richard. 1994. "Trace mineral analysis and psychoneuroimmunology." Journal of Orthomolecular Medicine, Vol. 9, No. 2, pp. 79–93.

Marshall, Robert. 1998. "No healing without quality food." Acres USA, April, pp. 24–29.

Martinez, et al. 1976. "La Estructvan del consumo de alimentes en el medio rural pobre." Publ. 1–29, Division cle nutricion, Instituto Nacional de la Nutrition: Mexico City.

Martins, Mary. 1999. "Soil organic matter." Acres USA, August, pp. 10–13.

McCarrison, Robert. 1921. *Studies in deficiency disease.* Oxford Medical Publications, Henry Frowde, Hodder and Stoughton, London.

MetaMetrix. 2000. "IgE and IgG1 and 4 food antibody interpretation." MetaMetrix Clinical Laboratory, Norcross, GA.

Meyerowitz, Steve. 1999. "Gutsy moves—natural ways to support digestion." Better Nutrition, July.

Miller, Janette *et al.* 1992. "Rice: A high or low glycemic index food?" American Journal of Clinical Nutrition, Vol. 56.

Miller, Janette, Kaye Foster-Dowell and Stephen Colagiuri. 1996. "The G.I. factor: the glycemic index solution." Hudder Headline, Australia Dty Ltd.

Milton, Katherine. 1986. "Digestive physiology of primates." News in Physiological Sciences, Vol. 1, pp. 76–79.

Milton, Katherine. 1987. "Primate diets and gut morphology: implications for hominid evolution." pp. 93–115. IN Harris, M. and E. B. Ross (Eds.) *Food and Evolution.* Temple University Press, Philadelphia, PA.

Morris, Desmond. 1994. *The human animal.* Crown Publishers (Random House, Inc.) New York.

Mount, James. 1975. *The food and health of western man.* John Wiley and Sons, New York.

Mowat, Farley. 1963. *Never cry wolf.* Dell Publications, now Bantam Books (Random House), Chicago, IL.

Nesmith, Jeff. 1999. "Low levels of protective gene may explain Gulf War illness." Atlanta Journal-Constitution, June 17.

Nesse, Randolf and George Williams. 1994. *Why we get sick.* Vintage Books, Random House, New York.

Nesse, Randolf. 1998. "Evolution and the origins of disease." Scientific American, November.

Nomi, Toshitaka and Alexander Besher. 1983. *You are your blood type.* Pocket Books, Simon and Schuster, New York.

Ornstein, Robert and David Sobel. 1987. *The healing brain.* Simon and Schuster, New York.

Osborne, Sally. 1998. "Eat right 4 your type hype." Health and Healing. Wilson, Vol. 22, No. 4. Price-Pottenger Nutrition Foundation, La Mesa, CA.

Outerbridge, Thomas. 1987. "The disappearing chinampas of Xochimilco." The Ecologist, Vol. 17, No. 2.

Page, Melvin. 1949. *Degeneration-regeneration.* Biochemical Research Foundation, St. Petersburg, FL.

Page, Melvin. 1954. *Body chemistry in health and disease.* The Page Foundation, St. Petersburg, FL.

Page, Melvin and Leon Abrams, Jr. 1972. *Your body is your best doctor.* Keats Publishing Co., New Canaan, CT.

Palin, Michael. 1997. Full Circle, PBS television series.

Pereira, Winin. 1991. "Traditional rice growing in India." The Ecologist, Vol. 21, No. 2.

Pert, Candace. 1986. "The wisdom of the receptors: neuropeptides, the emotions, and bodymind." Advances, Institute for the Advancement of Health, Vol. 3, No. 3, pp. 8–16.

Pert, Candace, Henry Dreher and Michael Ruff. 1998. "The psychosomatic network: foundations of mind-body medicine." Alternative Therapies, Vol. 4, No. 4.

Pettersson, B. D. 1978. "A comparison between conventional and biodynamic farming systems as indicated by yields and quality." Proceed. International Research Conference IFOAM. Wirz Verlag, Aarau.

Pfeiffer, Ehrenfried. 1947. *Soil fertility, renewal and preservation.* The Lanthorn Press, Sussex, England (1983 edition).

Price, Weston. 1941. "Race decline and race regeneration." Journal of the American Dental Association, Vol. 28, pp. 548–558.

Price, Weston. 1948. (5th Ed.) *Nutrition and physical degeneration.* The American Academy of Applied Nutrition, Los Angeles, CA. Republished (1982) by The Price-Pottenger Nutrition Foundation, Inc., La Mesa, CA.

Prideaux, Tom and Editors of Time-Life. 1973. *Cro-magnon man—The emergence of man series.* Time-Life Books, New York.

Pringle, Heather. 1998. "New women of the Ice Age." Discover Magazine, April, pp. 62–69.

Pottenger, Francis, Jr. 1944. (6th Ed.) *Symptoms of visceral disease.* C. V. Mosby Co., St. Louis, MO.

Pottenger, Francis, Jr. 1946. "The effect of heat-processed foods and metabolized vitamin D milk on the dentofacial structures of experimental animals." American Journal of Orthodontics and Oral Surgery, Vol. 32, No. 8, pp. 467–485.

Pottenger, Francis, Jr. 1983. *Pottenger's cats. A study in nutrition.* Price-Pottenger Nutrition Foundation, Inc., La Mesa, CA.

Quinn, Daniel. 1992. *Ishmael.* Bantam/Turner, New York.

Radetsky, Peter. 1995. "Gut thinking." Discover Magazine, May, pp. 76–81.

Rateaver, Bargyla. 1987. "Fighting phytate fears." Acres USA, March, pp. 22–24.

Reading, Chris and Ross Meillon. 1988. *Your family tree connection.* Keats Publishing Co., New Canaan, CT.

Rifkin, Jeremy. 1992. *Beyond beef.* Dutton, New York.

Rivici, Emmanuel. 1961. "Research in physiopathology as a basis for guided chemotherapy." (Not available.) Library of Congress catalog card No. 60–53061.

Rogers, Sherry. 1988. *You are what you ate.* Prestige Publishers, Syracuse, NY.

Rogers, Sherry. 1990. *Tired or toxic? A blueprint for health.* Prestige Publishers, Syracuse, NY.

Rogers, Sherry. 1991. *The cure is in the kitchen: the strict healing phase for the macrobiotic diet.* Prestige Publishers, Syracuse, NY.

Rogers, Sherry. 1994. *Wellness against all odds.* Prestige Publishers, Syracuse, NY.

Rogers, Sherry. 1996. *The E.I. syndrome revised.* SK Publishing, Sarasota, FL.

Rogers, Sherry. 1999. "Total Wellness" (newsletter). February. Prestige Publishers, Syracuse, NY.

Rogers, Sherry. 1999. "Total Wellness" (newsletter). August. Prestige Publishers, Syracuse, NY.

Rogers, Sherry. 2000. *No more heartburn.* Kensington Publishing Corp., New York.

Ross, Eric. 1987. "An overview of trends in dietary variations from hunter-gatherers to modern capitalist societies." Chap. I IN Marvin Harris and Eric Ross (Eds.) *Food and evolution.* Temple University Press, Philadelphia, PA.

Rowan, Robert. 1999. "Kristal and Wolcott metabolic typing effective." Letter to the editor, Townsend Letter for Doctors and Patients. June.

Rozin, Paul. 1987. "Psychological perspectives on food preferences and avoidances." Chap. 7 IN Marvin Harris and Eric Ross (Eds.) *Food and evolution.* Temple University Press, Philadelphia, PA.

Rubin, Herman. 1952. *Glands, sex and personality.* Funk, Inc.

Sagan, Carl. 1977. *The dragons of Eden.* Ballantine Books, Random House, New York.

Salunkhe, D. K. and B. B. Desai. 1988. "Effects of agricultural practices, handling, processing and storage on vegetables." IN E. Karmas and R. S. Harris (Eds.). *Nutritional evaluation of food processing* (3rd Edition). Van Nostrand Reinhold, New York. pp. 23–71.

Schenker, Guy. 1995. "An analytical system of clinical nutrition." Nutri-Spec, Mifflintown, PA.

Schmid, Ronald. 1994. *Native nutrition.* Healing Arts Press, Rochester, VT.

Schuphan, W. 1976. "Mensch und Nahrungspflanze. Der biologische wert der nahrungspflanze von pestizideinsatz, bodenqualitat und düngung." Dr. W. Junk, B. V. Verlag, Den Haag.

Schuphan, W. 1974. "Nutritional value of crops as influenced by organic and inorganic fertilizer treatments—results of 12 years' experiments with vegetables." Quality Plant, 23, pp. 333–358.

Schwartz, G. R. 1988. *In bad taste: the MSG syndrome.* Health Press, Santa Fe, NM.

Sears, Barry. 1995. *The zone, a dietary road map.* Regan Books, Harper-Collins, New York.

Sears, Barry. 1999. *The anti aging zone.* Rogan Books, Harper-Collins, New York.

Sell, S. 1987. (4th Ed.) *Immunology, immunopathology and immunity.* Elsevier, New York. pp. 314–321.

Senanayake, Ranil. 1983. "The ecological, energetic and agronomic systems of ancient and modern Sri Lanka." The Ecologist, Vol. 13, No. 4.

Sharon, Nathan. 1977. "Lectins." Scientific American, June, pp. 108–119.

Sheldon, W. H., S. S. Stevens and W. B. Tucker. 1940. *The varieties of human physique.* Harper and Bros., New York and London.

Shreeve, James. 1999. "Secrets of the gene." National Geographic, Vol. 196, No. 4, pp. 42–75. October. National Geographic Society, Washington, DC.

Sierra. 2000. "Getting it right." Vol. 9, No. 1 (January).

Simoons, Frederick. 1981. "Celiac disease as a geographic problem." Chap. 17 IN Walcher and Kretchmer (Eds.). *Food, nutrition and evolution.* Masson Publishers USA, New York.

Smith, Bruce. 1995. *The emergence of agriculture.* Scientific American Library, W. H. Freeman and Co., New York.

Smith, N. E. and R. L. Baldwin. 1973. "Effects of breed, pregnancy and lactation on weight of organs and tissues in dairy cattle." Journal of Dairy Science, Vol. 57, No. 9, pp. 1055–1060.

Sportelesis. 1999. "The Sportelesis program." Sportelesis, Santa Ana, CA.

Spruce, Neal. 1997. "Apex fitness program." Apex Fitness Group, Inc., Thousand Oaks, CA.

Stefansson, V. 1962. *My life with the Eskimos.* (Originally published in 1913.) Collier, New York.

Steinkraus, Keith (Ed.) and Roger Cullen, Carl Pederson, Lois Nellis and Ben Gavitt (Assoc./Asst. Eds.). 1983. *Handbook of indigenous fermented foods.* Marcel Dekker, Inc., New York.

Stini, William. 1981. "Body composition and nutrient reserves in evolutionary perspective." Chap. 10 IN Walcher and Kretchmer (Eds.). *Food, nutrition and evolution.* Masson Publishers USA, Inc., New York.

Stout, Jeff. 2000. "Beta-endorphins. the bodybuilder's high." Muscle and Fitness, Vol. 61, No. 5 (February). Weider Publications, Inc.

Strong, A. D. *et al.* 1999. "Prevalence and extent of atherosclerosis in adolescents and young adults." Journal of the American Medical Association 281, pp. 727–735.

Tannahill, Reay. 1988. *Food in history.* Crown Publishing Inc., New York.

Taub, E. L. 1978. *Food allergy and the allergic patient.* Springfield, MA. Thomas.

Treves, Frederick. 1885. "Lectures on the anatomy of the intestinal canal and peritoneum in man." The British Medical Journal, Vol. 1 (May) pp. 415–419, 470–474, 588–583, 527, 580.

Underhill, Betty. 1955. "Intestinal length in man." The British Medical Journal, November 19.

Valentine, Tom and Carole Valentine. 1986. *Metabolic typing. medicine's missing link.* Thorsons Publishing Group, Wellingborough, NY.

Walford, Roy and Lisa Walford. 1994. *The anti-aging plan.* Four Walls, Eight Windows, New York.

Wallach, Joel. 1993. "The argument for expensive urine." Acres USA, November, p. 24.

Wardle, David, M. A. Huston, J. P. Grime, F. Berendse, E. Garnier, W. K. Lauenroth, H. Setälä, and S. D. Wilson. 2000. "Biodiversity and ecosystem function: an issue in ecology." Bulletin of the Ecological Society of America, Vol. 81, No. 3, pp. 235–239.

Watson, George. 1965. "Differences in intermediary metabolism in mental illness." Psychological Reports 17, pp. 563–582.

Watson, George. 1972. *Nutrition and your mind.* Harper and Row, New York, San Fransisco and London.

Watson, George. 1979. *Personality strength and psycho-chemical energy.* Harper and Row, New York, San Francisco and London.

Watts, David. 1989. "Calcium and virus activation." Newsletter, Vol. 3, No. 5, pp. 47–48. Trace Elements, Inc., Addison, TX.

Watts, David. 1990. "Nutrients interrelationships—minerals-vitamins-endocrines." Journal of Orthomolecular Medicine, Vol. 5, No. 1, pp. 11–19.

Watts, David. 1991. "Osteoporosis-contraindications of vitamin D and calcium." Newsletter, Vol. 5, No. 1. Trace Elements, Inc., Addison, TX.

Watts, David. 1993. *Mineral imbalance, endocrines and hair tissue mineral analysis.* Trace Elements, Inc., Addison, TX. pp. 89–93.

Watts, David. 1994. *Balancing body chemistry.* Trace Elements, Inc., Addison, TX.

Watts, David. 1995. *Trace elements and other essential nutrients.* Trace Elements, Dallas, TX.

Watts, David. 1999a. "Trace elements and glucose disorders." Newsletter, Vol. 11, No. 2. Trace Elements, Inc., Addison, TX.

Watts, David 1999b. "Hormones and nutrition." Newsletter, Vol. 11, No. 3. Trace Elements, Inc., Addison, TX.

Weil, Andrew. 1995. *Spontaneous healing.* Ballantine Books (Random House), New York.

Wharton, Charles. 1966. "Man, fire and wild cattle in North Cambodia." Proceed. 5th Annual Tall Timbers Fire Ecology Conference, March 24–25. Tallahassee, FL. pp. 23–65.

Wharton, Charles. 1968. "Man, fire and wild cattle in Southeast Asia." Proceed. Annual Fire Ecology Conference, March 14–15. Tallahassee, FL. pp. 107–167.

Wharton, Charles. 1978. *The natural environments of Georgia.* Bulletin 114, Georgia Geological Survey, Georgia Department of Natural Resources. Atlanta, GA.

White, Randall and Erica Frank. 1994. "Health effects and prevalence of vegetarianism." West Journal of Medicine, 160, pp. 465–471.

Whittaker, Julian. 1999. "Health and healing." Vol. IX, No. 1 (January). Phillips Publishing, Inc., Potomac, MD.

Wiley, Rudolf. 1987. "The effect of acid/alkaline nutrition on psycho-physiological function." International Journal of Biosocial Research, Vol. 9, No. 2, pp. 182–202.

Wiley, Rudolf. 1989. *Biobalance—the acid/alkaline solution to the food-mood-health puzzle.* Life Sciences Press, Tacoma, WA.

Wiley, Rudolf. 1991. *The biobalance workbook.* Phoenix Press, Panama City, FL.

Williams, R. J. 1956. *Biochemical individuality, the basis for the gene-totrophic concept.* University of Texas Press, Austin and London (7th Printing, 1979).

Williams, R. J. 1967. *You are extra-ordinary.* Pyramid Publications (Harcourt Brace Jovanovich, Inc.), New York.

WNYC. 1999. "The infinite mind." PBS. Lichtenstein Creative Media.

Wolcott, William. 1993. "The H.O.P.E. report" (Section 2). Healthexcel, Inc., Winthrop, MA.

Wrench, G. T. 1938. *The wheel of health.* C. W. Daniel Co., Ltd., London.

Wright, Herbert. 1977. "Environmental change and the origin of agriculture in the old and new worlds." IN Reed, Charles (Ed.) *Origins of agriculture.* The Hague: Mouton.

Wurtman, J. and R. Wurtman. 1983. "Studies on the appetite for carbo-hydrates in rats and humans." Journal of Psychiatric Research, 17, pp. 213–221.

Wurtman, Richard. 1982. "Nutrients that modify brain function." Scientific American, April, pp. 50–59.

Yesner, David. 1987. "Life in the 'garden of eden': causes and consequences of the adoption of marine diets by human societies." Chap. 11 IN Marvin Harris and Eric Ross (Eds.) *Food and evolution.* Temple University Press, Philadelphia, PA.

Zuckerman, Marvin. 1998. "The infinite mind." PBS, March 30. Lichtenstein Creative Media.

APPENDIX A

Kelley's Metabolic Types

(After Kelley 1977, 1999)

Group A: *Sympathetic dominant, vegetarian (Types I, IV, VI):* Strong anterior pituitary, thyroid, parathyroid, adrenal medulla and gonadal glands. Nutritional support: Vitamins D, K and C, biotin, folic acid, PABA, niacin, minerals magnesium, manganese, zinc, chromium; HCL and pancreatic enzymes; prone to acidosis.

Type I: Strict vegetarian (100% raw diet). No animal products needed.

Type IV: Non-strict vegetarians (60% raw diet). Some animal products; Mediterranean types.

Type VI: Poor metabolizers assimilating only 20% of their food and needing 60% cooked food, much supplemental support.

Group B: *Parasympathetic dominants, carnivores (Types I, V, VII):* Strong posterior pituitary, pineal, thymus, adrenal cortex and gastrointestinal organs. Requires different suite of foods and supplements: Vitamins E, B12, niacinimide, pantothenic acid, choline, inositol, minerals: calcium, phosphorus, zinc, RNA, bioflavinoids. Should avoid green, leafy vegetables and high doses of B vitamins. Prone to Alkalosis.

Type II: Burn carbohydrates rapidly, must have meat (up to 14 oz/day) which slows carbohydrate metabolism. Should limit B and K vitamins. Usually of northern European origin.

Type V: Can eat a more balanced diet with meat two or three times a week.

Type VII: Often sickly, with inefficient metabolism. Needs more than normal supplementation.

Group C: Sympathetic-parasympathetic dominance, balanced (Types III, VIII, IX, X): Thrives on food from both vegetarian and meat-eating groups. Enjoys great dietary freedom, neither oxidizing too fast or too slow. Needs: Vitamins A, B1, B2, B6, B12, C, E, niacin, niacinimide, folic acid, biotin, pantothenic acid, PABA; minerals: calcium, phosphorus, magnesium, manganese, chromium, zinc, extra HCL, pancreatic enzymes.

Type III: Have crippled metabolisms using only 10–15% of food and supplements; need easily digested foods and larger quantities of supplements than any other type. May feel bad enough to have death wishes. (Stress of modern living can put other metabolic types in categories III, VI and VII.)

Type VIII: Has the greatest number of people of any of the 10 categories; can eat a wide variety of food and supplements. Generally healthy, these fortunate individuals can handle high levels of stress.

Type IX: Cannot do well on raw foods, need 70% cooked foods. This type does best on visiting a smorgasbord 3 or 4 times per week. They hate raw food.

Type X: These are balanced and super-efficient metabolizers needing a wide variety of foods but no large quantities of anything. They eat half as much as any other of the 10 types, need little sleep and feel terrific.

APPENDIX B

Watson's Psychochemical Types

TYPE 1—SLOW OXIDIZERS: Burn carbohydrates inefficiently, can't use heavy fat/protein since they need carbs to break them down. Blood sugar may be high but can't burn it down sufficiently. Glycolytic cycle not producing enough pyruvate (pyruvic acid) and oxalo-acetate necessary to convert acetyl-coenzyme A to produce energy in the Krebs citric acid cycle. End result is insufficient acetate (Acetyl-coenzyme A). Need supplements to assist in breakdown of pyruvate and oxalo-acetate (oxalo-acetic acid).

Need: High carbohydrate (grains, veggies, fruits), low purine-rich proteins and fats (can use dairy, eggs, coffee, and tea).

Use sparingly: Beans, lentils, peas, avocado, cauliflower, spinach, asparagus; high purine proteins, alcohol, high fat, low flour pastries (cheesecake, Danish).

Supplements: A (must be fish liver oil), B1, B2, B6, C, D, niacin, PABA, potassium, magnesium, copper, iron, manganese.

TYPE 2—FAST OXIDIZERS: Burn carbohydrates too fast and in too large amounts. Use up acetate; produce pyruvate and oxalo-acetate faster than acetate. Abnormal psychological reactions to too much carbohydrate because of insufficient acetate. High blood sugar gives "high." Person is physically and psychologically hypersensitive. To increase availability of acetate needs high-purine proteins and high fat, low carb diet.

Need: High-purine proteins (herring, liver, mussels, sardines, salmon), fats, limited carbohydrates. Avoid dairy. Can eat mid-purine foods: meat, fowl, seafood, spinach, whole grains, beans, lentils, peas, peanuts.

337

Use sparingly: Potatoes, rice, spaghetti, bread, cereal, salads, dairy, most fish, eggs, soft drinks, coffee, tea and alcohol. (According to Watson, alcohol tolerance reflects one's biochemical health, i.e., "The more one can drink without adverse effect, the worse off he is.")

Supplements: A (must be palmitate, NOT fish oil), E, B12, C, niacinimide, choline, inositol, calcium, phosphorus, iodine, zinc.

TYPE 3—SUB-OXIDIZERS. Can eat most foods but may handle carbohydrates and fats inadequately. Need to strive for optimum nutrition including supplements and high purine proteins. Can be made more aggressive and daring by diet changes.

Need: Optimum protein intake plus whole grain cereals, sufficient fruits and vegetables to furnish calories not provided by protein.

Supplements: A, E, B1, B2, B6, B12, niacinimide, pantothenic acid, PABA, C, choline, inositol, calcium, phosphorus, iodine, zinc, magnesium, iron.

TYPE 4—VARIABLE OXIDIZERS. Can switch between Type 1 and Type 2, even on a daily basis. Must learn by careful observation and experimentation. Supper may even interfere with the effects of breakfast next morning. Obviously a difficult type to manage successfully.

APPENDIX C

Page's Autonomic Types

SYMPATHETIC DOMINANT. Catabolic or "breakdown" glands.

Dominant endocrine ("speed up") glands: Anterior pituitary, thyroid, adrenal medulla, male gonad. If Overactive—phosphorus is too high, calcium low (posterior pituitary secretion is deficient).

Characteristics: high blood pressure, above normal temperature, controls the phosphorus level of the blood, stimulates conversion of glycogen back to sugar.

Disease predisposition: angina, coronary thrombosis, cancer, diabetes (practically confined to this type), acute stage of arthritis; heals slowly with infections, nightly muscle cramps prevalent.

Body type: Heavy above waist, often with large breasts in female.

Other observations: mentally alert, generally extrovert, irritable, generally has nervous energy and ambition.

Adjunct therapy: 2 or 3 units of insulin (normal pancreatic output 15-18 units daily).

PARASYMPATHETIC DOMINANT. Anabolic "build up" glands.

Dominant endocrine ("slow up") glands: pancreas; Isles of Langerhans that secrete insulin, posterior pituitary, estrin producing glands, parathyroid, adrenal cortex. If overactive - calcium is too high.

Characteristics: low blood pressure, subnormal temperature, controls calcium level of the blood, converts excess sugar to glycogen, adrenal cortex functions with parathyroid to raise calcium levels.

Disease predisposition: Calcareous deposits, chronic arthritis, cataracts, calculus on teeth, deposits in kidneys and arterial walls.

Body type: Weight below waist. A curvaceous female, especially if hypo-posterior pituitary.

Adjunct therapy: tiny amounts of thyroid or pituitary extract.

APPENDIX D

Abravanel's Metabolic Body Types

ADRENAL DOMINANT

BODY FORM: Solidly built, broad shoulders, thick waist, powerful; female: flat rear end, sensual roundness, great legs.

TYPE FOOD DESIRED: High protein, salty, red meat, salami, and alcohol.

TYPE FOOD NEEDED: Pituitary stimulants like dairy.

DISADVANTAGES: Tendency to overweight, pot belly, cardiovascular problems, diabetes, thyroid under-active (thyroid hormone needed to regulate cholesterol).

ADVANTAGES: Good creativity, seldom has respiratory diseases or colitis, steady, hard worker, hearty, warm, and eats anything, needs little sleep.

SUPPLEMENTS: Needs high A, B1, B3, B6, and E.

THYROID DOMINANT

BODY FORM: Slim, lithe, shapely, delicate, slender arms and legs, slim hands and feet, built for speed. Female: wide shoulders, slender hips, definite waist, sharp voluptuous curves, and stomach not flat like gonadal type. Males have small rear ends.

TYPE FOOD DESIRED: Sugar, carbohydrates, caffeine, uses coffee and Danish to stimulate thyroid.

TYPE FOOD NEEDED: High protein (adrenal stimulants), minimum carbohydrate.

DISADVANTAGES: Fat around middle, "jelly roll," ("spare tire") skin irritations, allergies, low resistance to respiratory infections.

ADVANTAGES: Can eat without gaining weight.

SUPPLEMENTS: Needs high choline, inositol, B12, magnesium, zinc.

PITUITARY DOMINANT: (rare, 10% of population, fewer females than males).

BODY FORM: Head appears a little large for body, fat stored all over, stomach rounded like a child, body same as at age 12-14, no "saddlebag" thighs, rear end tending to be small.

TYPE FOOD DESIRED: Dairy products

TYPE FOOD NEEDED: Needs highest protein of any type: eggs, red meat, organ meats (to stimulate adrenals and sex glands).

DISADVANTAGES: Baby fat everywhere, pudgy, allergies, weak sexual function, overweight, mental obsessions, frequent colds, "life stops below neck." Tends to stimulate posterior pituitary while anterior pituitary is under-stimulated.

ADVANTAGES: Excellent creative thought, deep, good at discussion, curious and lively intelligence.

SUPPLEMENTS: No especially high levels of nutrients specified (compared to other types).

APPENDIX E

Lawder's Biochemical Types

FAST OXIDIZER: More carnivorous, but only about 5% are true carnivores.

> PARASYMPATHETIC DOMINANTS: More stimulation goes to thymus, gastrointestinal tract and adrenal cortex.

> OXIDIZES FOOD RAPIDLY: Carbohydrates processed too quickly.

> BLOOD pH: Slightly below normal, calcium levels high.

> NEEDS: Ideal ratio C30%, P40%, F30%.

> NEEDS: Three square meals daily with protein each meal; traditional English breakfast good. Needs slowly oxidizing foods like meat, eggs, dairy, chicken and fish. Cauliflower, root vegetables, corn, squash are good choices. Avoid most fruits; apples OK.

> DESCRIPTION: Slow, almost phlegmatic, blood pressure and temperature tending towards subnormal.

> PROBLEMS: Susceptible to asthma, hypoglycemia, edema, and diverticulosis, viral infections, arthritis and arteriosclerosis, binge eating.

SLOW OXIDIZER: Only 15% are true vegetarians (most Afro-Americans are slow oxidizers).

> SYMPATHETIC DOMINANTS: More stimulation goes to adrenal medulla, pituitary, pineal and gonads. Adrenaline keeps intestines slow.

> OXIDIZES FOODS SLOWLY: Does better on carbohydrates because of their rapid assimilation. Proteins digest too

slowly-stomach may act as a 115-degree oven, releasing toxins from undigested proteins (see Dr. Bieler's work).

BLOOD pH: Nearer normal (expels CO2 more quickly); calcium levels lower, phosphorus levels high.

NEEDS: Ideal ratio C60%, P20%, F20%.

NEEDS: Diet lower in protein, higher in carbohydrate; needs added bulk of fruits and vegetables to prevent constipation; digestive tract motility is suppressed creating greater danger of toxins from nitrites, nitrates and MSG.

DESCRIPTION: Higher levels of activity, frequent mood swings, ambitious, strong emotions.

PROBLEMS: Prone to arteriosclerosis, high cholesterol, diabetes, and hypertension.

MID OXIDIZER: Omnivores with tendencies toward either carnivory or herbivory. Only 2% of people are perfect, balanced mid-oxidizers. Other 68% either lean toward fast or slow type.

NEEDS: Ideal diet: C45%, P30%,F25%. Most difficult group because most of these individuals are not clearly fast or slow oxidizers.

PROBLEMS: Slow mid-oxidizer: may have hereditary hyperlipidemia. Gas, bloating and other problems associated with inactive gut. Fast mid-oxidizer: weight problems, hypoglycemia, chronic fatigue, and uncontrolled hunger.

APPENDIX F

Wiley's Biochemical Types

ACID TYPE:

BURNS GLUCOSE AND FAT FAST: (Fast Oxidizer)

DIURNAL pH: Blood plasma values below 7.46.

IDEAL DAILY PROTEIN INTAKE (in ounces): Body weight (pounds) divided by 15.

DAILY CALORIC INTAKE: Ideal weight (pounds) x 18

IDEAL FAT INTAKE: 20% of total caloric intake.

PROBLEMS: Hypoglycemia—carbohydrates make individuals *more* acidic.

NEEDS: Organ meats, red meats, dark-meat poultry, salmon, dark meat tuna, sardines, herring, fish roe, shellfish, legumes, most vegetables (avoid tomatoes, lettuce, greens, broccoli, cabbage, zucchini). Eat avocados, olives, apples, pears (avoid other fruits like citrus, peaches, grapes, cherries, etc.) whole dairy or cheese, eggs, limit whole grains to a daily side dish for regularity, nuts, seeds, olive oil, butter, lard, ice cream, cheesecake, pastries.

VITAMIN/MINERALS: A, E, B12, niacinimide, pantothenic acid, inositol, choline, calcium, phosphorus, iron and zinc.

ALKALINE TYPE:

BURNS GLUCOSE SLOWLY (Slow Oxidizer)

DIURNAL pH: Blood plasma values above 7.46.

IDEAL DAILY PROTEIN INTAKE (in ounces) = ideal weight (pounds) divided by 20.

IDEAL FAT INTAKE: 15% of total caloric intake.

PROBLEMS: Too high (250-1500mg/day) calcium may be detrimental. Most diabetics, those with gout, elevated cholesterol, triglycerides, and LDL lipids are alkaline (may be a too-alkaline acidic type).

NEEDS: Light-meated fish, skinned fowl (never eat meat or fish for breakfast), salads, most vegetables (avoid legumes and soy, spinach, cauliflower and asparagus). Most fruits, some low-fat (less than 1.5%) dairy and some eggs, all whole grains with exception of corn (avoid nuts, seeds), regular coffee (not decaf), zero to low fat sherbets.

VITAMINS/MINERALS: A, D, C, B1, B6, niacin, PABA, folic acid, biotin, potassium, magnesium, iron, copper, manganese, chromium.

MIXED TYPES:

IDEAL DAILY PROTEIN INTAKE (in ounces): Ideal weight (pounds) divided by 15.

FAT INTAKE: 20% of total caloric intake.

NEEDS: Regarding meats, vegetables, fruits and desserts use as primary source those permitted acid types above, as well as a secondary source those permitted alkaline types above. Primary (acid type) meats optional for breakfast, but lunch and dinner *must* contain a primary/secondary blend of meat, fish or poultry.

VITAMINS/MINERALS: No manufacturer known to Wiley supplies the combination of supplements needed for mixed types.

APPENDIX G

Principal Body Types (Doshas) of the Ayurveda Mind / Body System and their Attributes in Balance and Imbalance

(After Chopra 1991).

	Vata	Pitta	Kapha
Dominant mental Attribute	Changeable mind	Orderly mind	Steady mind
Other major attributes	Thin, eats and doesn't gain, tires easily, short sleeper, oversensitive nervous system, changeable	Medium build, fair, ruddy, large appetite, cannot skip meals, intense	Heavy-set, steady energy flow, long sleeper, slow, mildly hungry, skin oily, relaxed
Mental attributes exaggerated by imbalance	Worries, anxiety, overactive mind, short attention span, impatience, depression	Anger, hostility, tension, self-critical, irritable, resentful	Dull, mental inertia, lassitude, stuporous, depressed, over-attachment

Behavioral attributes exaggerated by imbalance	Insomnia, fatigue, restless, can't relax, low appetite, impulsive	Short-tempered, argumentative, critical, intolerant, aggressive, bold	Procrastinator, cannot accept change, greedy, over-sleeper, balky, lethargic, possessive
Physical attributes exaggerated by imbalance	Constipation, dry skin, low stamina, high blood pressure, cold intolerant, erratic digestion, sensitive to dryness	Skin inflammations, excessive hunger and thirst, bad breath, sour body odor, heartburn/ulcers, heat intolerant, digestive problems, patchy, florid complexion	Cold/damp intolerant, nasal/sinus problems, mucus discharge, congestion, skin pallor, fluid retention, high cholesterol, obesity, allergies, diabetes
Positive qualities	Cheerful, optimistic, stimulating, enthusiastic, resilient, imaginative, spontaneous	Content, pleasant, chivalrous, inclined to moderation, sweet natured, joyous, sharp-witted, confident, outspoken, energetic, innate drive	Steady, calm, strong, forgiving, courageous, affectionate, serene, loving, "jolly fat man"
Dominant sensory attributes	Hearing, touch	Sight	Taste, smell
Exercise needs	Light as with walking, aerobics, 1/2 hour per day sufficient	Moderate: swimming, brisk walk, skiing, jogging	Moderately heavy, weight lifting, running, rowing

Dietary negatives	"Summer foods" like raw greens, cool drinks, pungent, bitter and astringent foods, "light foods," dry foods like popcorn	Too much salty, sour, pungent spicy or fermented foods, hot, light, oily foods, too much food	Too much sweet, salty, fatty foods, susceptible to toxins
Dietary positives	Warm food, added butter and fat, sensitive to "atmosphere" in dining, hot "winter foods," salt, sour, sweet foods soothing and satisfying, balanced by heavy oily and hot foods*	Cool or warm foods, but not steamy hot, needs bitter, sweet and astringent foods like salads, less butter/fat, cool drinks, balanced by cold, heavy, dry foods*	Needs "light" meals, dry food without much water, minimum of butter, oil, sugar, needs pungent, bitter and astringent foods, needs stimulating foods, balanced by light, dry, hot food*
Key to "normalizing" mind-body	Regular habits: quiet, ample rest, abundant fluids, decreased stress, regular meals, avoid cold, light food	Moderation: coolness, ample leisure, exposure to natural beauty, decreased stimulation, balance of rest/activity, avoid strenuous exercise and heat, sleep and drink cool, meditate	Stimulation: regular exercise, weight control, seek variety of stimulation, reduce intake of sweets, avoid cold/damp, drink warm fluids

*Footnote: Heavy foods: wheat, beef, cheese

Light foods: barley, chicken, and skim milk

Oily foods: milk, soybeans, coconut

Dry foods: honey, lentils, cabbage

Hot foods: peppers, honey, eggs

Cold foods: mint, sugar, milk

APPENDIX H

Synopsis of Wolcott's Major Metabolic Types in Relation to Nutrients, Venous Blood pH and Blood Sugar

(After Wolcott 1993, 1998B).

Metabolic Type	Blood pH—Food Needs	Food Group Needed	Effect of Food Group on Venous Blood pH and Blood Sugar

Autonomic System Dominant

Sympathetic (1a)(5)	Acid; must eat, fruit, veggies (2)	Group I (3)	Alkalizes-raises (normalizes)
Balanced (1a)	pH close to 7.4; balanced diet best	Group III	Normal
Parasympathetic (1a)(6)	Alkaline; must eat heavy meat/fat	Group II (4)	Acidifies-lowers (normalizes)

Oxidative System Dominant

Fast oxidizer (1b)	Acid; must eat heavy meat/fat	Group II (4)	Alkalizes-raises (normalizes)
Mixed oxidizer (1b)	pH close to 7.4; balanced diet best	Group III	Normal
Slow oxidizer (1b)	Alkaline; must eat fruit, veggies	Group I (3)	Acidifies-lowers (normalizes)

(1a) Each of these types has slow, mixed and fast oxidative dominant categories.

(1b) Each of these types has sympathetic, balanced and parasympathetic autonomic dominant categories. Together, this totals 18 metabolic types. If you add the four glands (pituitary, adrenal, thyroid and gonads), each of which can be dominant, you arrive at a grand total of 72 possible metabolic types.

(2) Oddly, hard exercise can apparently shift this person's metabolism to a fast oxidative dominant type (needing the opposite nutrient group).

(3) Group I foods (low purine proteins, fruits, vegetables, minimal fat, restricted dairy) either increase oxidation rate (increases hyperactivity, acidity) and/or stimulate the parasympathetic system (increase hypoactivity, alkalinity).

(4) Group II foods (heavy meat/fat, all dairy, root vegetables, barley, sprouted grains; fruit and most grains restricted) either decrease oxidation rate (increase hypoactivity, alkalinity) and/or stimulate the sympathetic system (increase hyperactivity, acidity).

(5) External physical characteristics: taller, thinner, narrow shoulders, wide hips, large bones, dry skin, angular or long skull, large pupils. Psychological characteristics: stronger left brain activity, hyperactive, highly motivated "go-getters," get angry easily.

(6) External physical characteristics: shorter and wider, broad shoulders, narrow hips, stronger than average, poor muscle definition, round face and skull, small pupils, often overweight. Psychological characteristics: stronger right brain activity, emotional and intuitive, warm, outgoing, emotionally stable, cautious, slow to anger.

APPENDIX I

Synoptic Classification of the Metabolic Types Based Largely on Tissue Mineral Analysis (TMA)

(After Watts, 1990, 1993, 1994, 1995).

FAST METABOLIZER: Sympathetic dominant, fast oxidation rate.

DOMINANT ENDOCRINE GLANDS: (with basic catabolic effects) are thyroid, adrenal cortex (glucocorticoids—catabolic steroids), adrenal medulla (epinephrine-catabolic steroid), anterior pituitary.

GLYCOLYTIC CYCLE: Rapid, pyruvate, oxaloacetic acid and citric acid adequate, acetate inadequate.

TISSUE ACIDITY: Dominant, metabolic rate high, thymus and lymphatics reduced, sedative minerals (calcium, magnesium) levels low, stimulatory minerals (sodium, potassium, phosphorus) high. Body apple-shaped.

Type I: Increased adrenal cortical, adrenal medulla, thyroid and anterior pituitary activity.

Type 2: Increased adrenal cortical function, decreased thyroid function (as in alarm stage of stress).

Type 3: Decreased adrenal cortical function, increased thyroid function, tendency to depression, irritability.

Type 4: Decrease in both adrenal cortex and thyroid function. Extreme fatigue, depression, anxiety.

Avoid stimulative nutrients: A, B1, B3, B5, B6, B10, E, potassium, sodium, potassium, iron, manganese, selenium, soft H20; high protein diet well tolerated. Give thyroid-inhibiting foods such as brassicas (mustards), cruciferous plants (broccoli, cauliflower, cabbage eaten raw) cassava, apricots, prunes, cherries, bamboo shoots.

SLOW METABOLIZER: Parasympathetic dominant, slow oxidation rate.

DOMINANT ENDOCRINE GLANDS: (with basic anabolic effects) are pancreas, parathyroid, adrenal cortex (anabolic steroids like growth hormone), posterior pituitary.

GLYCOLYTIC CYCLE: Pyruvates, oxaloacetic acid and citric acid not adequate.

TISSUE ALKALINITY DOMINANT: metabolic rate low; sedative minerals (calcium, magnesium) high, stimulatory minerals (sodium, potassium, phosphorus) low. Body pear-shaped.

Type 1: Decreased adrenal and thyroid function. Energy production suboptimum.

Type 2: Increased adrenal cortical function, decreased thyroid function. Energy fluctuation pronounced, mood swings.

Type 3: Decreased adrenal cortical function, increased thyroid function. If chronic, depression , irritability.

Type 4: Both adrenal cortical and thyroid functions elevated. Acute alarm/resistance stages of the stress syndrome.

Avoid sedative nutrients: B2, B12, D, calcium, magnesium, zinc, copper, chromium; high protein diet poorly tolerated.

APPENDIX J

Effect of Certain Vitamins, Minerals and Glandular Activity on Increase or Decrease of Other Nutrients and Hormones.

(After Watts 1990, 1993, 1994)

Too Much	Increases	Decreases
Calcium	Insulin	Zinc, iron, phosphorus, magnesium, potassium, sodium
Iron		Copper, cobalt (reduces B12)
Copper	Insulin, Calcium	Iron, zinc, Vitamin C
Zinc	Potassium	Copper
Magnesium		Calcium, sodium
Over active Thyroid	Phosphorus	Calcium, magnesium, copper
Overactive Parathyroid	Calcium	Potassium, magnesium
Vitamin D	Calcium	Magnesium, potassium, phosphorus
Lead		Magnesium, calcium, iron, zinc, manganese, chromium
Manganese, Iron		Magnesium, zinc
Niacin		Copper
Vitamin A	Zinc	Calcium, Vitamins E, D
Vitamin E	Sodium	Vitamin A, magnesium
Vitamin C	Iron	Copper
Phosphorus		Calcium
Vanadium		Vitamin C, Sulfur Amino Acids, chromium
Potassium	Calcium	
Sodium	Magnesium	
Cadmium		Zinc, iron, manganese

APPENDIX K

Minerals and Mineral Ratios and Their Effect on Behavior and Neuroendocrine Systems in Health and Disease

(After Malter 1994).

Minerals (s)	Status	Symptom and effects
Calcium/Magnesium Ideal ratio: 7:1 (42 to 6mg%)	Both low	Hyperactivity, high anxiety, nervous energy, aggressive, volatile, emotions on surface. Sympathetic dominant tends to have *absolute* deficiency of tissue magnesium relative to TMA (tissue mineral analysis) ideal.
	High Calcium/ low Magnesium	Small deviation associated with hypoglycemia—a large one with dysinsulinism or diabetes. Both sympathetic and parasympathetic dominants may have *relative* magnesium deficiency (Parasympathetic dominants can be magnesium deficient with normal tissue levels).
	Both high	Often an emotional block; deadening of feelings, barrier to "outside" stimuli and emotions

	High Calcium	Tends to block energy production with feelings of depression, low self-esteem, pessimism, blood sugar, and neuromuscular problems.
	Chronic high Calcium/ Magnesium ratio	Denial, cover-ups, alcohol and sugar cravings, obsessive-compulsive behavior, high anxiety, heavy depression, extremely judgmental and vulnerable to others' judgment.
	Chronic Magnesium loss	Occurs in both fast and slow oxidative types; out of control, unstable feelings; High sodium/ potassium ratio; excess muscle tension, cramping; soft tissue deposition of calcium. TMA usually reflects magnesium loss, NOT an excess of magnesium over calcium. Calcium supplementation can be dangerous; supplement with magnesium.
Sodium/Potassium Ideal ratio: 2.4:1 (24mg to 10mg%)	Ratio high 63:1	May have rage and panic attacks instead of fight or flight reaction. Associated with chronic pain and inflammation. May be supplemented with magnesium, potassium and zinc.
	Sodium retention increased	Adrenals increase aldosterone production, loss of magnesium and zinc (temporary or chronic).
	Ratio increased	Alarm stage of stress-fear and anger. Magnesium loss. Person hostile and dominating or fearful, anxious and submissive (generally not focused on another person(s).
	Low Sodium/ Potassium ratio ("inversion')	Anger suppressed, passively aggressive, indecisive, chronic prolonged stress may occur with adrenal exhaustion; susceptibility to cancer, kidney problems and diabetes.

Copper (critical role in energy production; toxic in excess)	High Copper/low Potassium	Slower metabolism; highly emotional and volatile—either blind rage or intense fear/panic for no discernable reason.
	Decrease in Zinc/Copper ratio (TMA may record "dumping")	Child with heavy metal load can change from hyperactive fast oxidizer to a slow oxidizer with more calm and self-control. Ideal zinc/copper ratio: 8:1.
	High copper with high cadmium, aluminum; low zinc	Seizures at age 1-1/2; begins dumping at age 5, excess copper at age 5, possibly due to zinc supplements.
	Accumulation of Copper and toxic metals	Intensified by birth control pill and estrogen replacement therapy.
High copper (usually stored in liver, brain)		May have severe psychological and physical problems: obsessive-compulsive behavior, severe depression, mood swings, memory and concentration problems; suicidal tendencies. Affects MAO* and serotonin levels. Reoccurring infections, especially of ear. Children can apparently be born with toxic metal overload.
Calcium/Phosphorus; Ideal ratio: 2.63:1 (42 to 16mg%)	Ratio increases. Example: 20: 5 or calcium/ magnesium 10/10: sodium/ potassium: 2/2	Person may experience parasympathetic and posterior pituitary dominance and is slow oxidizer. Metabolism slow.
	Ratio decreases. Example: 2:10 or calcium/ magnesium: 2/2: sodium/ potassium 10/10	Person may experience sympathetic and anterior pituitary dominance and is fast oxidizer. Metabolism fast. May be either adrenal or thyroid dominant.

Sodium/Magnesium* * Ideal ratio: 4:1 (24 to 6mg%)	Ratio increases	Adrenal glands become over active.
	Ratio decreases	Adrenal activity slows.
	Very low ratio	Adrenal insufficiency and possible exhaustion ("burnout").
Calcium/Potassium** Ideal ratio: 4.2:1(42 to 10mg%)	Ratio increases	Symptoms of under active thyroid
	Ratio decreases	Symptoms of over active thyroid.

*Accumulation of MAO (monoamine oxidase) inhibitors given as anti-depressants in tissues strongly related to excess tissue copper.

**Comparing the magnitude of sodium/magnesium with that of calcium/potassium allows determination of whether dominance is adrenal or thyroid.

APPENDIX L

Attributes of the Four Major Blood Types

(following D'Adamo 1996).

	O	A	B	AB
Personality	Strong, reliable, leader	Settled, cooperative, orderly	Balanced, flexible, creative	Rare, charismatic, mysterious
General adaptability	Intolerant to new dietary and environmental changes	Well-adapted to dietary and environmental changes	Versatile adaption to changes	"Designed" for modern conditions
Adaptability to disease	Susceptible to plagues that trouble crowded cultures. Resists infection	Resistant to plagues that trouble crowded cultures	No natural weaknesses. Strong immune system	Reacts negatively to both A and B conditions
Vulnerable to specific diseases	Blood-clotting disorders arthritis, allergies, autoimmune diseases	Cardio-vascular disease, cancer, liver and gallbladder disorders, anemia, diabetes	Type I diabetes, rare viruses, neurological disorders, autoimmune disease, CFS	Heart disease, cancer, anemia
General dietary program	Carnivore, needs high animal protein, avoid grains and dairy	Vegetarian, poorly adapted to most legumes and meats	Balanced omnivore, adapted to dairy and high carbohydrate	Mixed diet in moderation
Specific foods to avoid (sensitivity to their lectins (examples only)	Dairy products, whole wheat products, corn based cereals, white potatoes	Almost all meats, seafoods, some legumes, unsoured or unfermented dairy products, most wheat products	Chicken (turkey OK), shellfish, wheat, rye, corn, tomato	Lima beans, pasta, red meat, pork, non-sour, non-fermented dairy
Needed supplements	B-complex, Vitamin K, calcium, iodine	Vitamin B-2, Vitamin C, Vitamin E, folic acid, iron	Magnesium, lecithin	Vitamin C, zinc
Supplements to avoid (or use with caution)	Vitamin A, Vitame E (use food sources)	Excessive Vitamin A, beta carotene		As with Type A

Gittleman's Metabolic Types

(after Gittleman 1996)

SLOW BURNER: Does not burn carbohydrates fast enough. Thyroids and adrenals under active, tending to hyperinsulinemia.

NEEDS: Low fat (fat slows down metabolic rate); some lean proteins (chicken, turkey, light-meat fish) to speed up metabolic rate and produce hormone glucagon which blocks fat-storage promoting insulin hormone; a diet high in complex carbohydrates (squash, sweet potatoes, peas, corn, etc.), not processed or simple carbohydrates (honey, sugar, soft drinks, pasta, bagels, breads); more potassium to accelerate metabolic rate.

DIETS SOMEWHAT SUCCESSFUL FOR THIS TYPE: Weight Watchers, Diet Center, Lean Bodies, Overeaters Anonymous. Variations of slow burner diet: Pritikin, Ornish, McDougall.

CAVEATS: Possible gluten sensitivity, insulin sensitivity; some slow burners may need additional protein and essential fatty acids. Avoid foods low in the glycemic index; use high index foods only as quick lift when working out; strenuous exercise works best.

SUPPLEMENTS: B1, B2, niacin, B6, PABA, C, D, potassium, magnesium, manganese, iron.

FAST BURNER: Burns carbohydrate too fast. Thyroids and adrenals overactive, tending to hypoglycemia.

NEEDS: Heavy protein, especially red meats, and other purine-rich proteins: wild game, herring, sardines, organ meats (and even caviar); foods high in calcium; relatively high fat levels (fat slows metabolic rate), including avocado and nut butter; foods high in calcium (slows metabolic rate) (broccoli, sea veggies, sesame). Full-fat dairy products can be beneficial (calcium, fat and tryptophan in them slows metabolism). Needs diet low in complex carbohydrates (as well as simple ones).

DIETS THAT ARE SUCCESSFUL FOR THIS TYPE: Atkins, Scarsdale, Stillman, Carbohydrate Addict, Endocrine Control.

CAVEATS: Avoid foods high in glycemic index unless combined with fats or protein. Avoid strenuous exercise (running, cycling, aerobics). Walking, gardening, swimming, tai chi best.

SUPPLEMENTS: A, Niacinimide, Pantothenic Acid, B12, choline, inositol, C, E, bioflavinoids, calcium, zinc, iodine, EPA.

APPENDIX N

Some Characteristics of Cooper's Metabolic Types Classified According to the Dominant Endocrine Gland.

Compiled (and modified) from Cooper and Lance (1999).

STRONG TYPES: Long gut, slow metabolism, traditional vegetarian diet, cold/raw foods OK.

ADRENAL (WARRIOR) TYPE: Energy levels Pitta (fiery, intense). Stocky, mesomorphic, broad shoulders, chest, stubby fingers.

CRAVES: Meat, fat, salt, alcohol.

NEEDS: Plant foods, starches, some lean meat and dairy.

BODY FAT LOCATION: Upper body, mostly pot belly.

EXERCISE: Aerobic, not muscle building kinds.

PERSONALITY: Assertive, decisive, task-oriented, extrovert.

OVARIAN (NURTURER) TYPE: Energy level Endomorphic/Kapha, some Vata. Lower body "substantial," curvy, upper body smaller or leaner.

CRAVES: Creamy, spicy foods.

NEEDS: Fruits, most vegetables, lean dairy, spices.

BODY FAT LOCATION: Buttocks, thighs.

EXERCISE: Needs aerobic, muscle building on upper half only.

PERSONALITY: Warm, caring, service oriented, extrovert.

SLEEK TYPES: Short gut, metabolism moderate to fast, needs more protein-rich diet, and warm, cooked foods.

THYROID (COMMUNICATOR) TYPE: Energy level, vata (changeable). Ectomorphy, symmetrical, but long arms, legs, hands, feet, oval head.

CRAVES: Sweets, flour-based foods, caffeine.

NEEDS: High quality animal protein, vegetables, eggs, nuts, monounsaturated fats.

BODY FAT LOCATION: Spare tire area.

EXERCISE: Needs light aerobic, must strength train.

PERSONALITY: Creative, easily bored, lively, extrovert.

PITUITARY (VISIONARY) TYPE: Energy level either Vata or Kapha (slow, steady). Ectomorph or endomorph, teen-age body, medium to large head, often thin and straight.

CRAVES: Dairy foods, pungent, spicy foods.

NEEDS: "light" protein, vegetables (cooked), whole grains (Asian type diet), should not skip breakfast.

BODY FAT LOCATION: Evenly all over, pouch below navel.

EXERCISE: Does not come naturally, strength exercise most important.

PERSONALITY: Either a calm, intellectual introvert or a childlike, witty extrovert.

APPENDIX O

Two Major Metabolic Types and the Characteristics of each Generally Agreed Upon by Most Writers on the Topic.

Which Branch of the Autonomic Nervous System is in Control (or overactive) Seems to be the Main Area of Disagreement.

FAST OXIDIZER	SLOW OXIDIZER
Burns carbohydrates too fast.	Burns carbohydrates too slowly.
Dominant endocrine glands (1): Thyroid, adrenal medulla, adrenal cortex (glucocorticoids), pancreas (glucagon secretion)	Dominant organ systems/endocrine glands (1): Gastrointestinal system, pancreas (digestive enzymes), pancreas (insulin secretion), parathyroid (keeps calcium high).
Adrenals overactive	Adrenals under active
Glycogen converting to glucose	Glucose converting to glycogen
Needs calcium (sedative mineral) (2)	Needs potassium (stimulative mineral) (3)
Predominantly acid	Predominantly alkaline
Catabolic state dominant (6)	Anabolic state dominant (6)
Needs high protein/fat (2)(5)-low complex Carbohydrate	Needs high complex carbohydrate-low protein/fat (3) (Omit alkaline-inducing legumes).
Tendency to Hypoglycemia	Tendency to Hyperinsulinemia
Predominantly carnivorous	Predominantly herbivorous (vegetarian)
Sympathetic branch of autonomic nervous system most active (4)	Parasympathetic branch of autonomic nervous system most active (4)

1. Abravanal and Cooper consider adrenal/ovarian dominants to be slow oxidizers and thyroid/pituitary dominants to be fast oxidizers. Bieler considers the adrenals dominant in slow and the thyroid dominant in fast oxidizers.

2. To slow metabolism of carbohydrates (includes legumes).

3. To speed up metabolism.

4. Kelley and Lawder consider that fast oxidizers (presumably carnivores) are parasympathetic dominants and slow oxidizers (presumably herbivores) are sympathetic dominants. Page, Watts and Baum hold an opposing view. Wolcott holds that carnivores (high protein/fat eaters) either have over-active parasympathetic systems or over-active oxidation (fast oxidizers) while herbivores (high carbohydrate eaters) either have an over-active sympathetic system in control or their metabolism is dominated by under active oxidation (slow oxidizers).

5. These in general, according to Wiley, have an alkalizing effect on venous plasma pH. Wiley (1999) cautions that basing food choices on ash content determination of acid or base can cause serious metabolic damage (Wiley states that meat and legumes produce an acid ash, but are *alkalizing* in the body.)

6. Wolcott calls the catabolic/anabolic balance the "lipo-oxidative system," while the oxidative system he terms the "carbo-oxidative" system. Anabolic imbalance (control) results in decreased cell membrane permeability and a shift towards anaerobic metabolism. Conversely, a catabolic imbalance favors increased cell membrane permeability, a shift towards acrobic metabolism and uncontrolled oxidation, Wolcott (2000).

APPENDIX P

A Summary of Foods from Part II, Appropriate for Fast and Slow Oxidizers.

(For details see Gittleman 1996)

FAST OXIDIZERS (1):   (Carnivore types)
                                             {Wolcott's Protein Type}

NEED: High protein/fat—low carbohydrate diet consisting of: Red meats, high purine foods,* dark-meat poultry, full fat dairy, eggs, olives, complex carbohydrates **(5)** limited to legumes (beans and peas), some whole-grain products, breads from *sprouted* grains **(6),** some root vegetables, nuts, high-fat seeds (pumpkin, sunflower, etc.) Restrict or avoid fruits, especially citrus (high potassium speeds metabolism even more). Avoid or limit stimulating caffeine (coffee, tea, chocolate) and processed complex carbohydrates **(3),** simple carbohydrates **(4)** and high glycemic index foods **(7).**

---

*High purine foods: Sardines, salmon, herring, organ meats such as liver, shellfish, wild game (most authors); pinto beans, lentils, garbanzo beans, black-eyed peas; onions (Benjamin Frank); asparagus, mushrooms, cauliflower, spinach. It is customary for gout patients to avoid high purine foods (could they be slow oxidizers?).

SLOW OXIDIZERS (2):   (Herbivore or vegetarian types)
{Wolcott's Carbo Type}

NEED: Low to moderate protein/low fat—high carbohydrate
diet consisting of: Low purine, lean meats such as skinned
white meat fowl, very lean beef and veal, light meat fish
(flounder, haddock, white tuna, cod, most fresh water fish);
limited low fat dairy (calcium in milk products slows down
metabolism even more); complex carbohydrates such as
squash, peas, corn and sweet potatoes; all whole grains, salads, most fruits, coffee and tea (caffeine stimulates metabolic
rate); potassium-rich foods (to speed up metabolism) such as
citrus, bananas, tomatoes, squash, "seaweed." Avoid or limit
nuts, oily seeds, legumes (beans, peas), soy, simple carbohydrates **(4)** and processed complex carbohydrates **(3).**

(1) Needs substantial breakfast. Most authors agree that
fast oxidizers need to limit the B-complex vitamins that
are involved with energy release.

(2) Can forego breakfast. This is the so-called "light" diet and
suitable only for alkaline (slow oxidizer) types. For alkaline females Wiley claims that sunlight, vitamin D, folic
acid, calcium-rich foods and anaerobic exercise (weights
and resistance machines) are far more valuable in reducing osteoporosis than high-potency calcium supplements.
In addition, excessive calcium further slows an already
slow metabolism.

(3) Processed complex carbohydrates from grains, such as
pasta, bagels, white flour breads, rice cakes and puffed cereals react in the body as simple sugars, increasing insulin and lowering glycogen, which means more body fat.
They lead to carbohydrate "addiction" or insulin resistance.

(4) Simple carbohydrates are sugars: honey, molasses, corn
syrup, fructose (fruit sugar), lactose (milk sugar).

(5) Complex carbohydrates are starches: whole grains, potatoes, beans, peas and many other vegetables. Fast oxidizers should eat them with fats (butter, oil, cheese).

(6) Phytates in unsprouted grains lower calcium which fast oxidizers need.

(7) High glycemic index foods like brown rice, carrots, oat bran, white potatoes, and whole wheat bread need to be eaten with protein and/or fat to slow down glucose release (ice cream, remarkably, is very low on the glycemic index because of its high fat content or additives).

Index